Immunotherapies for Acute Myeloid Leukemia

Immunotherapies for Acute Myeloid Leukemia

Special Issue Editor
Jochen Greiner

MDPI • Basel • Beijing • Wuhan • Barcelona • Belgrade • Manchester • Tokyo • Cluj • Tianjin

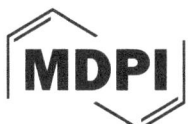

Special Issue Editor
Jochen Greiner
Department of Internal Medicine,
Diakonie Hospital Stuttgart
Germany

Editorial Office
MDPI
St. Alban-Anlage 66
4052 Basel, Switzerland

This is a reprint of articles from the Special Issue published online in the open access journal *Journal of Clinical Medicine* (ISSN 2077-0383) (available at: https://www.mdpi.com/journal/jcm/special_issues/Immuno_Acute_Myeloid_Leukemia).

For citation purposes, cite each article independently as indicated on the article page online and as indicated below:

LastName, A.A.; LastName, B.B.; LastName, C.C. Article Title. *Journal Name* **Year**, *Article Number*, Page Range.

ISBN 978-3-03936-110-6 (Hbk)
ISBN 978-3-03936-111-3 (PDF)

© 2020 by the authors. Articles in this book are Open Access and distributed under the Creative Commons Attribution (CC BY) license, which allows users to download, copy and build upon published articles, as long as the author and publisher are properly credited, which ensures maximum dissemination and a wider impact of our publications.

The book as a whole is distributed by MDPI under the terms and conditions of the Creative Commons license CC BY-NC-ND.

Contents

About the Special Issue Editor vii

Preface to "Immunotherapies for Acute Myeloid Leukemia" ix

Jochen Greiner
The Important Role of Immunotherapies in Acute Myeloid Leukemia
Reprinted from: *J. Clin. Med.* **2019**, *8*, 2054, doi:10.3390/jcm8122054 1

Håkon Reikvam, Elise Aasebø, Annette K. Brenner, Sushma Bartaula-Brevik, Ida Sofie Grønningsæter, Rakel Brendsdal Forthun, Randi Hovland and Øystein Bruserud
High Constitutive Cytokine Release by Primary Human Acute Myeloid Leukemia Cells Is Associated with a Specific Intercellular Communication Phenotype
Reprinted from: *J. Clin. Med.* **2019**, *8*, 970, doi:10.3390/jcm8070970 5

Jochen Greiner, Marlies Götz, Donald Bunjes, Susanne Hofmann and Verena Wais
Immunological and Clinical Impact of Manipulated and Unmanipulated DLI after Allogeneic Stem Cell Transplantation of AML Patients
Reprinted from: *J. Clin. Med.* **2020**, *9*, 39, doi:10.3390/jcm9010039 25

Weerapat Owattanapanich, Patompong Ungprasert, Verena Wais, Smith Kungwankiattichai, Donald Bunjes and Florian Kuchenbauer
FLAMSA-RIC for Stem Cell Transplantation in Patients with Acute Myeloid Leukemia and Myelodysplastic Syndromes: A Systematic Review and Meta-Analysis
Reprinted from: *J. Clin. Med.* **2019**, *8*, 1437, doi:10.3390/jcm8091437 47

Brent A. Williams, Arjun Law, Judit Hunyadkurti, Stephanie Desilets, Jeffrey V. Leyton and Armand Keating
Antibody Therapies for Acute Myeloid Leukemia: Unconjugated, Toxin-Conjugated, Radio-Conjugated and Multivalent Formats
Reprinted from: *J. Clin. Med.* **2019**, *8*, 1261, doi:10.3390/jcm8081261 61

Heleen H. Van Acker, Maarten Versteven, Felix S. Lichtenegger, Gils Roex, Diana Campillo-Davo, Eva Lion, Marion Subklewe, Viggo F. Van Tendeloo, Zwi N. Berneman and Sébastien Anguille
Dendritic Cell-Based Immunotherapy of Acute Myeloid Leukemia
Reprinted from: *J. Clin. Med.* **2019**, *8*, 579, doi:10.3390/jcm8050579 93

Krzysztof Giannopoulos
Targeting Immune Signaling Checkpoints in Acute Myeloid Leukemia
Reprinted from: *J. Clin. Med.* **2019**, *8*, 236, doi:10.3390/jcm8020236 107

Susanne Hofmann, Maria-Luisa Schubert, Lei Wang, Bailin He, Brigitte Neuber, Peter Dreger, Carsten Müller-Tidow and Michael Schmitt
Chimeric Antigen Receptor (CAR) T Cell Therapy in Acute Myeloid Leukemia (AML)
Reprinted from: *J. Clin. Med.* **2019**, *8*, 200, doi:10.3390/jcm8020200 119

Ghazala Naz Khan, Kim Orchard and Barbara-ann Guinn
Antigenic Targets for the Immunotherapy of Acute Myeloid Leukaemia
Reprinted from: *J. Clin. Med.* **2019**, *8*, 134, doi:10.3390/jcm8020134 133

About the Special Issue Editor

Jochen Greiner, Prof. Dr., started his research career as a postdoctoral researcher at the Institute of Internal Medicine III, University of Ulm, Germany, where he became member and head of the Tumorimmunology Group. His research focuses on immune responses of cytotoxic T cells against malignant cells. This includes the definition of new antigens for immunotherapeutic approaches, the development of vaccines for the clinical treatment of haematological malignancies, especially of acute myeloid leukemia and other haematological malignancies and solid tumors, as well as the evaluation of immune responses against leukemias after allogeneic stem cell transplantation. The activities of the group include in vitro T cell assays, preclinical studies, and clinical trials. He and his group investigate immune responses and possibilities to increase T cell responses against leukemic stem cells. He has published 74 research articles, 45 of which as first or last author in peer-reviewed journals such as *Journal of Clinical Oncology*, *Blood*, *Leukemia*, and *Clinical Cancer Research*. Currently, Professor Greiner is Medical Director of the Department of Hematology and Oncology at Diakonie-Klinikum Stuttgart. He is also still active as a scientist and the head of the Tumor Immunology Laboratory at the University of Ulm.

Preface to "Immunotherapies for Acute Myeloid Leukemia"

This series on immunotherapies in acute myeloid leukemia (AML) aims to provide readers with new insights on established and emerging immunotherapeutic approaches for AML patients. The therapeutic landscape in AML is rapidly changing, and several drugs have been developed and their use has been authorized. Thus, median overall survival for AML patients has increased; however, it remains relatively low.

Immunotherapeutic approaches might be an option to prevent disease relapse and to eliminate leukemic cells or leukemic stem cells (LSC) that survive intensive treatment approaches. The efficacy of immunotherapeutic approaches has become ever more evident in solid tumors, especially immune checkpoint inhibitors that are routinely used in several solid tumor entities, but also in lymphoma. In this Special Issue, our focus is on different strategies of immunotherapeutic approaches in AML.

Jochen Greiner
Special Issue Editor

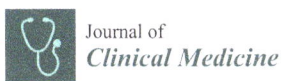

Editorial

The Important Role of Immunotherapies in Acute Myeloid Leukemia

Jochen Greiner [1,2]

1. Department of Internal Medicine, Diakonie Hospital, 70176 Stuttgart, Germany; greiner@diak-stuttgart.de
2. Department of Internal Medicine III, University Hospital of Ulm, 89081 Ulm, Germany

Received: 18 November 2019; Accepted: 20 November 2019; Published: 22 November 2019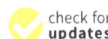

This series on immunotherapies in acute myeloid leukemia (AML) aims to give readers new insights on established but also emerging immunotherapeutic approaches for AML patients. The therapeutic landscape in AML is rapidly changing, and several drugs have been developed and approved such as first and second generation FLT3 inhibitors [1–3], IDH1 and 2-inhibitors [4,5], demethylating agents, liposomal cytarabine and daunorubicin (CPX-351) [6], venetoclax [7,8] and the hedgehog pathway inhibitor glasdegib. However, relapse after intensive chemotherapy or allogeneic hematopoietic stem cell transplantation is one of the major obstacles impeding the complete elimination of all AML cells [9]. Thus, although the median overall survival for AML patients has increased, it still remains relatively low [10].

Therefore, immunotherapeutic approaches might be an option to prevent disease relapse and to eliminate leukemic cells or leukemic stem cells (LSC) that survive intensive treatment approaches. The efficacy of immunotherapeutic approaches has become ever more evident in solid tumors, especially immune-checkpoint inhibitors that are routinely used in several solid tumor entities, but also lymphoma [11,12].

Our focus in this special issue is different strategies of immunotherapeutic approaches in AML.

Some of the immunotherapies in the treatment of AML, such as allogeneic hematopoietic stem cell transplantation (HSCT) and donor lymphocyte infusion (DLI), have been part of routine clinical practice in the treatment of AML for a long time, whereas other immunotherapeutic approaches have only recently entered clinical practice or need to be further developed. A key aspect is the mechanisms underlying the cure of AML patients, which are based on the graft-versus-leukemia (GvL) effect, in which allogeneic T cells recognize target antigens on malignant cells by T cell approaches including DLI. An effective and well-tolerated regimen for HSCT in patients with AML and MDS is the FLAMSA-RIC regimen, and therefore novel data of this approach are presented in this issue [13].

It is very appropriate to utilize DLI after allogeneic HSCT to prevent relapse, to prolong progression-free survival, to establish full donor chimerism, and to restore the GvL effect in patients with hematological malignancies. There are different strategies to use DLI in a therapeutic setting for the treatment of morphological relapse, and also for prophylactic use in AML/MDS and DLI administered preemptively. There is also the approach of antigen-directed immunogenic and specifically stimulated and modified DLI as well as virus-specific donor T cells and third-party DLI [14].

DC-based immunotherapies also have the potential to bring about demonstrable clinical responses in AML patients, although there has not been a complete breakthrough for this type of therapy until today. Van Acker et al. have highlighted different DC strategies in AML [15].

Leukemia-associated antigens (LAAs) represent immunogenic structures to target LSC [16,17], and LAA might be relevant for the elimination of malignant cells by cytotoxic T lymphocytes. Therefore, LAAs might be a good target for specific immunotherapeutic approaches. Several LAAs have been identified in the context of malignant hematological diseases [16,18,19], and in clinical phase I/II peptide vaccination trials, some LAAs showed immunological as well as clinical responses [20–23].

In this special issue, we also elucidate antibody-based therapies in AML, such as T cell activating antibodies including immune-checkpoint inhibitors and diverse monoclonal antibodies [11,12,24]. Immune-checkpoint inhibitors have changed clinical treatment algorithms of malignant diseases such as malignant melanoma, lung cancer, as well as lymphoma. Today, immune-checkpoint inhibitors are not yet established in the routine treatment of AML but should be considered as further immunotherapeutic options in the future, especially in the context of allogeneic stem cell transplantation [24]. Further antibody-directed approaches such as unconjugated, toxin-conjugated, radio-conjugated, and multivalent formats of antibody-based therapy, are demonstrating the potential of a diverse leukemia-derived antibody strategy which is already established in acute lymphoblastic leukemia and are summarized in one section of this issue [25].

Chimeric antigen receptor T cells (CARs) are highly effective in the treatment of refractory and relapsed acute lymphoblastic leukemia, to some lower extent in aggressive lymphoma, but also in multiple myeloma [26]. However, early CAR-T cell approaches are also being tested in AML with interesting target structures, and these strategies are described in this issue [27]. Immune responses are complex and are also influenced by T cell cross-talk and communication by cytokines and the communication of leukemic cells with their microenvironment, as presented by Reikvam et al. [28] in this issue.

All of these aspects emphasize the high potential of immunotherapeutic approaches to improve the survival of AML patients in the future, where combination therapies utilizing immunotherapeutic drugs could represent further innovation strategies to further improve the treatment of AML.

Conflicts of Interest: The author declares no conflict of interest.

References

1. Stone, R.M.; Mandrekar, S.J.; Sanford, B.L.; Laumann, K.; Geyer, S.; Bloomfield, C.D.; Thiede, C.; Prior, T.W.; Dohner, K.; Marcucci, G.; et al. Midostaurin plus Chemotherapy for Acute Myeloid Leukemia with a FLT3 Mutation. *N. Engl. J. Med.* **2017**, *377*, 454–464. [CrossRef] [PubMed]
2. Perl, A.E.; Martinelli, G.; Cortes, J.E.; Neubauer, A.; Berman, E.; Paolini, S.; Montesinos, P.; Baer, M.R.; Larson, R.A.; Ustun, C.; et al. Gilteritinib or Chemotherapy for Relapsed or Refractory FLT3-Mutated AML. *N. Engl. J. Med.* **2019**, *381*, 1728–1740. [CrossRef] [PubMed]
3. Cortes, J.E.; Khaled, S.; Martinelli, G.; Perl, A.E.; Ganguly, S.; Russell, N.; Kramer, A.; Dombret, H.; Hogge, D.; Jonas, B.A.; et al. Quizartinib versus salvage chemotherapy in relapsed or refractory FLT3-ITD acute myeloid leukaemia (QuANTUM-R): A multicentre, randomised, controlled, open-label, phase 3 trial. *Lancet Oncol.* **2019**, *20*, 984–997. [CrossRef]
4. DiNardo, C.D.; Stein, E.M.; de Botton, S.; Roboz, G.J.; Altman, J.K.; Mims, A.S.; Swords, R.; Collins, R.H.; Mannis, G.N.; Pollyea, D.A.; et al. Durable Remissions with Ivosidenib in IDH1-Mutated Relapsed or Refractory AML. *N. Engl. J. Med.* **2018**, *378*, 2386–2398. [CrossRef]
5. Stein, E.M.; DiNardo, C.D.; Pollyea, D.A.; Fathi, A.T.; Roboz, G.J.; Altman, J.K.; Stone, R.M.; DeAngelo, D.J.; Levine, R.L.; Flinn, I.W.; et al. Enasidenib in mutant IDH2 relapsed or refractory acute myeloid leukemia. *Blood* **2017**, *130*, 722–731. [CrossRef]
6. Lancet, J.E.; Uy, G.L.; Cortes, J.E.; Newell, L.F.; Lin, T.L.; Ritchie, E.K.; Stuart, R.K.; Strickland, S.A.; Hogge, D.; Solomon, S.R.; et al. CPX-351 (cytarabine and daunorubicin) Liposome for Injection Versus Conventional Cytarabine Plus Daunorubicin in Older Patients With Newly Diagnosed Secondary Acute Myeloid Leukemia. *J. Clin. Oncol.* **2018**, *36*, 2684–2692. [CrossRef]
7. DiNardo, C.D.; Pratz, K.; Pullarkat, V.; Jonas, B.A.; Arellano, M.; Becker, P.S.; Frankfurt, O.; Konopleva, M.; Wei, A.H.; Kantarjian, H.M.; et al. Venetoclax combined with decitabine or azacitidine in treatment-naive, elderly patients with acute myeloid leukemia. *Blood* **2019**, *133*, 7–17. [CrossRef]
8. Wei, A.H.; Strickland, S.A., Jr.; Hou, J.Z.; Fiedler, W.; Lin, T.L.; Walter, R.B.; Enjeti, A.; Tiong, I.S.; Savona, M.; Lee, S.; et al. Venetoclax Combined With Low-Dose Cytarabine for Previously Untreated Patients With Acute Myeloid Leukemia: Results From a Phase Ib/II Study. *J. Clin. Oncol.* **2019**, *37*, 1277–1284. [CrossRef]

9. Lee, C.J.; Savani, B.N.; Mohty, M.; Gorin, N.C.; Labopin, M.; Ruggeri, A.; Schmid, C.; Baron, F.; Esteve, J.; Giebel, S.; et al. Post-remission strategies for the prevention of relapse following allogeneic hematopoietic cell transplantation for high-risk acute myeloid leukemia: Expert review from the Acute Leukemia Working Party of the European Society for Blood and Marrow Transplantation. *Bone Marrow Transplant.* **2018**. [CrossRef]
10. Dohner, H.; Estey, E.; Grimwade, D.; Amadori, S.; Appelbaum, F.R.; Buchner, T.; Dombret, H.; Ebert, B.L.; Fenaux, P.; Larson, R.A.; et al. Diagnosis and management of AML in adults: 2017 ELN recommendations from an international expert panel. *Blood* **2017**, *129*, 424–447. [CrossRef] [PubMed]
11. Annibali, O.; Crescenzi, A.; Tomarchio, V.; Pagano, A.; Bianchi, A.; Grifoni, A.; Avvisati, G. PD-1/PD-L1 checkpoint in hematological malignancies. *Leuk. Res.* **2018**, *67*, 45–55. [CrossRef] [PubMed]
12. Gravbrot, N.; Gilbert-Gard, K.; Mehta, P.; Ghotmi, Y.; Banerjee, M.; Mazis, C.; Sundararajan, S. Therapeutic Monoclonal Antibodies Targeting Immune Checkpoints for the Treatment of Solid Tumors. *Antibodies* **2019**, *8*, 51. [CrossRef] [PubMed]
13. Owattanapanich, W.; Ungprasert, P.; Wais, V.; Kungwankiattichai, S.; Bunjes, D.; Kuchenbauer, F. FLAMSA-RIC for Stem Cell Transplantation in Patients with Acute Myeloid Leukemia and Myelodysplastic Syndromes: A Systematic Review and Meta-Analysis. *J. Clin. Med.* **2019**, *8*, 1437. [CrossRef] [PubMed]
14. Greiner, J.; Götz, M.; Bunjes, D.; Hofmann, S.; Wais, V. Immunological and clinical impact of manipulated and unmanipulated DLI after allogeneic stem cell transplantation (allo-SCT) of AML patients. *J. Clin. Med.* **2019**, submitted for publication.
15. Van Acker, H.H.; Versteven, M.; Lichtenegger, F.S.; Roex, G.; Campillo-Davo, D.; Lion, E.; Subklewe, M.; Van Tendeloo, V.F.; Berneman, Z.N.; Anguille, S. Dendritic Cell-Based Immunotherapy of Acute Myeloid Leukemia. *J. Clin. Med.* **2019**, *8*, 579. [CrossRef]
16. Anguille, S.; Van Tendeloo, V.F.; Berneman, Z.N. Leukemia-associated antigens and their relevance to the immunotherapy of acute myeloid leukemia. *Leukemia* **2012**, *26*, 2186–2196. [CrossRef]
17. Schneider, V.; Zhang, L.; Rojewski, M.; Fekete, N.; Schrezenmeier, H.; Erle, A.; Bullinger, L.; Hofmann, S.; Gotz, M.; Dohner, K.; et al. Leukemic progenitor cells are susceptible to targeting by stimulated cytotoxic T cells against immunogenic leukemia-associated antigens. *Int. J. Cancer* **2015**, *137*, 2083–2092. [CrossRef]
18. Greiner, J.; Schmitt, M.; Li, L.; Giannopoulos, K.; Bosch, K.; Schmitt, A.; Dohner, K.; Schlenk, R.F.; Pollack, J.R.; Dohner, H.; et al. Expression of tumor-associated antigens in acute myeloid leukemia: Implications for specific immunotherapeutic approaches. *Blood* **2006**, *108*, 4109–4117. [CrossRef]
19. Greiner, J.; Ono, Y.; Hofmann, S.; Schmitt, A.; Mehring, E.; Gotz, M.; Guillaume, P.; Dohner, K.; Mytilineos, J.; Dohner, H.; et al. Mutated regions of nucleophosmin 1 elicit both CD4(+) and CD8(+) T-cell responses in patients with acute myeloid leukemia. *Blood* **2012**, *120*, 1282–1289. [CrossRef]
20. Schmitt, M.; Schmitt, A.; Rojewski, M.T.; Chen, J.; Giannopoulos, K.; Fei, F.; Yu, Y.; Gotz, M.; Heyduk, M.; Ritter, G.; et al. RHAMM-R3 peptide vaccination in patients with acute myeloid leukemia, myelodysplastic syndrome, and multiple myeloma elicits immunologic and clinical responses. *Blood* **2008**, *111*, 1357–1365. [CrossRef]
21. Rezvani, K.; Yong, A.S.; Mielke, S.; Savani, B.N.; Musse, L.; Superata, J.; Jafarpour, B.; Boss, C.; Barrett, A.J. Leukemia-associated antigen-specific T-cell responses following combined PR1 and WT1 peptide vaccination in patients with myeloid malignancies. *Blood* **2008**, *111*, 236–242. [CrossRef] [PubMed]
22. Greiner, J.; Schmitt, A.; Giannopoulos, K.; Rojewski, M.T.; Gotz, M.; Funk, I.; Ringhoffer, M.; Bunjes, D.; Hofmann, S.; Ritter, G.; et al. High-dose RHAMM-R3 peptide vaccination for patients with acute myeloid leukemia, myelodysplastic syndrome and multiple myeloma. *Haematologica* **2010**, *95*, 1191–1197. [CrossRef] [PubMed]
23. Rezvani, K.; Yong, A.S.; Mielke, S.; Jafarpour, B.; Savani, B.N.; Le, R.Q.; Eniafe, R.; Musse, L.; Boss, C.; Kurlander, R.; et al. Repeated PR1 and WT1 peptide vaccination in Montanide-adjuvant fails to induce sustained high-avidity, epitope-specific CD8+ T cells in myeloid malignancies. *Haematologica* **2011**, *96*, 432–440. [CrossRef] [PubMed]
24. Giannopoulos, K. Targeting Immune Signaling Checkpoints in Acute Myeloid Leukemia. *J. Clin. Med.* **2019**, *8*, 236. [CrossRef]
25. Williams, B.A.; Law, A.; Hunyadkurti, J.; Desilets, S.; Leyton, J.V.; Keating, A. Antibody Therapies for Acute Myeloid Leukemia: Unconjugated, Toxin-Conjugated, Radio-Conjugated and Multivalent Formats. *J. Clin. Med.* **2019**, *8*, 1261. [CrossRef]

26. Majzner, R.G.; Mackall, C.L. Clinical lessons learned from the first leg of the CAR T cell journey. *Nat. Med.* **2019**, *25*, 1341–1355. [CrossRef]
27. Hofmann, S.; Schubert, M.L.; Wang, L.; He, B.; Neuber, B.; Dreger, P.; Muller-Tidow, C.; Schmitt, M. Chimeric Antigen Receptor (CAR) T Cell Therapy in Acute Myeloid Leukemia (AML). *J. Clin. Med.* **2019**, *8*, 200. [CrossRef]
28. Reikvam, H.; Aasebo, E.; Brenner, A.K.; Bartaula-Brevik, S.; Gronningsaeter, I.S.; Forthun, R.B.; Hovland, R.; Bruserud, O. High Constitutive Cytokine Release by Primary Human Acute Myeloid Leukemia Cells Is Associated with a Specific Intercellular Communication Phenotype. *J. Clin. Med.* **2019**, *8*, 970. [CrossRef]

© 2019 by the author. Licensee MDPI, Basel, Switzerland. This article is an open access article distributed under the terms and conditions of the Creative Commons Attribution (CC BY) license (http://creativecommons.org/licenses/by/4.0/).

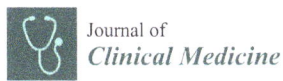

Article

High Constitutive Cytokine Release by Primary Human Acute Myeloid Leukemia Cells Is Associated with a Specific Intercellular Communication Phenotype

Håkon Reikvam [1,2,*], Elise Aasebø [1], Annette K. Brenner [2], Sushma Bartaula-Brevik [1], Ida Sofie Grønningsæter [2], Rakel Brendsdal Forthun [2], Randi Hovland [3,4] and Øystein Bruserud [1,2]

1 Department of Clinical Science, University of Bergen, 5020,Bergen, Norway
2 Department of Medicine, Haukeland University Hospital, 5021 Bergen, Norway
3 Department of Medical Genetics, Haukeland University Hospital, 5021 Bergen, Norway
4 Institute of Biomedicine, University of Bergen, 5020 Bergen, Norway
* Correspondence: Hakon.Reikvam@med.uib.no; Tel.: +55-97-50-00

Received: 23 May 2019; Accepted: 1 July 2019; Published: 4 July 2019

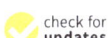

Abstract: Acute myeloid leukemia (AML) is a heterogeneous disease, and this heterogeneity includes the capacity of constitutive release of extracellular soluble mediators by AML cells. We investigated whether this capacity is associated with molecular genetic abnormalities, and we compared the proteomic profiles of AML cells with high and low release. AML cells were derived from 71 consecutive patients that showed an expected frequency of cytogenetic and molecular genetic abnormalities. The constitutive extracellular release of 34 soluble mediators (CCL and CXCL chemokines, interleukins, proteases, and protease regulators) was investigated for an unselected subset of 62 patients, and they could be classified into high/intermediate/low release subsets based on their general capacity of constitutive secretion. *FLT3*-ITD was more frequent among patients with high constitutive mediator release, but our present study showed no additional associations between the capacity of constitutive release and 53 other molecular genetic abnormalities. We compared the proteomic profiles of two contrasting patient subsets showing either generally high or low constitutive release. A network analysis among cells with high release levels demonstrated high expression of intracellular proteins interacting with integrins, RAC1, and SYK signaling. In contrast, cells with low release showed high expression of several transcriptional regulators. We conclude that AML cell capacity of constitutive mediator release is characterized by different expression of potential intracellular therapeutic targets.

Keywords: acute myeloid leukemia; gene mutations; differentiation; cytokines; proteomic profile; integrin; RAC1; SYK

1. Introduction

Acute myeloid leukemia (AML) is a heterogeneous hematological malignancy characterized by clonal proliferation of a hierarchically organized leukemia cell population that arises from hematopoietic progenitors in the bone marrow [1–3]. AML is distinguished from other related blood disorders by the presence of at least 20% myeloblasts in the bone marrow [1–3]. However, despite this common characteristic, AML is very heterogeneous [1], and patients differ, for example, with regard to genetic abnormalities [4–7], transcriptional [8] and cell cycle regulation [9], autocrine and paracrine growth regulation [10–13], as well as the cellular metabolomic [14] and proteomic profiles [15–17]. This cell population heterogeneity is also reflected in the biological characteristics of AML stem cells [8,10].

Most relapses occur within 2–3 years after diagnosis and the overall five-year leukemia-free survival for younger AML patients able to receive intensive chemotherapy possibly combined with stem cell transplantation is only 45–50%, and a major cause of death is chemoresistant AML relapse thought to originate from remaining AML or preleukemic cells that recapitulate disease development [18–21]. Cure is not possible for the large group of elderly/unfit patients who cannot receive such intensive therapy due to an unacceptable high risk of severe treatment-related morbidity or treatment-related mortality [2]. Thus, there is a need for identification of new therapeutic targets and development of new therapeutic strategies that are more efficient and better tolerated [22]. Targeting of the bidirectional communication between AML cells and their neighboring leukemia-supporting stromal cells is a possible approach [23–28]. In a previous study investigating another patient cohort, we described that high constitutive mediator release is associated with better long-term overall survival compared with low constitutive release [29]. The aims of the present study were, therefore, to characterize the in vitro secretome of primary human AML cells, to investigate possible associations between the capacity of constitutive mediator secretion and molecular genetic abnormalities, and to compare the proteomic profiles for primary AML cells with generally high and low capacity of releasing extracellular soluble mediators.

2. Materials and Methods

2.1. AML Patients and Preparation of Primary AML Cells

The study was approved by the Regional Ethics Committee (REK) (REK III 060.02, 10th of June 2002; REK Vest 215.03, 12th of March 04; REK III 231.06, 15th of March 2007; REK Vest 2013/634, 19th of March 2013; REK Vest 2015/1410, 19th of June 2015), The Norwegian Data Protection Authority 02/1118-5, 22 October 2002, and The Norwegian Ministry of Health 03/05340 HRA/ASD, 16 February 2004. All samples were collected after written informed consent.

The study population included 71 consecutive AML patients with high peripheral blood blast counts (>5 × 10^9/L) and a high percentage of leukemic blasts among peripheral blood leukocytes (Table 1). Highly enriched AML cell populations (at least 95% leukemic blasts) could thereby be prepared by density gradient separation alone (Lymphoprep, Axis-Shield, Oslo, Norway). The cells were stored in liquid nitrogen until used in the experiments [30].

Table 1. The clinical and biological characteristics of the 71 acute myeloid leukemia (AML) patients included in the study.

Age and gender		Etiology	
Median (years)	64	Previous chemo-radiotherapy	1
Range (years)	18–90	CML	1
Females	31	Li–Fraumeni's syndrome	1
Males	40	Polycythemia vera	1
		MDS	8
		Relapse	10
		de novo	49
FAB[1] classification		Cytogenetic abnormalities[3]	
M0/1	26	Adverse	17
M2	14	Favorable	5
M4/5	22	Intermediate	43
M6	1	Normal	40[4]
Unknown	8	Unknown	6
CD34 expression			
Negative (<20%)	28[2]		
Positive (>20%)	43		

[1] The French–American–British classification. [2] The percentage of positive cells in flow cytometric analysis. [3] The European Leukemia Net classification was used [2]. [4] The 43 patients classified as intermediate cytogenetics included 40 patients with normal karyotype. Abbreviations: CML, chronic myeloid leukemia; MDS, myelodysplastic syndrome.

2.2. Mutation Profiling, Flow Cytometric Analyses, and Analysis of Global Gene Expression Profiles

Submicroscopic mutation profiling of 54 genes frequently mutated in AML was done by using the Illumina TruSight Myeloid Gene Panel and sequenced using the MiSeq system and reagent kit v3 (all from Illumina, San Diego, CA, USA). A detailed description of the methodology and the 54 genes is given in a previous publication [31]. Fragment analysis of *FLT3* exon 14–15, *NPM1* exon 12, and sequencing of *CEBPA* were performed as described previously [32].

Immunophenotyping was performed as a part of the standard diagnostic workup using freshly isolated cells [2], and analyses were performed by multiparametric flow cytometry (BD FACS Canto; Franklin Lakes, NJ, USA).

Our methods for analysis of global mRNA profiles have been described previously [31]. All these analyses were performed using the Illumina iScan Reader and based upon fluorescence detection of biotin-labeled cRNA. For each sample, 300 ng of total RNA was reversely transcribed, amplified, and biotin-16-UTP-labeled (Illumina TotalPrep RNA Amplification Kit; Applied Biosystems/Ambion; San Diego, CA, USA). The amount and quality of the biotin-labeled cRNA was controlled by the NanoDrop spectrophotometer and Agilent 2100 Bioanalyzer (Agilent Technologies, Inc.; Santa Clara, CA, USA). Biotin-labeled cRNA (750 ng) was hybridized to the HumanHT-12 V4 Expression BeadChip. The Human HT-12 V4 BeadChip targets 47,231 probes that are mainly derived from genes in the NCBI RefSeq database (Release 38). Data from the array scanning were investigated in GenomeStudio and J-Express 2012. All arrays within each experiment were quantile normalized before being compiled into an expression profile data matrix.

2.3. Analysis of Constitutive Mediator Release by Primary Human AML Cells

The studies of constitutive mediator release included a consecutive subset of 46 patients from the original study population (see Section 2.1 and Table 1). AML cells (1×10^6/mL) were cultured for 48 h in Stem Span SFEM^{TM} medium in flat-bottomed 24-well (2 mL/well) culture plates (Nunc Micro-Well; Sigma-Aldrich, Saint-Louis, MO, USA) before supernatants were collected and stored at −80 °C until analyzed. The levels of the following 34 mediators were determined by Luminex analyses (R&D Systems; Minnesota, MN, USA) or enzyme-linked immunosorbent assays (ELISA) (R&D Systems; Minnesota, MN, USA): (i) the chemokines CCL2-5 and CXCL1/2/5/8/10/11; (ii) the interleukins IL-1β/1RA/6/10/33; (iii) the matrix metalloproteinases MMP-1/2/9 together with the protease/protease regulators tissue inhibitor of metalloproteinases 1 (TIMP-1), Cystatin B and C, polymorphonuclear (PMN) elastase, serpin C1 and E, and CD147, plasminogen activator (PA), and complement factor D (CFD); (iv) the immunomodulatory tumor necrosis factor-α (TNF); (v) the growth factors granulocyte-macrophage colony-stimulating factor (GM-CSF), hepatocyte growth factor (HGF), heparin-binding EGF-like growth factor (HB-EGF), basic fibroblast growth factor (bFGF), and vascular endothelial growth factor (VEGF); and (vi) the soluble angiopoietin-1 receptor tyrosine kinase with immunoglobulin-like and EGF-like domain 2 (Tie-2).

2.4. Proteomic Profiling: Selection of Patients, Sample Preparation, and Proteomic Analysis

The present study is based on mutational analysis of the leukemic cells for 71 consecutive and thereby unselected AML patients with a high number and/or percentage of AML blasts in the peripheral blood (Table 2). This selection based on the peripheral blood blast level (see Section 2.1) was used to reduce the risk of inducing molecular alterations in the leukemia cells due to more extensive separation procedures. The karyotyping (Table 1) as well as the mutational analyses showed an expected frequency of both cytogenetic and molecular genetic abnormalities, suggesting that despite the separation-dependent selection of patients, they are representative for AML in general. Constitutive cytokine release was investigated for a consecutive and thereby unselected subset of 46 patients from the original study population. Global proteomic profiling of enriched AML cells was performed for 16 of the 46 patients included in the constitutive release study; and these 16 patients represent all patients in the secretomic cohort completing intensive antileukemic treatment with induction chemotherapy followed by either 2–4 consolidation cycles or allogeneic stem cell transplantation as the final consolidation. Thus, they represent an unselected subset of relatively young and fit patients (Tables S1,S2).

Table 2. An overview of the mutational landscape of 71 consecutive AML patients. The table presents the main classification and the number of mutations. For each main class the term total group refers to the total number of mutations in this class (first number) together with the number of patients with mutations belonging to this main class (second number). Those mutations that should be included as a part of the prognostic evaluation in routine clinical practice are marked with arrows (↑ increased survival; ↓ decreased survival) [2].

Classification	Mutation	Number with Mutation	Classification	Mutation	Number with Mutation
NPM1	↑NPM1	20	Chromatin modification	↓ASXL1	12
	Total group	20–20		EZH2	3
Signaling	↓FLT3-ITD	20		GATA2	4
	FLT3-TKD	8		KDM6A	1
	HRAS	1		Total group	20–15
	JAK2	1	Myeloid transcription factors	↑CEBPA	8
	KIT	1		↓RUNX1	13
	KRAS	5		Total group	21–18
	NRAS	10	Spliceosome/ transcription repressors	BCOR	4
	PTPN11	3		BCORL1	4
	Total group	49–42		SF3B1	2
Tumor suppressors	CDKN2A	1		SRSF2	8
	CUX1	1		ZRSB2	1
	IKZF1	7		Total group	19–15
	PHF6	3	Cohesin	RAD21	2
	TP53↓	7		SMC1A	1
	WT1	5		STAG2	8
	Total group	24–21		Total group	11–11
DNA methylation	DNMT3A	19	Others	CSF3R	3
	IDH1	5		NOTCH1	2
	IDH2	11		SETBP1	1
	KMT2A/MLL	2		Total group	6–5
	TET2	12			
	Total group	49–39			

We followed the step-by-step procedure published previously for proteomic sample preparation and analysis of primary AML cells [15], except for the following two modifications: the 20 µg cell lysates were analyzed as label-free samples in contrast to being spiked with an internal standard, and no peptide fractionation was performed. The samples were analyzed on a QExactive HF Orbitrap mass spectrometer (Thermo Fisher Scientific; Waltham, MA, USA) coupled to an Ultimate 3000 Rapid Separation LC system (Thermo Fisher Scientific) [33,34]. The raw LC–MS files were searched against a concatenated reverse-decoy Swiss-Prot *Homo sapiens* fasta file (downloaded 05.03.18, containing 42,352 entries) in MaxQuant version 1.6.1.0 [35,36].

2.5. Bioinformatical and Statistical Analyses and Presentation of the Data

All statistical analyses were performed in GraphPad Prism 5 (GraphPad Software, Inc., San Diego, CA, USA). Unless otherwise stated, p-values <0.05 were regarded as statistically significant. The Fisher's Exact test was used to compare different groups (two-tailed p-values). Bioinformatical analyses were performed using the J-Express 2009 analysis suite (MolMine AS, Bergen, Norway) [37]. Concentrations were then median normalized and transformed to logarithmic values before differences were analyzed. Unsupervised hierarchical clustering was performed with Euclidian correlation and complete distance measure for all analyses in J-Express. The Panther classification system (version PANTHER14.0) was used to identify distinct functional classes [38].

The proteomics data processing of the raw data (i.e., filtering for reverse hits, contaminants and proteins only identified by site, and log$_2$ transformation of label-free quantification (LFQ) intensities), and statistical analysis of two groups using Welch's t-test was performed in Perseus version 1.6.1.1. [39]. Furthermore, Z-statistics were used to find the proteins with the most abundant fold changes (FCs), i.e., the proteins with highest or lowest FC when comparing the high-release with the low-release group and calculating the FCs from the median log$_2$ intensity per group as described by others [40]. Unsupervised hierarchical clustering was performed with Euclidian correlation and complete distance measure for all analyses in J-Express [37], and gene ontology analysis in DAVID version 6.8 [41]. Gene ontology (GO) terms with false discovery rate (FDR) < 0.05, the number of proteins associated to the term, and the fold enrichment were presented. The significantly different proteins were imported to the STRING database version 11.0 [42] to obtain protein–protein interaction networks, using experiments and databases as interaction sources at highest confidence (0.9). The networks were imported and visualized in Cytoscape version 3.3.0 [43]. Venny 2.1 (http://bioinfogp.cnb.csic.es/tools/venny/) was used to create Venn diagrams.

To summarize, due to the previously described AML heterogeneity and the fact that we sometimes have unequal numbers of quantified values of a protein in the two groups, we assumed an unequal variation in the groups and first applied the Welch t-test to identify proteins with significantly ($p < 0.05$) different mean tests. Thereafter we used Z-statistics as an additional test to identify those proteins with the most extreme/significant fold changes (fold change defined as the median intensity for high-release patients relative to the median intensity for low-release patients; the intensities were then log2-transformed).

3. Results

3.1. The Genetic Heterogeneity of AML Patients: TP53 Mutations are Associated with High-Risk Karyotypes and NPM1 Mutations are Associated with Mutations in DNA Methylation Genes

We analyzed the submicroscopic mutational profile for all 71 patients. The profile included 54 frequent mutated genes in myeloid malignancies, 37 of them carried non-benign mutations in our patients (Figure 1). At least one mutation was detected for 69 of the 71 patients, and one of patients without detected mutations had a balanced translocation. The median number of mutations per patient was 3.5 (range 0–7). The most frequently detected mutations were *NPM1* exon 12 insertion and the *FLT3*-ITD mutation (20 patients for each), followed by mutations in the *DNMT3A* (19), *TET2* (13), and *RUNX1* (13) genes (Figure S1).

We used the same (and now generally accepted) classification of AML-associated mutations in our present study as was used in two large previous studies, including 1540 and 200 patients, respectively [6,7]. The following mutations were detected in our patients: (i) *NPM1* insertion (detected in 20 out of the 71 patients), (ii) mutations causing activation of intracellular signaling (9 genes, 42 patients), (iii) mutated tumor suppressor genes (8 genes, 21 patients), (iv) mutations in genes involved in DNA methylation (5 genes, 39 patients) or (v) chromatin modification (3 genes, 15 patients), (vi) mutations in genes encoding myeloid transcription factors (3 genes, 20 patients), (vii) mutated genes important for the spliceosome (5 genes, 15 patients), (vii) mutated genes encoding cohesion proteins (3 genes, 9 patients), and (viii) the three genes *CSF3R*, *NOTCH1*, and *SETBP1* that were mutated in 5 patients (Table 2). The median number of different class mutations per patient was 2.5 (range 0–5); 24% of the patients had mutations from two different main classes and 34% from three main classes of mutations (Table S1).

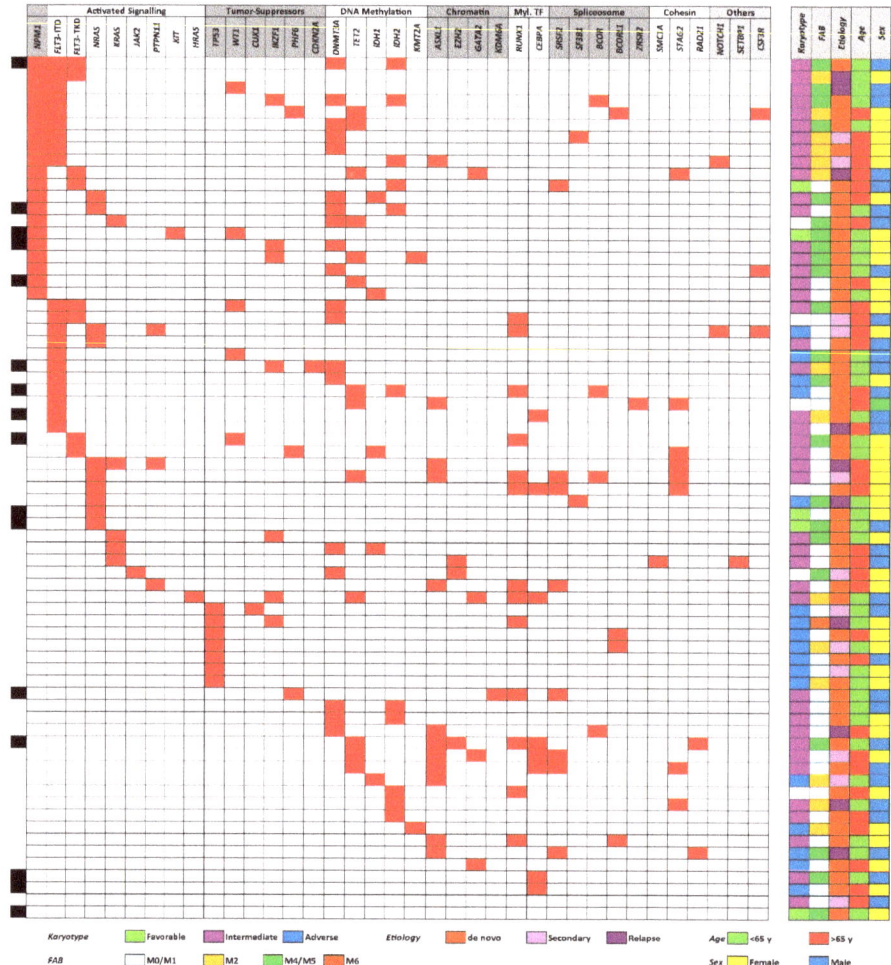

Figure 1. The total genomic profile and organization of mutations into defined categories; an overview of the data for the 71 AML patients included in our study. The figure shows the somatic mutations identified from a 54 gene mutation panel, the mutations being classified as described previously [6,7]. A majority of 69 patients had at least one detectable mutation. Risk classification of the karyotypes, morphological signs of differentiation (i.e., FAB-classification), etiology, age, and gender are presented in the right part of the figure. The patients selected for proteomic analyses are indexed with black in the left part of the figure.

We compared the mutational status with karyotype, French–American–British (FAB) classification (i.e., morphological differentiation), de novo versus secondary leukemia, age, and gender (Figure 1); these statistical analyses are summarized in Table S3. Firstly, we observed a highly significant association between *NPM1* and DNA methylation gene mutations (Fisher's Exact test, p = 0.0015), whereas the association between *FLT3*-ITD and *NPM1* mutations did not reach significance. Secondly, there was a negative association between *NPM1* and myeloid transcription factor mutations (Fisher's Exact test, p = 0.0001), and also between *NPM1* and chromatin modifier mutations that occurred together only for two patients. Thirdly, all patients with *TP53* mutations had high-risk cytogenetic abnormalities (Fisher's Exact test, p < 0.0001). Fourthly, *NPM1* mutations were associated with morphological signs of differentiation, i.e., FAB classification M2/M4/M5/M6 (Fisher's Exact test, $p = 0.0233$). Finally, even in this relatively small patient cohort, we observed that no patients with TET2 mutations (13 patients) had IDH mutation (5 patients); this inverse correlation has been described in previous cohorts [6], but did not reach statistical significance in our smaller cohort. We did not detect any significant associations between individual mutation or mutational main classes and age, gender, or AML etiology (de novo/secondary). A trend toward higher number of identified mutations in patients >65 years was detected, (median 4 mutations >65 years, and median 3 mutations <65 years), although did not reach statistical significance in this patient cohort. To summarize, the frequencies of individual mutations and the various associations are similar to what has been described previously [7,44]; the observations thus suggest that our patient cohort of consecutive patients with relatively high peripheral blood blast counts is representative for AML in general.

3.2. Expression of Molecular Differentiation Markers by Primary AML Cells: The Expression of the CD34 Stem Cell Markers Differs between Mutational Subsets

The AML cell expression of eight common differentiation markers (CD13, CD14, CD15, CD33, CD34, CD45, CD117, and HLA-DR) was available for 62 unselected AML patients. We first did an unsupervised hierarchical cluster analysis based on this expression profile (Figure S2). We could then identify four main patient subsets, but no single mutation or mutational class showed significant associations with any of the four main patient clusters.

We investigated whether there were any significant correlations between the CD34 stem cell marker and any of the other differentiation markers, but no significant associations were then detected.

We finally investigated whether any of the mutations that are used as prognostic markers in routine clinical practice [2] showed significant correlations with the expression of single differentiation markers. These statistical analyses are summarized in Table S3. Firstly, *NPM1* mutations showed a significant correlation with CD33 expression (Fisher's Exact test, $p = 0.0107$) and a negative association with CD34 expression (Fisher's Exact test, $p < 0.0001$). These *NPM1* associations are similar to the observations in a previous large study of 184 unselected patients [45], and they are consistent with the observation that *NPM1* mutations are frequently associated with morphological signs of differentiation (see above). Secondly, neither *FLT3*-ITD nor *DNMT3A* mutations showed any association with CD34 expression. *NPM1* mutations are frequently combined with *FLT3*-ITD and DNA-methylation mutations [6], but only the negative *NPM1* association reached significance in our relatively small cohort. Thirdly, patients with mutations in chromatin modifier genes showed an increased frequency of CD34 expression by their AML cells (Fisher's Exact test $p = 0.0159$). We detected the combination of *NPM1* and chromatin modifier mutations for only two patients, and this was similar to the observations in previous studies [7]. Thus, these mutational subsets also differ in their expression of differentiation markers, especially CD34 expression.

3.3. AML Patients Can Be Subclassified Based on Their Constitutive Release of Extracellular Mediators, but this Capacity Shows no Association with the Mutational Profile

Primary AML cells from 46 of the patients were available for additional studies of constitutive cytokine release during in vitro culture. This patient subset represents a constitutive and thereby unselected subset among the 71 patients included in our present study. We investigated the constitutive release of 34 soluble mediators, including several cytokines (interleukins, CCL and CXCL chemokines, immunoregulatory cytokines, growth factors), proteases, and protease regulators/inhibitors. A clustering analysis identified a subset of patients with generally high constitutive mediator release; the other patients showed generally low or intermediate release (Figure 2). Neither any single mutation nor mutational main class differed significantly when comparing the three patient subsets identified in this clustering analysis.

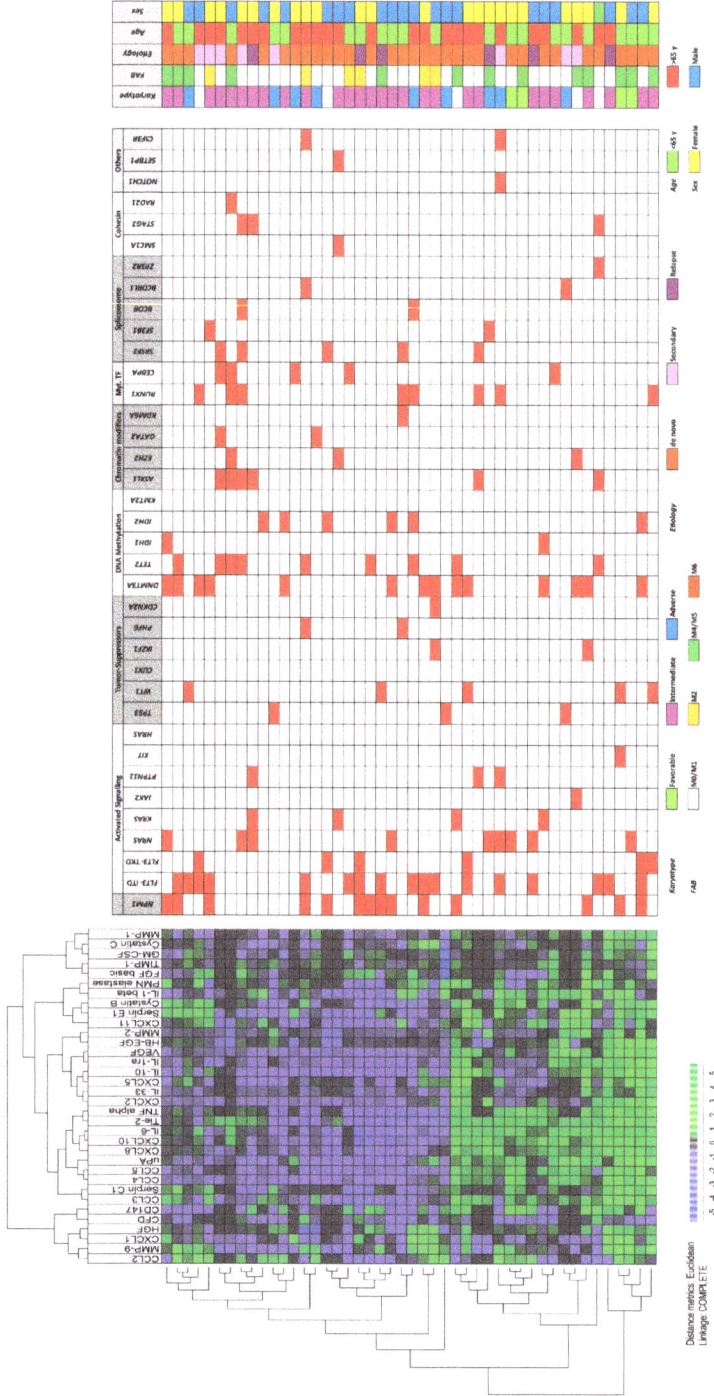

Figure 2. The secretome and genomic profile for 46 AML patients. Primary AML cells derived from a consecutive subset of 46 patients were cultured in vitro for 48 h and the supernatant levels of 34 soluble mediators were then determined. We performed an unsupervised hierarchical cluster analysis (Euclidean measure, and complete distance) based on these results and were then able to identify two distinct patient clusters corresponding to patients with generally high or intermediate/low supernatant level.

3.4. Comparison of Global Gene Expression Profiles for Patients with Generally High and Low Constitutive Release of Extracellular Mediators

We have previously described differences in global gene expression profiles between AML cells with generally high and low constitutive mediator release [46]. We performed a similar comparison for the patients included in the present studies based on the differentially expressed genes, and we could then identify two main patient subsets based on this expression (d-score >3.5; 149 genes identified). However, these two subsets did not differ significantly with regard to the distribution of single mutations or the overall mutational profiles of the AML cell populations (Figure S3).

3.5. Comparison of Proteomic Profiles for AML Cell Populations Showing Generally High and Low Constitutive Release of Extracellular Mediators

Our proteomic analyses identified 5852 proteins, but 5586 proteins were left after leaving out protein contaminants, reverse hits, and proteins only identified by site. Our further analyses were based on 4350 proteins that could be detected in at least five patients for each of the two compared groups. A significant difference ($p < 0.05$) in protein abundance between the two groups was detected for 256 of these proteins (182 proteins increased in patients showing high constitutive release, 74 proteins being increased in the others), i.e., determined by Welch's t-test and Z-statistics (a list of selected proteins are described more in detail in Table S4 and the complete list of all 256 proteins is given in Table S5).

We first performed an unsupervised hierarchical cluster analysis (Euclidean measure, and complete distance) based on the 256 differentially expressed proteins (Figure 3). Our analysis identified two main clusters/subsets of patients corresponding to patients with generally high and low constitutive release by their AML cells; only one of the high release patients clustered as an outlier. Furthermore, we performed GO term overrepresentation analyses based on the 256 differentially abundant proteins. The analysis of those proteins showing increased expression ($n = 74$) in patients with low constitutive mediator release and returned significantly increased GO terms, which reflected an altered regulation of nuclear functions/transcription/RNA metabolism (Table 3 and Table S4). It can be seen that a major part of these genes are important for transcriptional regulation/RNA expression/RNA metabolism.

We then analyzed those proteins showing increased expression in AML cells with high constitutive cytokine release; the most significant GO-terms are listed in Table 4. When analyzing the proteins with regard to cell compartment the four largest terms (extracellular exosomes, cytosol, membrane, and cytoplasm) were only partly overlapping with regard to individual proteins and included 153 of the 182 proteins that were significantly increased in high-release AML cells (Figure 4). These four GO terms reflect cytoplasmic/cytosolic structures/functions together with the terms actin filament and phagocytic vesicle membrane. One of the terms reflects metabolic functions (NADPH oxidase complex), whereas the two last terms reflect cell surface functions/cellular communication (focal adhesion, membrane rafts). Analysis of biological processes and molecular functions included several relatively small GO terms that also reflect intracellular signaling, protein interactions, or cell surface receptor signaling (Table 4). Table S4 gives a more detailed description of those proteins that were identified both in the GO term analyses (Table 4, Figure 4) and in the network analysis (Figure 5; proteins in the large network to the left in the figure with increased levels in high-secreting cells).

The proteins with increased expression in patients with generally high constitutive release are presented in Figure 4 (all proteins included in the GO-terms GO:0070062—extracellular exosome, GO:0005829—cytosol, GO:0016020—membrane, or GO:0005737—cytoplasm); Table 3 (classification of proteins showing $p < 0.01$); Table S4 (description of proteins from Table 3 with $p < 0.01$); and Table S5 (the complete list of all 256 differentially expressed proteins). These more detailed analyses and classifications of individual proteins from Table 3 and Table S4 also show that AML cells showing generally high or low constitutive release of extracellular mediators differ especially with regard to transcriptional regulation, cell surface molecular profile, intracellular signaling, intracellular trafficking, and cell adhesion/migration.

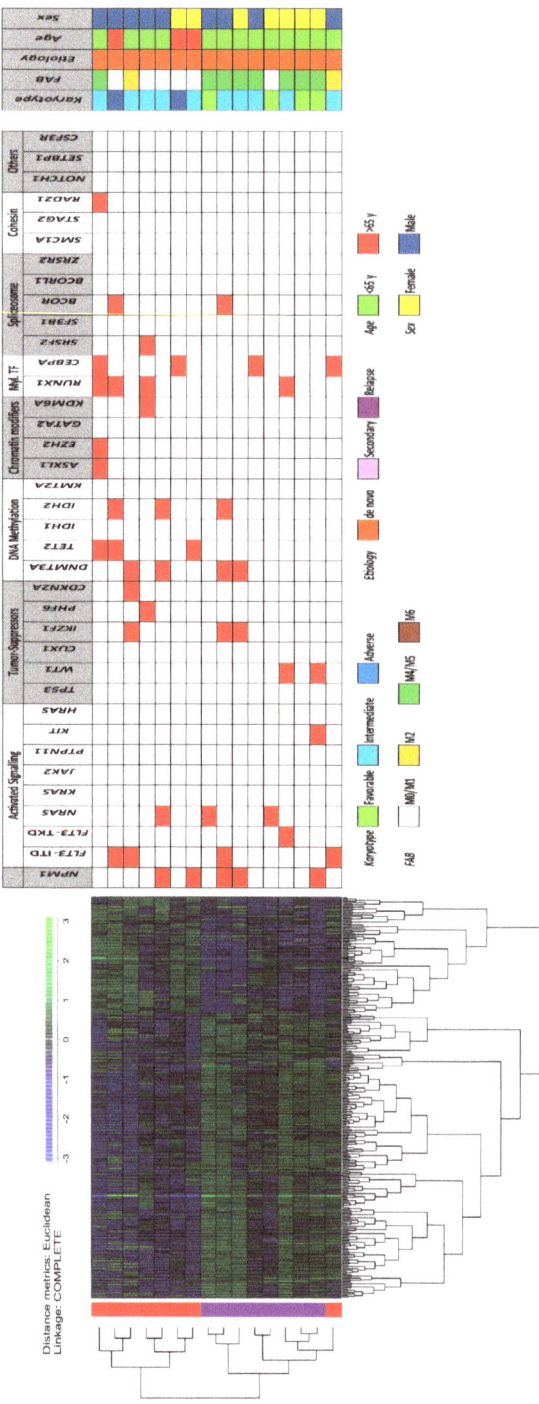

Figure 3. Identification of two main patient subsets based on proteomic differences of AML cells with high and low constitutive release. Eight of the 16 patients included in the proteomic studies belonged to the cluster characterized by generally high constitutive mediator release and the eight others showed low/intermediate secretion (Figure 2); 256 proteins differed significantly between these two groups. We performed an unsupervised hierarchical cluster analyses (Euclidean measure, and complete distance) based on the levels of these proteins, and the left part demonstrates the dendrogram and heat map; blue indicates low protein levels and green high levels. Two main clusters were then identified corresponding to the high and low/intermediate secretion patients except for one outlier patient (left column, red color indicating high release). As expected, the two main clusters were heterogeneous with regard to mutational frequencies (middle panel) and did not differ with regard to clinical or biological characteristics either (right panel).

Table 3. Differentially expressed proteins in primary AML cell populations with high (left) and low (high) constitutive release of extracellular soluble mediators. The mediators are classified based on their main functional characteristics. The information is based on the Gene database and selected references from the PubMed database (Table S4). The proteins being increased in high-secreting AML cells are those proteins that were both included in the gene ontology (GO) terms GO:0070062—extracellular exosome, GO:0005829—cytosol, GO:0016020—membrane, and GO:0005737—cytoplasm (Figure 4), and also in the main interacting protein network in the left part of Figure 5 (Table S4). The proteins being increased in the low-secreting AML cells are those proteins included the GO terms GO:0000790—nuclear chromatin and GO:0005736—DNA-directed RNA polymerase I complex (Table 4).

Main Classification	Increased Protein Levels in Cells with High Constitutive Release	Increased Protein Levels in Cells with Low Constitutive Release
Nucleosome		MBD3
Chromatin, histone, transcription, RNA	TOLLIP, NFKB1	HIF0, HIST1H2AI, MTA1, SMARCE1, MEN1, MBD3, POLR1E, CLPX, POLR1A, POLR1B
DNA repair		CLPX, JUND, POG2
Oncogene	CBL, DBNL	
Cell cycle regulation	IL16	
Intracellular signaling	SYK, HCLS1, AKAP1, TLR2, TOLLIP, AGTRAP, ANXA2, CECR1, INPP5D, LPKN, JKBKB, TBK1	
Tyrosine kinase	SYK, HCLS1, FGR, PKN1	
SRC tyrosine kinases	HCLS1, FGR, HCK,	
PI3K-Akt-mTOR	NCF4	
RAC1	RAC1, NCF4, RHOT1, ARHGEF1, PKN1, RHOG, ARHGAP30, PREX1, GMIP, DOK2, AKAP1	
GTPase	DNM2, ARHGEF1, PKN1, RHOG, ARHGAP30, PREX1, GMIP, AKAP1, ARHGAP, RAB27A	
G-protein coupled receptors	ARRB2, ARHGEF1, PREX1, GRK6	
Phagocytosis	CYBA, NCF2, NCF4, ELMO2	
Protein degradation	CBL, SERPINA1	
Intracellular trafficking	VAMP3, DNM2, PICALM, SNX18, ARAP1, ARAP1, TOLLIP, AP1G2, S100A10, S100A4, TOM1, SDCDP, DNAJC13, EPN1, APHGAP, RAB27A	
Microtubule, cytoskeleton, structure	DNM2, EPN1, SH3KBP1, PKN1, RHOG, AHNAK, SDCDP, S100A4, CKAP4, FAM49B	
Cell migration	PLXNB2, HCK, DNM2, RHOG, ELMO2, AHNAK	
Mitochondria, metabolism	FAM49B, FTL, IMPDH1, PDXK	CLPX
Lysosomes	CTSH, CTSS, CTSZ, LYZ, PSAP	
Cell metabolism, NADP	HCK, NCF4	
Cytokinesis	FMNL1	
Extracellular matrix, cell adhesion	EPN1, SH3KBP1	
Extracellular mediators	IL16, TLR2, TOLLIP	
Cell surface molecules	ITGAL, ITGAM, ITGB2, SYK, LILRB2, PKN1, LPXN	
Integrins	ITGAL, ITGAM, ITGB2, SYK, FGR, LPXN	
Viability, apoptosis	SH3KBP1, PKN1, ARAP1, TLR2	
AML	CBL, PICALM	
Differentiation	MNDA, NCF1, CECR1	

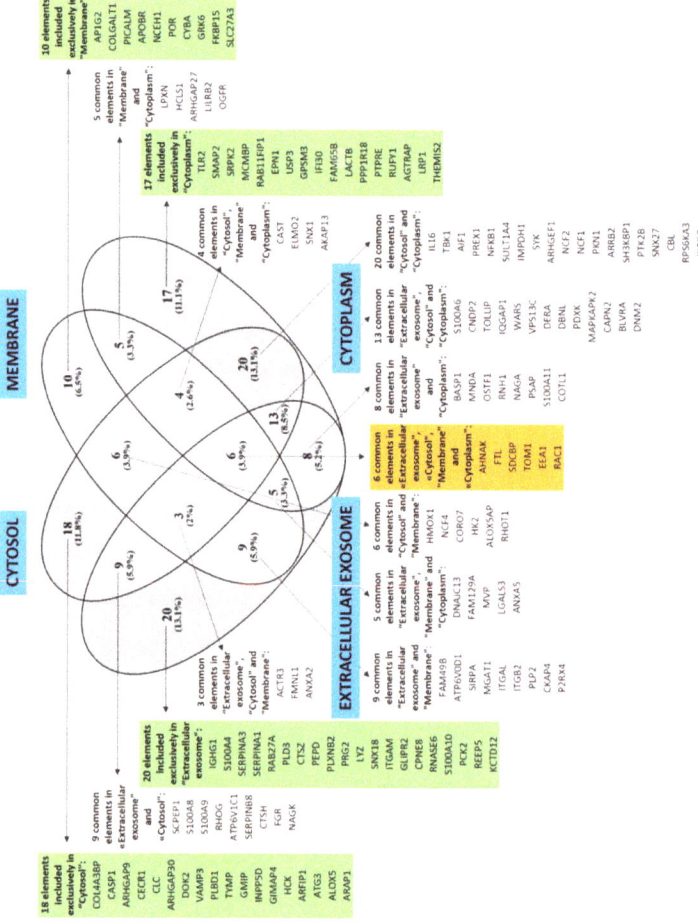

Figure 4. GO-terms including significantly increased proteins for AML cells with generally high constitutive release of extracellular soluble mediators. The over-representation analysis based on cellular compartment identified four GO terms with FDR < 0.05 and including at least 40 proteins, i.e., GO:0070062—extracellular exosome, GO:0005829—cytosol, GO:0016020—membrane, and GO:0005737—cytoplasm. These four GO-terms were partly overlapping (only six proteins included in all four); together they included 153 of the 186 proteins that were increased in AML cells with generally high constitutive release compared with AML cells with low/intermediate constitutive release.

Table 4. Significant GO-terms (i.e., FDR < 0.05) for proteins showing significantly increased levels in AML patients with intermediate/low and high constitutive mediator release.

Low constitutive mediator release; list of significant GO-terms		Protein number	Fold enrichment	FDR
Cell compartment	GO:0005654—nucleoplasm	31	2.8	2.3×10^{-5}
	GO:0000790—nuclear chromatin	8	11	0.0099
	GO:0005736—DNA-directed RNA polymerase I complex	4	80	0.017
Molecular function	GO:0003713—transcription coactivator activity	9	8.5	0.011
	GO:0001054—RNA polymerase I activity	4	78	0.018
High constitutive mediator release; list of significant GO-terms				
Biological processes	GO:0006954—inflammatory response	19	5.0	6.5×10^{-5}
	GO:0045087—innate immune response	20	4.7	8.3×10^{-5}
	GO:0048010—vascular endothelial growth factor receptor signaling pathway	9	13	8.6×10^{-4}
	GO:0007229—integrin-mediated signaling pathway	10	10	9.4×10^{-4}
	GO:0031623—receptor internalization	7	16	0.0062
	GO:0007165—signal transduction	29	2.5	0.015
	GO:0098609—cell–cell adhesion	13	4.8	0.026
Cell compartment	GO:0070062—extracellular exosome	73	2.7	1.4×10^{-13}
	GO:0005829—cytosol	79	2.5	5.7×10^{-13}
	GO:0016020—membrane	48	2.3	7.8×10^{-5}
	GO:0043020—NADPH oxidase complex	5	43	0.0048
	GO:0005737—cytoplasm	78	1.6	0.010
	GO:0030670—phagocytic vesicle membrane	7	12	0.026
	GO:0005925—focal adhesion	15	4.0	0.03
	GO:0045121—membrane raft	11	5.6	0.038
	GO:0005884—actin filament	7	11	0.046
Molecular function	GO:0005515—protein binding	129	1.4	5.8×10^{-6}
	GO:0017124—SH3 domain binding	11	8.9	5.8×10^{-4}
	GO:0035325—Toll-like receptor binding	4	96	0.0058

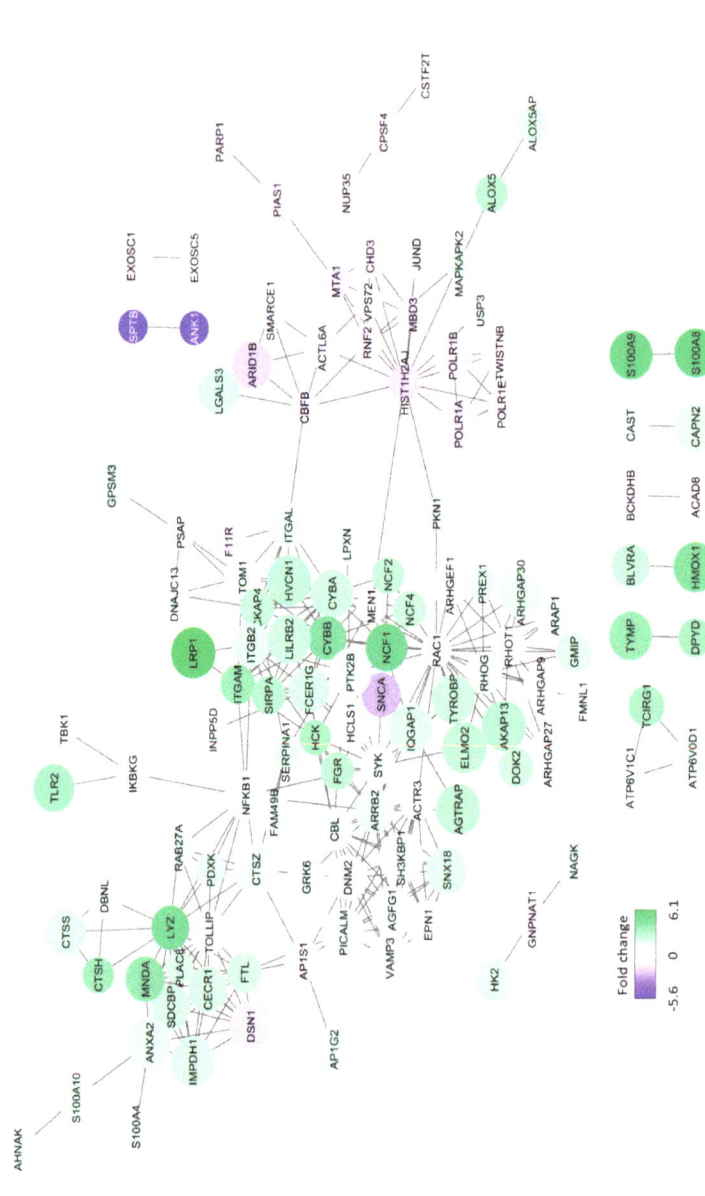

Figure 5. The network analysis of proteins showing differential expression in primary AML cells with generally high versus generally low constitutive release of extracellular mediators. The intensity of the color reflects the fold change (FC) significance when comparing the high- and low-release groups; thus a negative fold change indicates increased protein abundance in the low-release group (purple) and a positive fold change indicates increased protein abundance in the high-release group (green). This STRING-DB analysis was based only on the 256 proteins that were quantified and considered significantly different between the two groups; the figure thus shows proteins from our quantified data and no shells of interactors were considered.

We finally did a molecular network analysis based on the 256 differentially abundant proteins, and Figure 5 shows all molecular connections identified in this analysis (those molecules without any connections are left out). A total of 129 proteins were included in various networks; most of them appeared in a large network linked to the nodes spleen tyrosine kinase (SYK), NCF4 (a cytosolic regulator of superoxide-producing NADPH-oxidase), ARRB2 (regulator of G-protein-coupled receptor activity), ACTR3 (a major constituent of the ARP2/3 complex located at the cell surface and being essential for cell motility), and RAC1 (a GTPase belonging to the RAS superfamily of small GTP-binding proteins). Our overrepresentation analysis showed that exosomal proteins as well as proteins important for intracellular trafficking were differentially expressed; both these groups are important for communication from the leukemic cells to neighboring AML supporting stromal cells [47]. On the other hand, our network analysis showed that these AML cells had increased levels of several members of a signaling pathway, including cell surface integrins ($\alpha L\beta 2$, $\alpha M\beta 2$) known to mediate downstream signaling involving SYK and SRC kinase family members (FGR, HCK) [48–51]. Toll like receptor (TLR) 2 together with its downstream NFκB complex are also linked to this network [49]. Taken together these observations suggest that high constitutive extracellular release of soluble mediators is only a part of a more complex cellular phenotype that is characterized by differences in the bidirectional crosstalk between the leukemic cells and their neighboring AML-supporting cells. This bidirectional crosstalk involves cytokine-mediated signaling directed from the AML cells to the stromal cells. At the same time the stromal cells may influence the AML cells through soluble mediators or cell–cell contact with ligation of cell surface molecules, followed by downstream signaling (involving kinases and G-protein initiated signaling), and finally NFκB mediated modulation of cytokine/chemokine expression [48–52]. Finally, this crosstalk involves integrins that can mediate both inside–out and outside–in effects [48].

4. Discussion

AML is a heterogeneous disease, and this can also be seen from our present studies of primary human AML cells derived from a cohort of consecutive patients. In this study we focused on the molecular genetic abnormalities and the proteomic profiles of the leukemic cells [53]. Both the number and the nature of the molecular genetic abnormalities differed between the patients (number of detected mutations per patients 0–7, median 3.5 mutations). The frequencies of the various mutations were comparable to previous studies [6,7], *NPM1* mutations were associated with molecular and morphological signs of differentiation [45], and *TP53* mutations were associated with adverse karyotypes [54]. Taken together, these observations suggest that we investigated a representative AML patient population, even though we selected patients with relatively high peripheral blood blast counts/percentages.

In the present study, we included a group of consecutive and thereby unselected AML patients with a high percentage of leukemic blasts in peripheral blood. We used this selection of patients so that highly enriched AML cell populations could be prepared by density gradient separation alone; the risk of inducing molecular and/or functional alterations in the AML patients by more extensive cell separation procedures was thereby avoided [55]. Our results may therefore be representative only for this selected subset of patients, but several observations suggest that they possibly are representative for AML in general. Firstly, our patients showed an expected fraction of secondary versus de novo AML [56,57]. Secondly, as previously described in detail patients selected according to these criteria show a similar distribution of cytogenetic abnormalities as AML patients in general [30]. Thirdly, our present study shows that the distribution of various molecular genetic abnormalities is also similar to AML in general [6,7,44,58]. Finally, we have described in detail the selection of the 16 AML patients included in our proteomic studies (see Section 3.5), and they should then be regarded as representative for relatively young AML patients.

Extensive separation procedures will influence the functional characteristics of primary human AML cells, and one would expect that in vitro incubation in culture medium would have similar effects. However, previous studies have shown that the characteristics of even long-term cultured primary human AML cells are associated with patient survival [59], an observation suggesting that even in vitro cultured cells will reflect functional characteristics of clinical relevance.

Distinct immunophenotype profiles may be associated with specific mutations, and search for immunophenotype-based screening approaches have therefore been suggested [60,61]. We investigated the immunophenotype profiles of individual patients based on the expression of eight differentiation markers commonly used for classification of myeloid cells. We identified four different main clusters/patient subsets based on this profiling, but no single mutation or mutation main classes showed significant associations to any of these profiles. However, associations between mutations and single differentiation markers were observed, especially expression of the CD34 stem cell marker that was negatively associated with *NPM1* mutations as well as *FLT3*-ITD and *DNMT3* mutations, whereas chromatin modifier mutations were positively associated with CD34 expression. Such associations have also been described previously [45,62]. A possible explanation for this is that single mutations may have a major impact on the expression of single or related markers, whereas the overall mutational profile has a major impact on the overall differentiation profile.

In previous studies we showed that the constitutive release of a wide range of soluble mediators by primary AML cells varied considerably between patients, and a subset of patients then showed a generally high release compared with other patients that either showed intermediate or low release [11,52]. This capacity of constitutive mediator release was tested in a highly standardized in vitro model. We investigated the constitutive release for a consecutive subset of our patients, and again we found that a subset of patients showed generally higher release of most mediators compared with the other patients. We then selected those samples that were derived before the first time of diagnosis for all relatively young patients that completed intensive chemotherapy. We compared the proteomic profiles of the primary AML cells for eight patients showing high and another group of eight patients showing generally lower mediator release.

Several proteins were differentially expressed when comparing patients with generally high and low constitutive cytokine release. The high release patients showed high expression, especially of proteins involved in intracellular signaling, intracellular transport/trafficking and communication between cells (soluble mediators, exosomes, cell surface molecules, and intracellular mediators downstream to cell surface receptors). We did not identify any of the soluble mediators when analyzing differentially abundant cell proteins between the two patient subsets; this is not unexpected because there is often not a strong correlation between cellular levels and extracellular release of soluble mediators during culture [34].

The high constitutive mediator release should in our opinion be regarded as only a part of a more complex communication phenotype with neighboring non-leukemic stromal cells. In contrast, the cell populations with low constitutive release showed increased abundance proteins involved in or regulating gene transcription/RNA synthesis/RNA metabolism. A possible hypothesis may be that cells with high constitutive release have a higher dependency on neighboring AML-supporting stromal cells than leukemia cells showing low constitutive release. We would emphasize that primary AML cells have a wide range of secreted biomolecules, which can be useful in classification/prognostication and as therapeutic targets [11,52,63]. The mediators included in the present study are well-characterized and are released at detectable levels for most patients. For these reasons they should be regarded as biologically important in the disease, but they probably represent only a part of the AML cell secretome that is involved in the bidirectional crosstalk between leukemic and non-leukemic cells in their common bone marrow microenvironment.

5. Conclusions

We conclude that the high constitutive extracellular release of soluble mediators by primary human AML cells seems to reflect a complex functional phenotype with regard to communication between AML cells and their neighboring non-leukemic stromal cells in their common bone marrow microenvironment. Our proteomic comparison has identified high expression in this patient subset of several intracellular molecules that are regarded as possible therapeutic targets in human AML. Dual targeting of intracellular signaling and extracellular communication should therefore be considered for these patients.

Supplementary Materials: The following are available online at http://www.mdpi.com/2077-0383/8/7/970/s1, Figure S1: Mutation profile and mutation classes. Figure S2: The immunophenotypic profile and mutation profile. Figure S3: Transcriptomics data based on AML secretomic profile. Table S1: The biological and clinical characteristics of patients in the proteomic studies. Table S2: The mutational distribution for patients included in the proteomic studies. Table S3: Statistical comparisons of associations between various mutations and between mutations and signs of AML cell differentiation (morphology, CD34 expression). Table S4: Proteomic profiling based on AML secretome. Table S5: All proteins differently expressed between high and low secretome group.

Author Contributions: Conceptualization, H.R. and Ø.B.; methodology, H.R., E.A., A.K.B., S.B.B., I.S.G., R.B.F., and R.H.; software, H.R., E.A., and A.K.B.; validation, H.R. and Ø.B.; formal analysis, H.R., E.A., and A.K.B.; investigation, H.R., E.A., A.K.B., S.B.B., I.S.G., R.B.F., R.H., and Ø.B.; resources, H.R. and Ø.B.; data curation, H.R., E.A., and A.K.B.; writing—original draft preparation, H.R. and Ø.B.; writing—review and editing, H.R., E.A., A.K.B., S.B.B., I.S.G., R.B.F., R.H., and Ø.B; visualization, H.R., E.A., and A.K.B.; supervision, Ø.B.; project administration, H.R., and Ø.B.; funding acquisition, Ø.B.

Funding: This research was funded by The Norwegian Cancer Society (DNK 100933) and Helse-Vest.

Acknowledgments: Technical support from Karen Marie Hagen and Kristin Paulsen Rye is greatly appreciated.

Conflicts of Interest: The authors declare no conflict of interest.

References

1. Döhner, H.; Weisdorf, D.J.; Bloomfield, C.D. Acute myeloid leukemia. *N. Engl. J. Med.* **2015**, *373*, 1136–1152. [PubMed]
2. Döhner, H.; Estey, E.; Grimwade, D.; Amadori, S.; Appelbaum, F.R.; Buchner, T.; Dombret, H.; Ebert, B.L.; Fenaux, P.; Larson, R.A.; et al. Diagnosis and management of aml in adults: 2017 eln recommendations from an international expert panel. *Blood* **2017**, *129*, 424–447. [PubMed]
3. Arber, D.A.; Orazi, A.; Hasserjian, R.; Thiele, J.; Borowitz, M.J.; Le Beau, M.M.; Bloomfield, C.D.; Cazzola, M.; Vardiman, J.W. The 2016 revision to the world health organization classification of myeloid neoplasms and acute leukemia. *Blood* **2016**, *127*, 2391–2405. [PubMed]
4. Schlenk, R.F.; Dohner, K.; Krauter, J.; Frohling, S.; Corbacioglu, A.; Bullinger, L.; Habdank, M.; Spath, D.; Morgan, M.; Benner, A.; et al. Mutations and treatment outcome in cytogenetically normal acute myeloid leukemia. *N. Engl. J. Med.* **2008**, *358*, 1909–1918. [PubMed]
5. Valk, P.J.; Verhaak, R.G.; Beijen, M.A.; Erpelinck, C.A.; Barjesteh van Waalwijk van Doorn-Khosrovani, S.; Boer, J.M.; Beverloo, H.B.; Moorhouse, M.J.; van der Spek, P.J.; Lowenberg, B.; et al. Prognostically useful gene-expression profiles in acute myeloid leukemia. *N. Engl. J. Med.* **2004**, *350*, 1617–1628. [PubMed]
6. Papaemmanuil, E.; Gerstung, M.; Bullinger, L.; Gaidzik, V.I.; Paschka, P.; Roberts, N.D.; Potter, N.E.; Heuser, M.; Thol, F.; Bolli, N.; et al. Genomic classification and prognosis in acute myeloid leukemia. *N. Engl. J. Med.* **2016**, *374*, 2209–2221. [PubMed]
7. Cancer Genome Atlas Research, N.; Ley, T.J.; Miller, C.; Ding, L.; Raphael, B.J.; Mungall, A.J.; Robertson, A.; Hoadley, K.; Triche, T.J., Jr.; Laird, P.W.; et al. Genomic and epigenomic landscapes of adult de novo acute myeloid leukemia. *N. Engl. J. Med.* **2013**, *368*, 2059–2074.
8. Eppert, K.; Takenaka, K.; Lechman, E.R.; Waldron, L.; Nilsson, B.; van Galen, P.; Metzeler, K.H.; Poeppl, A.; Ling, V.; Beyene, J.; et al. Stem cell gene expression programs influence clinical outcome in human leukemia. *Nat. Med.* **2011**, *17*, 1086–1093.
9. Brenner, A.K.; Reikvam, H.; Lavecchia, A.; Bruserud, O. Therapeutic targeting the cell division cycle 25 (cdc25) phosphatases in human acute myeloid leukemia–the possibility to target several kinases through inhibition of the various cdc25 isoforms. *Molecules* **2014**, *19*, 18414–18447.
10. Hatfield, K.J.; Reikvam, H.; Bruserud, O. Identification of a subset of patients with acute myeloid leukemia characterized by long-term in vitro proliferation and altered cell cycle regulation of the leukemic cells. *Expert. Opin. Therap. Targets* **2014**, *18*, 1237–1251.

11. Brenner, A.K.; Reikvam, H.; Bruserud, O. A subset of patients with acute myeloid leukemia has leukemia cells characterized by chemokine responsiveness and altered expression of transcriptional as well as angiogenic regulators. *Front Immunol.* **2016**, *7*, 205. [PubMed]
12. Griessinger, E.; Anjos-Afonso, F.; Vargaftig, J.; Taussig, D.C.; Lassailly, F.; Prebet, T.; Imbert, V.; Nebout, M.; Vey, N.; Chabannon, C.; et al. Frequency and dynamics of leukemia-initiating cells during short-term ex vivo culture informs outcomes in acute myeloid leukemia patients. *Cancer Res.* **2016**, *76*, 2082–2086. [PubMed]
13. Griessinger, E.; Anjos-Afonso, F.; Pizzitola, I.; Rouault-Pierre, K.; Vargaftig, J.; Taussig, D.; Gribben, J.; Lassailly, F.; Bonnet, D. A niche-like culture system allowing the maintenance of primary human acute myeloid leukemia-initiating cells: A new tool to decipher their chemoresistance and self-renewal mechanisms. *Stem Cells Transl. Med.* **2014**, *3*, 520–529. [PubMed]
14. Hauge, M.; Bruserud, O.; Hatfield, K.J. Targeting of cell metabolism in human acute myeloid leukemia–more than targeting of isocitrate dehydrogenase mutations and pi3k/akt/mtor signaling? *Eur. J. Haematol.* **2016**, *96*, 211–221. [PubMed]
15. Hernandez-Valladares, M.; Aasebo, E.; Mjaavatten, O.; Vaudel, M.; Bruserud, O.; Berven, F.; Selheim, F. Reliable fasp-based procedures for optimal quantitative proteomic and phosphoproteomic analysis on samples from acute myeloid leukemia patients. *Biol. Proced. Online* **2016**, *18*, 13. [PubMed]
16. Aasebo, E.; Mjaavatten, O.; Vaudel, M.; Farag, Y.; Selheim, F.; Berven, F.; Bruserud, O.; Hernandez-Valladares, M. Freezing effects on the acute myeloid leukemia cell proteome and phosphoproteome revealed using optimal quantitative workflows. *J. Proteomics* **2016**, *145*, 214–225. [PubMed]
17. Aasebo, E.; Vaudel, M.; Mjaavatten, O.; Gausdal, G.; Van der Burgh, A.; Gjertsen, B.T.; Doskeland, S.O.; Bruserud, O.; Berven, F.S.; Selheim, F. Performance of super-silac based quantitative proteomics for comparison of different acute myeloid leukemia (aml) cell lines. *Proteomics* **2014**, *14*, 1971–1976. [PubMed]
18. Ossenkoppele, G.J.; Janssen, J.J.; van de Loosdrecht, A.A. Risk factors for relapse after allogeneic transplantation in acute myeloid leukemia. *Haematologica* **2016**, *101*, 20–25. [PubMed]
19. Terwijn, M.; Zeijlemaker, W.; Kelder, A.; Rutten, A.P.; Snel, A.N.; Scholten, W.J.; Pabst, T.; Verhoef, G.; Lowenberg, B.; Zweegman, S.; et al. Leukemic stem cell frequency: A strong biomarker for clinical outcome in acute myeloid leukemia. *PloS ONE* **2014**, *9*, e107587.
20. Wouters, R.; Cucchi, D.; Kaspers, G.J.; Schuurhuis, G.J.; Cloos, J. Relevance of leukemic stem cells in acute myeloid leukemia: Heterogeneity and influence on disease monitoring, prognosis and treatment design. *Expert. Rev. Hematol.* **2014**, *7*, 791–805.
21. Majeti, R. Clonal evolution of pre-leukemic hematopoietic stem cells precedes human acute myeloid leukemia. *Best Pract. Res. Clin. Haematol.* **2014**, *27*, 229–234.
22. Stapnes, C.; Gjertsen, B.T.; Reikvam, H.; Bruserud, O. Targeted therapy in acute myeloid leukaemia: Current status and future directions. *Expert. Opin. Investig. Drugs* **2009**, *18*, 433–455. [PubMed]
23. Binder, S.; Luciano, M.; Horejs-Hoeck, J. The cytokine network in acute myeloid leukemia (aml): A focus on pro- and anti-inflammatory mediators. *Cytokine Growth Factor Rev.* **2018**, *43*, 8–15. [PubMed]
24. Brenner, A.K.; Andersson Tvedt, T.H.; Bruserud, O. The complexity of targeting pi3k-akt-mtor signalling in human acute myeloid leukaemia: The importance of leukemic cell heterogeneity, neighbouring mesenchymal stem cells and immunocompetent cells. *Molecules* **2016**, *21*.
25. Reikvam, H.; Hatfield, K.J.; Fredly, H.; Nepstad, I.; Mosevoll, K.A.; Bruserud, O. The angioregulatory cytokine network in human acute myeloid leukemia-from leukemogenesis via remission induction to stem cell transplantation. *Eur. Cytokine Netw.* **2012**, *23*, 140–153. [PubMed]
26. Kupsa, T.; Horacek, J.M.; Jebavy, L. The role of cytokines in acute myeloid leukemia: A systematic review. *Biomed. Pap. Med. Fac. Univ. Palacky Olomouc Czech Repub.* **2012**, *156*, 291–301. [PubMed]
27. Cho, B.S.; Kim, H.J.; Konopleva, M. Targeting the cxcl12/cxcr4 axis in acute myeloid leukemia: From bench to bedside. *Korean J. Intern. Med.* **2017**, *32*, 248–257. [PubMed]
28. Bernasconi, P.; Farina, M.; Boni, M.; Dambruoso, I.; Calvello, C. Therapeutically targeting self-reinforcing leukemic niches in acute myeloid leukemia: A worthy endeavor? *Am. J. Hematol.* **2016**, *91*, 507–517. [PubMed]
29. Brenner, A.K.; Tvedt, T.H.; Nepstad, I.; Rye, K.P.; Hagen, K.M.; Reikvam, H.; Bruserud, O. Patients with acute myeloid leukemia can be subclassified based on the constitutive cytokine release of the leukemic cells; the possible clinical relevance and the importance of cellular iron metabolism. *Expert. Opin. Therap. Targets* **2017**, *21*, 357–369.

30. Bruserud, O.; Hovland, R.; Wergeland, L.; Huang, T.S.; Gjertsen, B.T. Flt3-mediated signaling in human acute myelogenous leukemia (aml) blasts: A functional characterization of flt3-ligand effects in aml cell populations with and without genetic flt3 abnormalities. *Haematologica* **2003**, *88*, 416–428.
31. Reikvam, H.; Hovland, R.; Forthun, R.B.; Erdal, S.; Gjertsen, B.T.; Fredly, H.; Bruserud, O. Disease-stabilizing treatment based on all-trans retinoic acid and valproic acid in acute myeloid leukemia-identification of responders by gene expression profiling of pretreatment leukemic cells. *BMC Cancer* **2017**, *17*, 630.
32. Staffas, A.; Kanduri, M.; Hovland, R.; Rosenquist, R.; Ommen, H.B.; Abrahamsson, J.; Forestier, E.; Jahnukainen, K.; Jonsson, O.G.; Zeller, B.; et al. Presence of flt3-itd and high baalc expression are independent prognostic markers in childhood acute myeloid leukemia. *Blood* **2011**, *118*, 5905–5913. [PubMed]
33. Wangen, R.; Aasebo, E.; Trentani, A.; Doskeland, S.O.; Bruserud, O.; Selheim, F.; Hernandez-Valladares, M. Preservation method and phosphate buffered saline washing affect the acute myeloid leukemia proteome. *Int. J. Mol. Sci.* **2018**, *19*, 296.
34. Aasebo, E.; Hernandez-Valladares, M.; Selheim, F.; Berven, F.S.; Brenner, A.K.; Bruserud, O. Proteomic profiling of primary human acute myeloid leukemia cells does not reflect their constitutive release of soluble mediators. *Proteomes* **2018**, *7*, 1.
35. Cox, J.; Mann, M. Maxquant enables high peptide identification rates, individualized p.P.B.-range mass accuracies and proteome-wide protein quantification. *Nat. Biotechnol.* **2008**, *26*, 1367–1372. [PubMed]
36. Cox, J.; Matic, I.; Hilger, M.; Nagaraj, N.; Selbach, M.; Olsen, J.V.; Mann, M. A practical guide to the maxquant computational platform for silac-based quantitative proteomics. *Nat. Protoc.* **2009**, *4*, 698–705. [PubMed]
37. Stavrum, A.K.; Petersen, K.; Jonassen, I.; Dysvik, B. Analysis of gene-expression data using j-express. *Curr. Protoc. Bioinformat.* **2008**, Chapter 7, Unit 7.3. [CrossRef]
38. Mi, H.; Muruganujan, A.; Casagrande, J.T.; Thomas, P.D. Large-scale gene function analysis with the panther classification system. *Nat. Protocols* **2013**, *8*, 1551. [PubMed]
39. Tyanova, S.; Temu, T.; Sinitcyn, P.; Carlson, A.; Hein, M.Y.; Geiger, T.; Mann, M.; Cox, J. The perseus computational platform for comprehensive analysis of (prote)omics data. *Nat. Methods* **2016**, *13*, 731–740.
40. Arntzen, M.O.; Koehler, C.J.; Barsnes, H.; Berven, F.S.; Treumann, A.; Thiede, B. Isobariq: Software for isobaric quantitative proteomics using iptl, itraq, and tmt. *J. Proteome Res.* **2011**, *10*, 913–920.
41. Huang, D.W.; Sherman, B.T.; Tan, Q.; Collins, J.R.; Alvord, W.G.; Roayaei, J.; Stephens, R.; Baseler, M.W.; Lane, H.C.; Lempicki, R.A. The david gene functional classification tool: A novel biological module-centric algorithm to functionally analyze large gene lists. *Genome Biol.* **2007**, *8*, R183. [CrossRef] [PubMed]
42. Szklarczyk, D.; Morris, J.H.; Cook, H.; Kuhn, M.; Wyder, S.; Simonovic, M.; Santos, A.; Doncheva, N.T.; Roth, A.; Bork, P.; et al. The string database in 2017: Quality-controlled protein-protein association networks, made broadly accessible. *Nucleic Acids Res.* **2017**, *45*, D362–D368. [CrossRef] [PubMed]
43. Shannon, P.; Markiel, A.; Ozier, O.; Baliga, N.S.; Wang, J.T.; Ramage, D.; Amin, N.; Schwikowski, B.; Ideker, T. Cytoscape: A software environment for integrated models of biomolecular interaction networks. *Genome Res.* **2003**, *13*, 2498–2504. [CrossRef] [PubMed]
44. Patel, J.L.; Schumacher, J.A.; Frizzell, K.; Sorrells, S.; Shen, W.; Clayton, A.; Jattani, R.; Kelley, T.W. Coexisting and cooperating mutations in npm1-mutated acute myeloid leukemia. *Leukemia Res* **2017**, *56*, 7–12. [CrossRef] [PubMed]
45. Tsykunova, G.; Reikvam, H.; Hovland, R.; Bruserud, O. The surface molecule signature of primary human acute myeloid leukemia (aml) cells is highly associated with npm1 mutation status. *Leukemia* **2012**, *26*, 557–559. [CrossRef] [PubMed]
46. Honnemyr, M.; Bruserud, O.; Brenner, A.K. The constitutive protease release by primary human acute myeloid leukemia cells. *J. Cancer Res. Clin. Oncol.* **2017**, *143*, 1985–1998. [CrossRef]
47. Brenner, A.K.; Nepstad, I.; Bruserud, O. Mesenchymal stem cells support survival and proliferation of primary human acute myeloid leukemia cells through heterogeneous molecular mechanisms. *Front Immunol.* **2017**, *8*, 106. [CrossRef]
48. Johansen, S.; Brenner, A.K.; Bartaula-Brevik, S.; Reikvam, H.; Bruserud, O. The possible importance of beta3 integrins for leukemogenesis and chemoresistance in acute myeloid leukemia. *Int. J. Mol. Sci.* **2018**, *19*, 251. [CrossRef]
49. Reikvam, H.; Olsnes, A.M.; Gjertsen, B.T.; Ersvar, E.; Bruserud, O. Nuclear factor-kappab signaling: A contributor in leukemogenesis and a target for pharmacological intervention in human acute myelogenous leukemia. *Crit. Rev. Oncog.* **2009**, *15*, 1–41. [CrossRef]

50. Schmitt, A.; Li, L.; Giannopoulos, K.; Greiner, J.; Reinhardt, P.; Wiesneth, M.; Schmitt, M. Quantitative expression of toll-like receptor-2, -4, and -9 in dendritic cells generated from blasts of patients with acute myeloid leukemia. *Transfusion* **2008**, *48*, 861–870. [CrossRef]
51. Bartaula-Brevik, S.; Lindstad Brattas, M.K.; Tvedt, T.H.A.; Reikvam, H.; Bruserud, O. Splenic tyrosine kinase (syk) inhibitors and their possible use in acute myeloid leukemia. *Expert Opin. Investig. Drugs* **2018**, *27*, 377–387. [CrossRef] [PubMed]
52. Bruserud, O.; Ryningen, A.; Olsnes, A.M.; Stordrange, L.; Oyan, A.M.; Kalland, K.H.; Gjertsen, B.T. Subclassification of patients with acute myelogenous leukemia based on chemokine responsiveness and constitutive chemokine release by their leukemic cells. *Haematologica* **2007**, *92*, 332–341. [CrossRef] [PubMed]
53. Godley, L.A. Profiles in leukemia. *N. Engl. J. Med* **2012**, *366*, 1152–1153. [CrossRef] [PubMed]
54. Rucker, F.G.; Schlenk, R.F.; Bullinger, L.; Kayser, S.; Teleanu, V.; Kett, H.; Habdank, M.; Kugler, C.M.; Holzmann, K.; Gaidzik, V.I.; et al. Tp53 alterations in acute myeloid leukemia with complex karyotype correlate with specific copy number alterations, monosomal karyotype, and dismal outcome. *Blood* **2012**, *119*, 2114–2121. [CrossRef] [PubMed]
55. Granfeldt Ostgard, L.S.; Medeiros, B.C.; Sengelov, H.; Norgaard, M.; Andersen, M.K.; Dufva, I.H.; Friis, L.S.; Kjeldsen, E.; Marcher, C.W.; Preiss, B.; et al. Epidemiology and clinical significance of secondary and therapy-related acute myeloid leukemia: A national population-based cohort study. *J. Clin. Oncol.* **2015**, *33*, 3641–3649. [CrossRef] [PubMed]
56. Bruserud, O.; Gjertsen, B.T.; Foss, B.; Huang, T.S. New strategies in the treatment of acute myelogenous leukemia (aml): In vitro culture of aml cells–the present use in experimental studies and the possible importance for future therapeutic approaches. *Stem Cells* **2001**, *19*, 1–11. [CrossRef] [PubMed]
57. Bruserud, O.; Gjertsen, B.T.; von Volkman, H.L. In vitro culture of human acute myelogenous leukemia (aml) cells in serum-free media: Studies of native aml blasts and aml cell lines. *J. Hemather. Stem Cell Res.* **2000**, *9*, 923–932. [CrossRef]
58. Patel, J.P.; Gonen, M.; Figueroa, M.E.; Fernandez, H.; Sun, Z.; Racevskis, J.; Van Vlierberghe, P.; Dolgalev, I.; Thomas, S.; Aminova, O.; et al. Prognostic relevance of integrated genetic profiling in acute myeloid leukemia. *N. Engl. J. Med.* **2012**, *366*, 1079–1089. [CrossRef]
59. Brenner, A.K.; Aasebo, E.; Hernandez-Valladares, M.; Selheim, F.; Berven, F.; Gronningsaeter, I.S.; Bartaula-Brevik, S.; Bruserud, O. The capacity of long-term in vitro proliferation of acute myeloid leukemia cells supported only by exogenous cytokines is associated with a patient subset with adverse outcome. *Cancers* **2019**, *11*, 73. [CrossRef]
60. Angelini, D.F.; Ottone, T.; Guerrera, G.; Lavorgna, S.; Cittadini, M.; Buccisano, F.; De Bardi, M.; Gargano, F.; Maurillo, L.; Divona, M.; et al. A leukemia-associated cd34/cd123/cd25/cd99+ immunophenotype identifies flt3-mutated clones in acute myeloid leukemia. *Clin. Cancer Res.* **2015**, *21*, 3977–3985. [CrossRef]
61. Mannelli, F.; Ponziani, V.; Bencini, S.; Bonetti, M.I.; Benelli, M.; Cutini, I.; Gianfaldoni, G.; Scappini, B.; Pancani, F.; Piccini, M.; et al. Cebpa-double-mutated acute myeloid leukemia displays a unique phenotypic profile: A reliable screening method and insight into biological features. *Haematologica* **2017**, *102*, 529–540. [CrossRef] [PubMed]
62. Falini, B.; Mecucci, C.; Tiacci, E.; Alcalay, M.; Rosati, R.; Pasqualucci, L.; La Starza, R.; Diverio, D.; Colombo, E.; Santucci, A.; et al. Cytoplasmic nucleophosmin in acute myelogenous leukemia with a normal karyotype. *N. Engl. J. Med.* **2005**, *352*, 254–266. [CrossRef] [PubMed]
63. Reikvam, H.; Fredly, H.; Kittang, A.O.; Bruserud, O. The possible diagnostic and prognostic use of systemic chemokine profiles in clinical medicine;the experience in acute myeloid leukemia from disease development and diagnosis via conventional chemotherapy to allogeneic stem cell transplantation. *Toxins* **2013**, *5*, 336–362. [CrossRef] [PubMed]

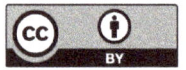

© 2019 by the authors. Licensee MDPI, Basel, Switzerland. This article is an open access article distributed under the terms and conditions of the Creative Commons Attribution (CC BY) license (http://creativecommons.org/licenses/by/4.0/).

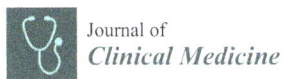

Review

Immunological and Clinical Impact of Manipulated and Unmanipulated DLI after Allogeneic Stem Cell Transplantation of AML Patients

Jochen Greiner [1,2,*], Marlies Götz [2], Donald Bunjes [2], Susanne Hofmann [3] and Verena Wais [2]

1. Department of Internal Medicine, Diakonie Hospital Stuttgart, 70176 Stuttgart, Germany
2. Department of Internal Medicine III, University of Ulm, 89081 Ulm, Germany; marlies.goetz@uni-ulm.de (M.G.); donald.bunjes@uniklinik-ulm.de (D.B.); Verena.Wais@uniklinik-ulm.de (V.W.)
3. Department of Internal Medicine V, University of Heidelberg, 69120 Heidelberg, Germany; susanne.hofmann@med.uni-heidelberg.de
* Correspondence: greiner@diak-stuttgart.de; Tel.: +49-731-150-6754

Received: 11 October 2019; Accepted: 17 December 2019; Published: 23 December 2019

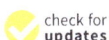

Abstract: Allogeneic stem cell transplantation (allo-SCT) is the preferred curative treatment for several hematological malignancies. The efficacy of allo-SCT depends on the graft-versus-leukemia (GvL) effect. However, the prognosis of patients with relapsed acute myeloid leukemia (AML) following allo-SCT is poor. Donor lymphocyte infusion (DLI) is utilized after allo-SCT in this setting to prevent relapse, to prolong progression free survival, to establish full donor chimerism and to restore the GvL effect in patients with hematological malignancies. Thus, there are different options for the administration of DLI in AML patients. DLI is currently used prophylactically and in the setting of an overt relapse. In addition, in the minimal residual disease (MRD) setting, DLI may be a possibility to improve overall survival. However, DLI might increase the risk of severe life-threatening complications such as graft-versus-host disease (GvHD) as well as severe infections. The transfusion of lymphocytes has been tested not only for the treatment of hematological malignancies but also chronic infections. In this context, manipulated DLI in a prophylactic or therapeutic approach are an option, e.g., virus-specific DLI using different selection methods or antigen-specific DLI such as peptide-specific CD8+ cytotoxic T lymphocytes (CTLs). In addition, T cells are also genetically engineered, using both chimeric antigen receptor (CAR) genetically modified T cells and T cell receptor (TCR) genetically modified T cells. T cell therapies in general have the potential to enhance antitumor immunity, augment vaccine efficacy, and limit graft-versus-host disease after allo-SCT. The focus of this review is to discuss the different strategies to use donor lymphocytes after allo-SCT. Our objective is to give an insight into the functional effects of DLI on immunogenic antigen recognition for a better understanding of the mechanisms of DLI. To ultimately increase the GvL potency without raising the risk of GvHD at the same time.

Keywords: allogeneic stem cell transplantation (allo-SCT); donor lymphocyte infusion (DLI); graft-versus-leukemia (GvL) effect; relapse; virus-specific T cells; α/β T depletion

1. Introduction

Donor lymphocyte infusion (DLI) holds curative potential for acute myeloid leukemia (AML) patients due to the augmentation of the graft-versus-leukemia (GvL) effect. However, DLI may cause graft-versus-host disease (GvHD), which could become life threatening. A better understanding of specific T cell responses against leukemic cells could escalate GvL potency without increasing the risk of GvHD.

DLI has been in use for approximately 30 years as a kind of adoptive T cell therapy and was first administered in chronic myeloid leukemia (CML) patients suffering from relapse after allogeneic stem cell transplantation (allo-SCT) [1]. DLI is a potent approach to enable remission after relapse, despite the risk of inducing GvHD (Figure 1). The best response rates were achieved in CML (80%), while in other hematological diseases, it was less effective [2]. Delayed DLI as a T cell boost as well as gradual dose escalation with repeated DLI is utilized to date in clinical practice to reduce GvHD risk [3]. Some technologies are under development and could play a significant role in the future. It has become clear that DLI can be administered at a much later time point. This allows for the manipulation of the T cell response, such as the selective depletion of alloreactive T cells or the introduction of molecular kill switches, which enable the termination of T cell activity in severe GvHD. These technologies could be particularly important in a haploid setting.

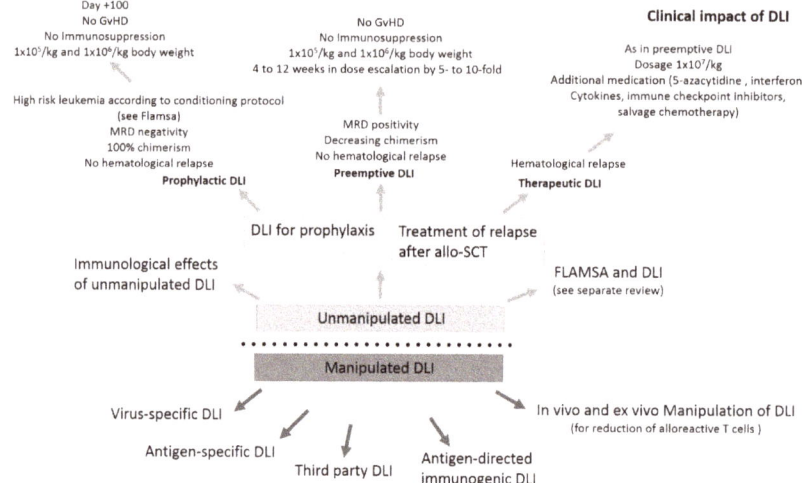

Figure 1. Different modalities and conditions of unmanipulated and manipulated donor lymphocyte infusion (DLI). Unmanipulated DLI is administered to prevent relapse in a prophylactic situation as well as to treat relapse. This has an immunological and, in the majority of cases, also a clinical impact. As to manipulated DLI, this manipulation may take place in vivo or ex vivo. GvHD, graft-versus-host disease; MRD, minimal residual disease; allo-SCT, Allogeneic stem cell transplantation.

Additional new immunotherapeutic T cell approaches are genetically modified affinity enhanced T cell receptor (TCR) against several leukemia-associated antigens (LAAs). LAAs such as New York esophageal squamous cell carcinoma-1 (NYESO-1) in multiple myeloma [4] or Wilms tumor antigen 1 (WT1)-TCR in AML and myelodysplastic syndrome (MDS) [5–7] have been clinically investigated and can be employed both in a autologous and in a allogeneic setting. Some were tested in clinical phase I/II peptide vaccination trials and showed immunological as well as clinical responses. Another approach includes T cell receptor (TCR)-gene modified T cells as well as chimeric antigen receptor (CAR) gene-modified T cells [8,9].

Many of these approaches may be applied to selected patients in the future, but there are several challenges. The best combinations and targets with high GvL potency and reduced GvHD risk have to be selected and the ideal cytokine milieu for therapy as well as the right T cell composition have to be discovered (Table 1).

Table 1. Prophylactic, preemptive and therapeutic studies in DLI. Conditions and response rates of studies and corresponding references.

Situation	Patients, Study Type	Strategy	Response	Reference
prophylactic	retrospective, matched n = 46, high-risk AML/MDS	DLI, +120 d post allo-SCT	7-yr OS, 67% vs 31% ($p < 0.001$) OS in the DLI group was significantly improved	Jedlickova et al. BMT, 2016
	retrospective, high-risk AML	DLI, post allo-SCT	OS in DLI group was improved 70% vs. 40% ($p = 0.027$)	Schmid et al. Br J Haematol, 2019
preemptive	n = 105, prospective standard-risk AML, ALL, MDS	49 low-dose IL-2 56 DLI	3-yr OS: DLI: 58%, IL-2: 28%	Yan et al. Blood, 2012
	n = 101, MDS/AML	preemptive chemotherapy in combination with DLI application	CIR, NRM and DFS 39.5%, 9.6%, and 51.7%	MO et al. Eur J Haematol, 2016
	prospective phase II study n = 20, MDS/AML	> 100 d post allo-SCT four azacytidine cycles (75 mg/m^2/d for 7 days)	hematological relapse in 13 patients (65%)	Platzbecker et al. Leukemia, 2012
therapeutic	retrospective, 399 patients	177 DLI, 228 no DLI	2 yr OS 21% with DLI, 9% without DLI ($p = 0.04$)	Schmid et al. J Clin Oncol, 2007
	n = 263, retrospective	cytoreductive therapy, followed by DLI or second HSCT	CR was reinduced in 32%; 2 yr OS was 14%	Schmid et al. Blood, 2012
	n = 57, prospective	cytarabine-based therapy and DLI	2 yr OS 19%	Levine et al. J Clin Oncol, 2002
	prospective phase I study AML	azacytidine post DLI	CR (6/8)	Ghobadi et al. Leuk Res, 2016
	retrospective, MDS/AML	azacytidine/DLI	Overall response was 33% OS after 2 yrs 29%	Schroeder et al. BBMT, 2015
	retrospective, AML	Sorafenib, in combination with hypomethylating agents and DLI	38% CR	De Freitas et al. Eur J Haematol, 2016

Legend: CIR=cumulative incidence of relapse; CR=complete remission; d=days; DLI=donor lymphocyte infusion; IL-2=interleukin-2; n=number; NRM=non-relapse mortality; OS=overall survival; yr=year.

A better comprehension of the interaction between DLI and the corresponding targets might facilitate the increase in GvL potency, without escalating the GvHD risk, which is of utmost importance.

2. Understanding the Functionality of DLI—Immunological Effects of Unmanipulated DLI

Although unmanipulated DLI is commonly used in the clinical setting, the immunological mechanisms have to be further elucidated. In particular, the role of antigen-specific T cell responses after DLI and a more extensive comprehension of leukemia elimination by T cells is mandatory in established immunotherapies such as allo-SCT and DLI. The main goal is to increase the GvL potency without raising the risk of GvHD at the same time. The most applied technique is the infusion of unmanipulated DLI after unmanipulated or in vivo T cell depleted transplantation from matched sibling or unrelated donors in patients with AML or MDS. After allo-SCT, tissue damage is gradually repaired. In this process, donor dendritic cells (DCs) replace the recipient DCs within the first 6 months after allo-SCT. Accordingly, the host and donor immune subsets do progressively adapt. This explains the clinical observation that a higher number of T cells can be administered without induction of severe GvHD (less than 10^5/kg body weight after 3 months, to 10^6/kg body weight at 6 months) [10]. Therefore, DLI should only be administered in the absence of tissue damage and inflammatory circumstances, for example without GvHD and uncontrolled infections. To date, these infusions are not guided by the diversity of the TCR repertoire or the subsets of lymphocytes [11,12].

For a better comprehension of the immunological function of DLI and for the recognition of immunogenic leukemia-associated antigens (LAAs), Hofmann et al. [13] assessed the frequency and diversity of LAA-specific cytotoxic T cells in a small patient cohort, before and after DLI. Patients were screened for LAA-specific cytotoxic T lymphocyte (CTL) responses, number of Tregs and cytokine levels before and after DLI. Several LAAs—among them, preferentially expressed antigen in melanoma (PRAME), WT1, receptor for hyaluronan acid-mediated motility (RHAMM), and NYESO-1—were tested for specific CTL responses before and after DLI. A significant increase in the number of LAAs recognized by CTLs in clinical responders after DLI and an enhanced LAA diversity in T cell responses were detected. Thus, clinical responses after allo-SCT and DLI might be dependent on an increase in the frequency and diversity of LAA-specific T cell responses. The assumption is that several LAAs play a role in CTL response after DLI and the increase in CTL specific LAA-detection is especially decisive for a successful clinical response to DLI. The diversity of antigen-specific T cells seems to have a strong influence on the GvL effect after allo-SCT and DLI. The conjunction of all these factors may contribute to the clinical outcome of patients treated with several DLI applications.

Moreover, clinical responders showed a significant decrease in the frequency of the highly immunosuppressive CD4+ Tregs. The quantity of Tregs remained stable in non-responders [13]. Tregs play a central role in the maintenance of self-tolerance and promote malignant cell progression by suppressing effective antitumor immunity [14], and thus it is truly striking that clinical responders in the analyzed patient cohort show a significant reduction of Treg. Further studies detected an association with a higher frequency of Treg and unfavorable clinical outcome in several other tumor entities including hematological malignancies [15–19].

These data imply that DLI may not only qualify for mono-therapeutic use but also for combined approaches. Thus, the reduction of Treg could improve the efficacy of other immunotherapies or immune checkpoint inhibitors [20].

In another analysis, patients with Nucleophosmin 1 (NPM1)-mutated AML were treated with DLI after allo-SCT. The authors detected immune responses against different LAAs, especially against NPM1-derived epitopes of the mutated region of NPM1. The detection of the immune responses was linked to minimal residual disease (MRD) negativity, therefore suggesting a correlation of GvL and LAA-specific CTL response [21]. Interestingly, in a cohort of 25 patients with NPM1-mutated AML, the presence of CTL responses against the immunogenic region of NPM1 was associated with a longer overall survival [22]. Due to a lack of tolerance against mutant-derived neoantigen epitopes, these are promising targets for immunotherapy and are currently particularly in the focus for checkpoint inhibitor therapies. Moreover, a correlation of mutational antigen load and clinical benefit was described for melanoma and non-small-cellular lung cancer [23,24]. Neoantigens derived from the mutated region of NPM1 are interesting targets in AML.

The cytokine milieu may influence the function of DLI. Moore et al. [25] show that interleukin-7 (IL-7) and IL-2 are homeostatic cytokines for naive CD4+ and CD8+ T cells. Furthermore, in high concentrations, IL-15 provides a setting for the directed expansion of in vitro-derived memory/effector CD8+ T cell populations that have been adoptively transferred. Yet, IL-15 has to be further tested in phase I trials.

Based on this concept, cytokine-induced killer (CIK) cells have been developed. CIK cells are memory T lymphocytes, which have acquired CD56 expression. In several experimental allogeneic models, CIK cells have demonstrated in vitro and in vivo antitumor activity, direct intratumor homing following intravenous administration and, more importantly, reduced GvHD activity. Finally, the study suggests that CIK cells may be effective in the treatment of post-transplant relapse [26]. Further scientific studies are necessary to improve the understanding of DLI and to increase the efficacy of DLI and DLI in combination with other drugs.

3. Clinical Impact of Unmanipulated DLI in AML

3.1. Therapeutic DLI for the Treatment of Morphological Relapse

Therapeutic DLI is well established in the treatment of clinical relapse in different hematological malignancies. The response rate and survival after DLI vary from entity to entity and depend on several factors, such as disease characteristics and the genotype of the disease, disease burden, the proliferative rate of the disease, donor origin, as well as the clinical situation of the patient.

In 1997, Collins et al. [27] published a retrospective study with 140 patients in 25 North American programs with relapsed malignancies (CML, AML, ALL, MDS and myeloma) after allo-SCT. In this study, a high percentage of patients with relapsed chronic-phase CML, DLI administration resulted in complete remission. While complete remission was observed less frequently in patients with advanced CML and acute leukemia [27]. Similar results were oberserved by Posthuma et al. [28], where DLI resulted in complete cytogenetic remission (CCR) of relapsed chronic-phase chronic myeloid leukemia (CML-CP) after allo-SCT in up to 80% of patients.

With GvHD as the main complication, in 1998, Verdonck et al. [29] evaluated the efficacy and toxicity of different doses of donor T cells. T cell doses varied from 0.1×10^7 to 33×10^7 T cells/kg body weight. They observed that higher T cell doses (> or = 10×10^7/kg) induced serious GvHD as well as marrow aplasia [29].

Based on this, Posthuma et al. [28] reduced the dosage of DLI in CML patients, which was associated with less GvHD but also with a longer interval between treatment and CCR. Posthuma also observed that DLI resulted in complete cytogenetic remission (CCR) of relapsed chronic-phase chronic myeloid leukemia (CML-CP) after allo-SCT in up to 80% of patients. Because of the longer interval between treatment and CCR, they postulated that combining alpha-interferon (alpha-IFN) with DLI would make it feasible to decrease the dose of DLI, thereby limiting GvHD, and at the same time decrease the interval between DLI and CCR for patients with either a hematologic or cytogenetic relapse. This concept is still used today in patients with AML as well as in other hematological malignancies. Further generated methods include chemotherapy, immunosuppressive medications, and the use of selected T cell subsets and/or modified T cells (for instance, suicide gene insertion) [26,30–32]. In addition, composition approaches have been used to try to improve the outcome of the treatment with DLI. There are strategies to combine DLI with other drugs that stimulate the immune system and T cells such as interferon derivates, cytokines or immune checkpoint inhibitors as well as combinations of DLI with other drugs such as hypomethylating substances and other immunomodulatory agents [30,33–35].

To evaluate the role of DLI in the treatment of relapsed AML in comparison to further strategies, Schmid et al. analyzed 399 patients retrospectively. In total, 177 patients were treated with DLI and

228 were the controls. The survival rate two years after allo-SCT was 21% for patients receiving DLI and 9% for patients without DLI treatment ($p = 0.04$). Among DLI recipients, a lower tumor burden at relapse (<35% of bone marrow blasts; $p = 0.006$) and favorable cytogenetics ($p = 0.004$) were predictive for survival in a multivariate analysis. Two-year survival was 15% ± 3% if DLI was administered in aplasia or in active disease [36].

The European Society for Blood and Marrow Transplantation (EBMT) Acute Leukemia Working Group conducted a retrospective study of AML patients in complete remission (CR) and relapse after allo-SCT. In 32%, CR could be reinduced, but long-term survival was almost exclusively achieved after successful induction of CR by cytoreductive therapy, followed either by DLI or by a second allo-SCT [37].

Retrospective studies found the combination of Sorafenib with DLI in FLT3-ITD+ AML with relapse after allo-SCT to be superior to treatment with DLI alone [38,39]. De Freitsas et al. retrospectively collected data of Sorafenib, partially in combination with hypomethylating agents and DLI. Hematological response was documented in 12 of 13 patients (92%), and five of 13 (38%) achieved CR. GvHD was frequently observed in association with DLI. Therefore, Sorafenib might represent a valid treatment option; however, prospective and larger studies are needed [40].

In particular, the combination of DLI with hypomethylating agents seems to be a very effective therapy for relapsed MDS and AML patients after allo-SCT [41–43]. In a phase I study [43], a phase II study [42] and several retrospective analyses [44–46], this was shown. A relevant number of the patients included showed significantly improved survival rates with acceptable toxicity [41–43]. For example, in a retrospective study with azacytidine and DLI, the overall response rate was 33% and the 2 year overall survival (OS) was 29% [45]. Nonetheless, it has to be considered that molecular relapse alone, diagnosis of MDS and low marrow blast count at the time of relapse are associated with better OS [38]. In a retrospective study, treatment with decitabine and DLI as alternative substance showed a response rate of 25%, including patients with previous azacytidine failure, and a 2 year OS of 11% [42]. There was no significant incidence of acute GvHD (aGvHD) or chronic GvHD (cGvHD). According to these data, hypomethylating agents in combination with DLI may be considered in patients who might not be eligible for a more aggressive remission induction [38]. For long-term disease control after relapse, a second allo-SCT has to be considered [38]. Patients with an MDS relapse or AML with low disease burden after allo-SCT seem to benefit more from azacytidine and DLI therapy, than patients with AML [45]. There are currently no specific data on these aspects.

If possible, in the case of bulky and fast-growing disease, intensive chemotherapy should be chosen rather than hypomethylating agents, as in a retrospective analysis, chemotherapy was superior, considering OS [47].

Especially in cases of high tumor burden, conventional chemotherapy should be considered. However, chemotherapy alone generally has no curative potential in this setting. To overcome the reduced effectiveness of DLI in these circumstances, Levine et al. used a chemotherapy strategy to debulk disease before administration of DLI. 65 patients were prospectively treated with cytarabine-based chemotherapy, followed by DLI. In total, 27 of 57 assessable patients achieved CR. GvHD was observed in 56% of the patients. Overall survival at 2 years for the entire cohort was 19%. Patients in CR were more likely to survive, with 1 and 2 year survival rates of 51% and 41%, respectively. In conclusion, treatment with chemotherapy before DLI can help patients with advanced myeloid relapse. However, patients with short remissions after allo-SCT are unlikely to benefit from this approach [48].

The possibility of combining DLI with chemotherapy was also evaluated in several other studies [49]. In the combination therapy, DLI is administered either at the time of the leukocyte nadir or after regeneration. DLI administration in the leukocyte nadir does not require sustained response but has a higher risk of toxicity. DLI after regeneration could reduce the GvHD risk but might not be appropriate in some patients without sustained response. Furthermore, in a retrospective study, it was demonstrated that intensive chemotherapy administered with a second allo-SCT or DLI is superior to chemotherapy alone in relapsed MDS after allo-SCT; OS was 32% in the immunotherapy group, 6% in the cyto-reductive chemotherapy only group, and 2% in the palliative care-only group ($p < 0.001$) [49]. Another option is chemotherapy followed by DLI and azacytidine, and for further insight, a phase I study was conducted in patients with AML relapse [43]. Nonetheless, prospective studies are needed [38].

Another concept for the treatment of AML relapse after allo-SCT is the initiation of epigenetic therapy, interspersed with low dose DLI. Therefore, a phase I/II feasibility study of panobinostat alone and the combination of panobinostat and decitabine prior to DLI in patients after allo-SCT with poor and very poor-risk AML was developed (Hovon 116-trial). This trial contained three dose levels consisting of either panobinostat (PNB) (20 mg at days 1, 4, 8, 11 of a 4 week-cycle) or PNB combined with decitabine (DCB, 10 or 20 mg/m^2 at days 1–3 of every 4 week-cycle). DLI consisted of 1×10^6 CD3 T cells/kg body weight at day 90 and 3×10^6 at day 180 in case of a matched sibling (sib) donor or of a 70% reduced dose in case of a matched unrelated donor (MUD). In the interim analysis, 54 patients were transplanted, and median follow up was 9 months (range: 2–25) after transplantation. In total, 41 of 54 patients received PNB alone, 13 PNB/DCB (20 mg/m^2), and 15 PNB/DCB (10 mg/m^2). Combining PNB with DCB at a dose of 20 mg/m^2 was not feasible due to resulting cytopenia. OS at 12 months from transplantation was 81% (±7). Five patients died due to non-relapse mortality and five died due to relapse. Relapse-free survival (RSF) at 12 months was 66% (±9). A historical HOVON control group of very poor-risk AML CR1 recipients of allo-SCT showed an OS of 52% ± 6 at 12 months and RFS of 43% ± 5. DLI could be administered in 34 patients, including 19 receiving two DLI, and nine patients three DLI. Out of 34 recipients of DLI, severe cGvHD occurred in five (15%) patients. Collectively, these results suggest an encouraging outcome with respect to relapse and OS in patients receiving PBN alone or PBN combined with DCB followed by DLI. An international prospective randomized study is in the pipeline [50].

At present, there are no valid data for treatment with chimeric antigen receptor (CAR) T cells for MDS and AML, but trials are ongoing.

In conclusion, therapeutic DLI is effective in AML/MDS and is currently used with or without other agents depending on the individual disease burden and GvHD risk (Table 1) [38]. Furthermore, the presented data suggest that chemotherapy is recommended in AML/MDS relapse after allo-SCT for patients who most likely tolerate the toxicity and are eligible for subsequent treatment with either DLI or second allo-SCT [38].

3.2. Biology of Therapeutic DLI

High tumor burden, proliferative rate and relapse, predominantly caused by immune escape mechanisms, limit the efficacy of DLI [33,51,52]. In particular, NK cells provide acute control over leukemic activity. However, by tolerance induction over time, NK cells lose their antileukemic reaction [53]. Other subsets such as gamma/delta (γ/δ) T cells appear to have a prolonged anti-leukemic effect [54].

In addition to the timing, frequency, setting and combination of DLI with other substances, there is still an ongoing discussion about the dosage of DLI.

Donor type and setting, as well as the frequency and interval between infusions of DLI, have an influence on the adequate dose of DLI. Considering these factors, the recommended range in literature is 0.001×10^8 to 8.8×10^8 CD3+-cells/kg body weight [55]. An approach with a smaller dosage for example of $0.1–1 \times 10^6$ CD3+/kg body weight, in the prophylactic setting seems reasonable. The infusion is to be repeated every four to eight weeks with an increase in the dosage by half a log level, e.g., 1. DLI: 1×10^6 CD3+/kg body weight, 2. DLI: 5×10^6 CD3+/kg body weight, 3. DLI: 1×10^7 CD3+/kg body weight, 4. DLI: 5×10^7 CD3+/kg body weight, etc. After every DLI administration, the incidence of GvHD and remission status have to be evaluated to reduce the risk of treatment-related mortality [56]. In case of preemptive or therapeutic DLI, the application of a higher starting dose is possible ($5–10 \times 10^6$ CD3+/kg body weight). However, the associated higher risk of GvHD has to be kept in mind [55].

Another aspect in this setting is the origin of DLI. Normally, DLI is collected from naïve donors as steady state lymphocytes. When donor lymphocytes are collected during stem cell apheresis, donors are pre-treated with granulocyte colony stimulating factor (G-CSF). However, the impact of G-CSF stimulation and the resulting composition of DLI on beneficial anti-leukemic responses and survival remains elusive. To evaluate the role of G-CSF-DLI, a retrospective analysis was conducted. The G-CSF-DLI patient cohort showed an improved conversion to full donor chimerism and a lower cumulative incidence of relapse or disease progression without a significantly increased cumulative incidence of GvHD [57]. DLI were examined by flow cytometry as to their cellular components. The results showed that infusion with a lower dose of CD14+ cells ($<0.33 \times 10^8$/kg body weight) was an independent risk factor for the occurrence of II–IV aGvHD (HR = 0.104, p = 0.032) in human leukocyte antigen (HLA)-identical transplant patients. In addition, a dose of CD14+ cells greater 0.33×10^8/kg body weight was associated with a lower incidence of hematological relapse and longer disease-free survival (DFS) (relapse: HR = 0.193, p = 0.007; DFS: HR = 0.259, p = 0.016). However, a greater number of CD14+ cells was an independent risk factor for II–IV aGvHD (HR = 1.758, p = 0.034) in haploidentical allo-SCT. These data show that the cell composition of DLI provides a novel approach for the development of cellular therapies by manipulating the components of infused cells [58].

Another interesting concept first identified by Vago et al. is the potential for leukemic cells to escape immunosurveillance through loss of the mismatched HLA [59]. Therefore, uniparental HLA would escape the immunotherapeutic effect of DLI. Currently, we do not routinely monitor for HLA loss in recurrent disease. However, this would potentially allow for more targeted utilization of DLI and possibly improve the efficacy [60].

Overall, it seems that DLI in the preemptive setting achieves a better response than DLI administered in case of dynamic relapse [61]. Yet, DLI alone may not be the preferred strategy for treatment of manifest relapse. Repetitive DLI can be considered based, e.g., on MRD positivity, 6–8 weeks after DLI administration. The cell doses used in this setting are usually one order of magnitude higher than in a prophylactic or preemptive situation (1×10^7/kg body weight) [51]. The main complication of DLI is GvHD.

3.3. Prophylactic Use of DLI in AML/MDS

Relapse is the most common cause of allo-SCT failure in AML. Accordingly, DLI has been routinely used in complete hematological remission without any sign of underlying disease, with full chimerism, for relapse prevention. The use of DLI in this setting is prophylactic. DLI application should be considered based on the expected risk of relapse and GvHD [38]. Generally, prophylactic DLI is administered at approximately day 100 after allo-SCT, if the patient is not under immunosuppression, and without signs of GvHD or infections.

In some studies, immunosuppressive drugs are applied concurrently with DLI [62]. However, there are discrepancies in the different results and therefore further trials are needed [38]. In case of preemptive and prophylactic use, the CD3+ dosage for the first infusion varies between 1×10^5/kg and 1×10^6/kg body weight and is dependent on donor type and timing [38]. In the absence of GvHD, most centers administer prophylactic DLI as a single-shot intervention, but also repetitive DLI [12,56], every 4 to 12 weeks in a dose escalation by 5- to 10-fold based on response, is feasible [38].

Jedlickova et al. analyzed DLI administration in high-risk AML and MDS (46 patients) at day 120 post allo-SCT with a matched control group (34 patients) in a retrospective study [12]. The OS in the DLI group compared with the control group was significantly better (7 year OS, 67% versus 31% ($p < 0.001$)). Ten patients (22%) relapsed in spite of DLI, compared with 53% in the control group. However, non-relapse mortality was low; GvHD was the main complication in the DLI group. Finally, 31/46 DLI recipients were alive and in CR at a median of 5.7 years after the first DLI.

Schmid et al. [63] described the evaluation of efficacy of prophylactic DLI in AML patients in a registry based matched-pair analysis. Patients received DLI in complete remission and controls were matched for parameters such as age, cytogenetics, diagnosis, stage, donor, gender, conditioning and T cell depletion therapy. In total, 89 matched pairs were used for further analysis. There was no difference in survival across the entire cohort, but, notably, the authors reported significantly improved overall survival in patients with high-risk AML. Thus, prophylactic DLI is effective and may contribute to improved outcome in high-risk AML patients [63].

Furthermore, in transplantation strategies using haploidentical donors, prophylactic DLI appear to be an option to prevent relapse with an acceptable risk of GvHD and GvHD-related mortality in hematological malignancies [64,65]. Several other colleagues recorded improved outcome after prophylactic DLI [12,63,66,67]. Therefore, prophylactic DLI seems to be an effective option to prevent relapse after allogeneic stem cell transplantation and the possibilities need to be further explored in clinical phase II and III studies.

FLAMSA-RIC and DLI

Leukemia relapse is a major obstacle in refractory leukemia undergoing allo-SCT. To improve outcome in this cohort, a sequential intensified conditioning (fludarabine 30 mg/m^2, high-dose cytarabine 2 g/m^2, and amsacrine 100 mg/m^2 from days −12 to −9 (FLAMSA-RIC)) and early rapid immunosuppressant withdrawal was invented. At this point, we will only provide a brief summary, for more information please see separate review in this special issue.

The outcome in this special risk group treated according the FLAMSA-RIC protocol is promising. The 5 year overall survival (OS) and 3 year relapse rate was 44.6% and 33.3%, respectively. To reduce the relapse risk further, prophylactic DLI was administered. Xuan and colleagues analyzed 153 refractory AML patients in a prospective study. Comparing the two groups (80 DLI versus 64 non-DLI), the relapse rate was less and OS was superior in patients receiving DLI than in those without DLI administration (22.7% vs. 33.9%, $p = 0.048$; 58.1% vs. 54.9%, $p = 0.043$). In a multivariate analysis, DLI and cGvHD were associated with less relapse and improved OS [68].

Another prospective study with FLAMSA-RIC DLI was conducted by Michallet et al. [69] in high-risk AML patients. At day +120 or 30 days after discontinuation of immunosuppressive therapy, patients received three increasing doses of donor DLI. There had to be no signs of GvHD or infections. The starting DLI dose was 1×10^6 CD3+ cells/kg body weight. In total, 66 AML patients were included with a median age of 52 years. In total, 17 patients developed cGvHD (10 limited and seven extensive), five of them after DLI, with a cumulative incidence of 48% at 2 years. Patients in CR at allo-SCT benefited most from sequential intensified conditioning followed by DLI. However high rates of deadly infections were observed; therefore, the authors recommend a prophylactic anti-infectious strategy [69].

3.4. Preemptive Use of DLI in AML/MDS

Preemptive DLI is administered in case of persistent MRD or at the first signs of relapse, such as MRD positivity or a decreasing donor chimerism. As in the prophylactic setting, there should be no signs of GvHD. Immunosuppressant drugs preferably should already have been tapered. The dosage for DLI can be chosen slightly higher than for prophylactic DLI, according to GvHD risk and donor type (1×10^5/kg and 1×10^6/kg body weight), followed by repetitive DLI administration in intervals of 4–12 weeks at an escalated dose schedule and increasing the cell doses by 5- to 10-fold with each infusion, if necessary. The timing of administration depends on reappearance of MRD or mixed chimerism. So far, there is the discussion whether DLI dosage needs to be adjusted in the setting of an unrelated, related or haploidentical donor. In this context, various retrospective studies have demonstrated the effificacy of preemptive DLI [56].

In a prospective analysis, 105 patients with standard-risk acute leukemia (AML, ALL or MDS) were MRD positive after allo-SCT—of which, 49 received low-dose IL-2 only, and 56 modified DLI, with or without low-dose IL-2. The cumulative risk of relapse was significantly lower and DFS was significantly higher in patients who received DLI compared to patients who were treated only with IL-2 ($p = 0.001$ and $p = 0.002$, respectively; 3-J-OS: DLI: 58%, IL-2: 28%). These data suggest that DLI administration in patients with standard-risk acute leukemia who are MRD positive after transplantation may improve transplantation outcomes [70]. Preemptive treatment with azacytidine in MDS and AML after allo-SCT is another aspect that needs to be evaluated. The up regulation of immune signaling in cancer through the viral defense pathway is the rationale behind the combination therapy of DLI and demethylation substances, such as the DNA methyltransferase inhibitors azacytidine und decitabine [71]. In a prospective phase II study, patients with a decrease in CD34+ donor chimerism to <80%, >100 days after allo-SCT received four azacytidine cycles (75 mg/m^2/day for 7 days) during complete hematologic remission. In total, 16 patients (80%) responded with either increasing CD34+ donor chimerism up to >80% (n = 10; 50%) or stabilization (n = 6; 30%) with the absence of relapse. Eventually, hematologic relapse occurred in 13 patients (65%), but was delayed until a median of 231 days (range, 56–558) after initial decrease in CD34+ donor chimerism to <80% [72].

Another prospective phase II study showed the efficacy of 5-azacytidine as well as 5-azacytidine in combination with DLI in patients with decreased chimerism or increasing MRD [73]. Based on these data, 5-azacytidine may be considered in patients with AML or MDS and decreasing donor chimerism [38]. Another approach in AML and MDS is DLI combined with maintenance therapies, using manipulated DLI to enhance the GvL effificacy while reducing the risk of GvHD [38]. In conclusion, pre-emptive azacytidine treatment can substantially prevent or delay hematologic relapse in patients with MDS or AML and MRD positivity after allo-SCT. Furthermore, a combination with DLI is possible.

The possibility of preemptive chemotherapy in combination with DLI application in patients with MDS and AML (n = 101) was analyzed in another study. The 3 year cumulative incidences of relapse, non-relapse mortality, and DFS after allo-SCT were 39.5%, 9.6%, and 51.7%, respectively. One month after Chemo-DLI 44 patients became MRD negative; their cumulative incidences of relapse and DFS significantly improved compared to those with persistent MRD one month after preemptive Chemo-DLI (relapse: 19.8% vs. 46.8%, p = 0.001; DFS: 69.6% vs. 46.4%, p = 0.004). Early onset MRD, persistent MRD after Chemo-DLI, and non-cGvHD after Chemo-DLI were associated with increased relapse and impaired DFS [74].

3.5. Biology of Preemptive/Prophylactic DLI

Nonetheless, it is still a challenge to separate GvL from GvHD and to find ways to enhance the GvL effect without inducing GvHD. Efforts have been made to reduce GvHD-associated morbidity and mortality by in vivo T cell depletion. This resulted in an impaired immune reconstitution, which lead to an increased incidence of opportunistic infections and a decreased GvL effect. The International Bone Marrow Transplant Registry (IBMTR) described in a retrospective study an increased leukemia relapse rate when the stem cell transplant was T cell depleted, underlining the importance of T cells as effector cells in GvL [75]. In addition, it was shown that increased natural killer T cells in the graft are associated with reduced GvHD incidence [76], whereas depletion of Tregs in DLI improves the GvL effect but on the other hand augments the risk of GvHD [77]. Thus, prophylactic and dose-escalated DLI was integrated in reduced intensity conditioning (RIC) protocols to reinforce the GvL effect and prevent disease relapse, however the risk of inducing GvHD remains [78].

The sensitivity of the underlying diseases to a DLI-mediated GvL effect is an additional factor. Response to DLI and DLI sensitivity was estimated by the relapse workshop of the National Cancer Institute [11]. CML, myelofibrosis and low-grade NHL were classified to be highly sensitive to DLI; AML, MDS, multiple myeloma and Hodgkin's disease intermediately; and ALL and DLBCL only as slightly sensitive. Additionally, freshly infused DLI may have a higher potency compared to frozen DLI depending on different viabilities and compositions [11,56,79].

Similarly, Gröger et al. observed long-term efficacy of prophylactic donor lymphocyte infusion in 61 patients with multiple myeloma [80]. Prophylactic DLI used in escalated doses in a selected cohort resulted in a low rate of grade II–IV GvHD and encouraging long-term results in these myeloma patients. These data support the relevance of a graft-versus-myeloma effect in long-term responders after allogeneic stem cell transplantation.

4. Antigen-Directed Immunogenic DLI

Already in 1999, Falkenburg et al. published the idea that relapse of CML in chronic phase after allo-SCT can be successfully treated by DLI [81]. Leukemia-reactive T cell lines that could effectively elicit an antileukemic response in vivo were selected and expanded in vitro. These T-lymphocyte (CTL) lines were generated from an HLA-identical donor. Three CTL lines were generated that were able to lyse the patient leukemic cells and inhibit the growth of leukemic progenitor cells. Intriguingly, these CTL did not react with lymphocytes from donor or recipient and did not affect donor hematopoietic progenitor cells. The three leukemia-reactive CTL lines were infused at 5 week intervals at a cumulative dose of 3.2×10^9 CTL. Complete eradication of the leukemic cells was observed shortly after the third infusion. The results showed that in vitro-cultured leukemia-reactive CTL lines selected for their ability to inhibit the proliferation of leukemic progenitor cells in vitro can be successfully applied to treat accelerated phase CML after allo-SCT. Based on this study further developments in AML patients after allo-SCT were possible.

Employing leukemia-specific enriched DLI could be another approach to improve the efficacy of DLI against leukemic cells, thus using immunogenic DLI directed against LAAs. These approaches may be used prospectively in selected patients to enforce GvL without inducing GvHD. The challenge will be to find the best combinations and targets to maximize the GvL- and minimize the GvHD effect, as well as the ideal cytokine milieu for therapy and the ideal T cell composition. A better understanding of the mechanisms of DLI with their targets would open doors to increase the GvL potency without raising the risk of GvHD at the same time.

One option to obtain LAA-specific T cells is the use of selection methods such as multimer approaches. Wang et al. reported about CD8+ T cells purified by streptamer technology [82]. The focus was on the immunogenic leukemia antigen WT1, the streptamer technology was employed and a 60-fold increase in WT1-specific CD8+ effector T cells after positive selection by magnetic cell separation was found. Thus, the streptamer technology allows selection of pure and antigen-specific effector T cells. These results further suggest that the functional status of CD8+ T cells purified by the streptamer technology is preserved and most purified cells are effector T cells. Therefore, these purified effector T cells could be suitable to provide immediate immune protection and might be useful for adoptive T cell transfer. However, the amount of LAA-specific T cells is low and therefore strategies for the ex vivo expansion of LAA-specific T cells have to be established. Bae et al. reported such an expansion strategy for BCMA-specific T cells in myeloma patients [83].

T cell receptor (TCR)-engineered T cells constitute another method among antigen-directed T cell approaches. Several clinical studies have been performed or are ongoing, targeting LAA like, e.g., WT-1 or PRAME. Tawara et al., demonstrated that WT-1 specific TCR-T cells manipulated ex vivo survived in vivo and induced immune responses in WT-1-positive HLA-A*24:02 positive AML and MDS patients. Furthermore, moderate clinical effects such as a decrease in blast counts in blood and bone marrow have been reported [84].

Combination strategies for these antigen-directed immunotherapeutic approaches with other immunotherapies such as immune checkpoint inhibitors might enhance or multiplicate the immune effects and are effective to eliminate leukemic cells and leukemic progenitor or even stem cells.

5. Specifically Stimulated and Modified DLI

5.1. Virus-Specific Donor T Cells for Cytomegalovirus (CMV)

CMV disease constitutes a serious complication after allo-SCT. Despite improved antiviral drug therapy used for the prophylaxis and/or treatment of CMV reactivation and disease, reactivation of CMV after allo-SCT occurs in more than 60% of CMV-seropositive patients. CMV reactivation remains a major cause for mortality and morbidity. Moreover, prolonged antiviral therapy can cause pronounced side effects, particularly myelosuppression and nephrotoxicity [85,86]. A novel prophylactic drug called letermovir showed a decrease in clinically significant CMV infection in a placebo-controlled randomized trial. Nevertheless, this prophylaxis is expensive and breakthrough infections, drug resistance as well as intolerance are still an issue [86]. Beyond humoral immune response, cell-mediated immune response is essential for the control of CMV infection and disease [87–90]. Studies demonstrated that patients are protected against CMV disease once a detectable T cell response against CMV has been mounted [91]. For prevention and therapy of CMV disease, the adoptive transfer of unmanipulated and virus-specific T cells has been evaluated in several clinical trials. [92–95]. The CMV-specific T cells are mostly derived from the donor, a third-party donor or even the patient himself prior to conditioning therapy. This specific treatment leads to virus clearance in patients after allo-SCT.

However, long-term in vitro culturing to select CMV-specific T cells is difficult and time consuming, therefore new strategies were necessary. For example, the cytokine capture assay is combined with the Miltenyi Clini MACS system to generate CMV-specific T cells. Accordingly, it was concluded that adoptive T cell therapy is a valid therapeutic option, which allowed patients to discontinue toxic antiviral drug therapy without further high-level reactivation of CMV.

An aggravation of GvHD was not observed. However, high-dose (>2 mg/kg body weight) corticosteroids could reduce the efficacy significantly.

5.2. Virus-Specific Donor T Cells for Epstein-Barr Virus (EBV)

EBV is widespread in all human populations and persists as a lifelong, asymptomatic infection.

Post transplantation lymphoproliferative disease (PTLD) associated with EBV is a life-threatening complication after allo-SCT [96]. In the past, the mortality from PTLD after allo-SCT was >80% [97]. Chemotherapy seems not to contribute to improved survival of patients with PTLD after allo-SCT and antiviral agents are not active against PTLD [97].

Fortunately, it was shown that by use of rituximab and the adoptive T cell transfer of EBV-specific T cells in high-risk patients, PTLD could be prevented [97], whereas EBV-specific T cells (in vitro generated donor derived or even third-party T cells) are administered in cases with EBV-DNA-emia in order to prevent EBV disease. If no response is achieved unselected DLI from EBV-positive donors are used in order to restore broad T cell reactivity including EBV-specific response (preemptive therapy 94–100% response; therapy of PTLD 71–75% response).

Another option is the treatment of established EBV-PTLD with EBV-specific T cells from the donor but there is the risk of a rapidly growing high-grade lymphoid tumor. In late-stage disease with multiorgan dysfunction at the time of T cell transfer, the results are poor [96]. In this case, the T cell therapy should be implemented as soon as possible. The main obstruction for the use of this approach is the limited availability of T cells and the urgency. To improve the availability of EBV-specific T cells in such urgent clinical situations, Moosmann et al. developed a rapid protocol for the isolation by overnight stimulation of donor blood cells with peptides derived from 11 EBV antigens, interferon-gamma surface capture and subsequent immunomagnetic separation. Therefore, protective EBV-specific T cell memory could be achieved after the infusion of a small number of EBV-specific T cells [96].

Another approach is the administration of Tabelecleucel (formerly known as ATA129) in patients with rituximab-refractory EBV-PTLD. Tabelecleucel is Atara's off-the-shelf T cell immunotherapy in development for the treatment of EBV-PTLD, as well as other EBV associated hematologic and solid tumors. To evaluate the efficacy, a global, multicenter, open-label phase 3 clinical study, called MATCH was designed. The recruitment for MATCH (NCT03392142) is ongoing until November 2020.

5.3. Third Party DLI

Tzannou et al. [98] state the improvement of overall survival for patients treated with allo-SCT will require efforts to decrease treatment-related mortality caused by severe viral infections. Broad antiviral protection to recipients of allo-SCT could be provided by adoptively transferred virus-specific T cells generated from eligible, third-party donors. In their study, third-party virus-specific T cells were administered to recipients of allo-SCT with drug-refractory infections. Infusions were safe and virus-specific T cell tracking by epitope profiling revealed persistence of functional virus-specific T cells of third-party origin for up to 12 weeks. In turn, Muranski et al. developed multi-virus-specific T cells not as therapeutic, but as prophylactic approach early after transplantation [99]. In a phase I study (NIH 14-H-0182) multi virus-specific T cells (MVSTs) with the target of immunodominant viral proteins such as CMV, EBV, human polyomavirus and adenovirus were administrated immediately (day +0 to +60) after allo-SCT. Elutriated lymphocytes from sibling donors were stimulated for 14 days with seven overlapping peptide libraries (pepmixes) pulsed onto autologous DCs in presence of IL-7, IL-15 and IL-2. Twelve patients were treated. There were no infusion toxicities detected, while minimal risk of aGvHD was observed, there was no correlation found with GvHD biomarkers. By serial CDR3 sequencing, it was shown that MVSTs contribute to the T cell repertoire. This approach suggests efficacy in reducing viral reactivation. A phase II study is warranted [99]. Further studies are warranted to establish third-party antiviral T cells for clinical use.

6. In Vivo and Ex Vivo Manipulation of DLI for the Reduction of Alloreactive T Cells

6.1. In Vivo T Cell Depletion

Donor T cells are not DLI in the common sense but are very important in the field of allo-SCT. Concerning in vivo T cell manipulation, there are different approaches, for example alemtuzumab, administered intravenously or administered during the transplantation itself as "campath-1H in the bag" [100,101] as well as antithymocyte globulin (ATG) [102]. In the field of in vivo T cell depletion, the haploidentical setting is the most interesting setting [103]. Because of post-transplant cyclophosphamide (PT-Cy) [104], further advances in graft cell processing and manipulation, as well as GvHD prophylaxis, haploidentical allo-SCT is a save option for nearly all patients with AML, since a significant reduction of treatment-related mortality is now possible. However, there are limited data with respect to DLI in the setting of haploidentical allo-SCT or considering early DLI with concurrent immunosuppression [38].

6.2. Ex Vivo T Cell Depletion

Alpha/beta T cells are the main cell population responsible for the success or failure of allo-SCT or DLI. Expression of the alpha/beta (α/β) TCR characterizes most mature T cells, which allows MHC-restricted recognition of peptides derived from non-self-proteins. The T cell repertoire after allo-SCT is influenced by the source of the graft and infectious challenges such as CMV and EBV, as well as GvHD and cellular intervention such as DLI. Depletion of naïve T cells from the graft is a promising approach to prevent GvHD while retaining a strong GvL effect [32]. Attempts are encouraging on the one hand against hematological tumor antigens for the treatment of overt leukemia relapse and on the other hand to enable a faster immunreconstitution after allo-SCT [105]. The repertoire of α/β T cells after allo-SCT has been studied in different allo-SCT settings and is still restricted 6 months after allo-SCT when compared to healthy individuals. Surprisingly cord blood grafts lead to a higher diversity of the α/β TCR repertoire at 6 and 12 months compared to other graft sources [106].

It has been shown that the main cell population responsible for the success or failure of allo-SCT or DLI is α/β T cells [53]. Since most alloreactive α/β T cells are present in the naïve repertoire of the donor, recipient-derived DCs are key players in producing an appropriate T cell activation [107]. DCs are derived from the hematopoietic system and therefore generate a recipient targeting immune response, including the malignant population, and therefore give rise to GvL [107]. The level of cross reactivity against antigens expressed on non-hematopoietic cells determines the likelihood and severity of GvHD.

In T cell-repleted allo-SCT, it is difficult to dissect the GvL and GvHD effect [108,109]. Consequently, many current transplantation techniques remove immune cells from the graft and administer DLI at a later time point as standard part of the transplantation regimen. Both a complete immune depletion by selection of CD34+ stem cells [110], and a partial depletion of alloreactive T cells through PT-Cy [111], are feasible. This upfront T cell depletion is associated with a lower risk of GvHD and allows early DLI administration for the majority of patients (e.g., 100 days) after allo-SCT. An improved segregation of the GvL- and GvHD effect is possible due to this approach. More recent transplantation strategies allow better consideration of the sophisticated variety of immune cells. These novel strategies utilize either a selective depletion of α/β T cells [112] or naïve subsets [32] to abrogate GvHD, while maintaining early immune surveillance directed against infections as well as leukemia.

One strategy to eliminate alloreactive T cells and at the same time protect virus-specific memory T cells is the ATIR101 program. is a new approach to reduce risk of GvHD after allo-SCT. It consists of a single DLI dose with functional, mature immune cells from a haploidentical family member. Thus, protective T cells are preserved to fight relapse and infections and reduce risk of GvHD. Alloreactive T cells are depleted ex vivo. So far, the results are promising; hence, this approach may increase the safety of allo-SCT from a haploidentical family donor.

7. Five-Year View

The T cell repertoire after allo-SCT is not as diverse as in healthy individuals [106,113]. GvHD is associated with both an increased [106] and a decreased diversity [114]. Selective GvL reactivity could be associated with lower diversity, lower magnitude and relatively specific tissue recognition of hematopoiesis by alloreactive α/β T cells [115]. The contribution of the diversity of the γ/δ TCR repertoire to the GvL after allo-SCT is not well described. The γ/δ T cell repertoire seems to be established quite early after 30–60 days after allo-SCT. CMV reactivation promotes the massive expansion of a few γ/δ T cell subtypes (belonging mainly to the delta-1 subset) resulting in a so-called repertoire focusing [116]. Henceforth, DLI administration for prophylactic, preemptive and overt relapse, as well as treatment of prophylaxis of infections, or immune reconstitution might not only depend on the type of the disease, or the timing but also on the size of the α/β and γ/δ T cell repertoire monitored at a given time point.

8. Conclusions

DLI after allo-SCT offers great opportunities with regard to the treatment or prophylaxis of relapse as well as preemptive treatment of a persistent MRD or decreased chimerism in AML/MDS patients. Furthermore, DLI may be administrated in the setting of treatment or prophylaxis of viral infections and provide substantial support with regard to immunreconstitution.

However, there are many aspects involved in the application of DLI. DLI application is a difficult intervention, whereby many factors have to be considered, for example individual patient-oriented factors prior to application, as well as possible combinations with further therapies during and after DLI application. Currently, there are many new developments, and this is quite necessary because DLI needs to be improved in terms of efficacy and toxicity reduction. This remains a major challenge with the goal to improve the outcome for AML patients after allo-SCT. Prospectively, *CAR* T cells may be an intriguing concept even in AML, with the possibility of leukemia rejection without eliminating healthy progenitor and stem cells. However, there is no feasible approach yet.

In this field, of manipulated and unmanipulated DLI after allo-SCT of AML patients, it remains most challenging to avoid substantial risks such as severe infections and several key points, such as dosage, donor origin, as well as the clinical situation of the patient, have to be considered prior to DLI administration. The pivotal point is to increase the GvL effect without escalating the risk of GvHD.

Author Contributions: Conceptualization, J.G. and V.W.; reviewing and editing, M.G.; validation of manuscript, D.B. and S.H., manuscript writing, J.G., V.W. and M.G.; interpretation of data D.B. and S.H. All authors have read and agreed to the published version of the manuscript.

Funding: This research received no external funding

Conflicts of Interest: The authors declare no conflict of interest.

References

1. Kolb, H.J.; Mittermuller, J.; Clemm, C.; Holler, E.; Ledderose, G.; Brehm, G.; Heim, M.; Wilmanns, W. Donor leukocyte transfusions for treatment of recurrent chronic myelogenous leukemia in marrow transplant patients. *Blood* **1990**, *76*, 2462–2465. [CrossRef] [PubMed]
2. Kolb, H.J.; Schattenberg, A.; Goldman, J.M.; Hertenstein, B.; Jacobsen, N.; Arcese, W.; Ljungman, P.; Ferrant, A.; Verdonck, L.; Niederwieser, D.; et al. Graft-versus-leukemia effect of donor lymphocyte transfusions in marrow grafted patients. *Blood* **1995**, *86*, 2041–2050. [CrossRef] [PubMed]
3. Barrett, A.J.; Mavroudis, D.; Tisdale, J.; Molldrem, J.; Clave, E.; Dunbar, C.; Cottler-Fox, M.; Phang, S.; Carter, C.; Okunnieff, P.; et al. T cell-depleted bone marrow transplantation and delayed T cell add-back to control acute GVHD and conserve a graft-versus-leukemia effect. *Bone Marrow Transplant.* **1998**, *21*, 543–551. [CrossRef] [PubMed]
4. Rapoport, A.P.; Stadtmauer, E.A.; Binder-Scholl, G.K.; Goloubeva, O.; Vogl, D.T.; Lacey, S.F.; Badros, A.Z.; Garfall, A.; Weiss, B.; Finklestein, J.; et al. NY-ESO-1-specific TCR-engineered T cells mediate sustained antigen-specific antitumor effects in myeloma. *Nat. Med.* **2015**, *21*, 914–921. [CrossRef]
5. Tawara, I.M.M.; Kageyama, S.; Nishida, T.; Terakura, S.; Murata, M.; Fujiwara, H.; Akatsuka, Y.; Ikeda, H.; Miyahara, Y.; Tomura, D.; et al. Adoptive Transfer of WT1-Specific TCR Gene-Transduced Lymphocytes in Patients with Myelodysplastic Syndrome and Acute Myeloid Leukemia. *Blood* **2015**, *126*, 97. [CrossRef]
6. Perret, R.; Valliant-Saunders, K.; Cao, J.W.; Greenberg, P.D. Expanding the scope of WT1-and cyclin A1-specific TCR gene therapy for AML and other cancers. *J. Immunol.* **2016**, *143*, 145.
7. Schmitt, T.M.; Aggen, D.H.; Stromnes, I.M.; Dossett, M.L.; Richman, S.A.; Kranz, D.M.; Greenberg, P.D. Enhanced-affinity murine T-cell receptors for tumor/self-antigens can be safe in gene therapy despite surpassing the threshold for thymic selection. *Blood* **2013**, *122*, 348–356. [CrossRef]
8. Kochenderfer, J.N.; Dudley, M.E.; Kassim, S.H.; Somerville, R.P.; Carpenter, R.O.; Stetler-Stevenson, M.; Yang, J.C.; Phan, G.Q.; Hughes, M.S.; Sherry, R.M.; et al. Chemotherapy-refractory diffuse large B-cell lymphoma and indolent B-cell malignancies can be effectively treated with autologous T cells expressing an anti-CD19 chimeric antigen receptor. *J. Clin. Oncol. Off. J. Am. Soc. Clin. Oncol.* **2015**, *33*, 540–549. [CrossRef]
9. Brudno, J.N.; Somerville, R.P.; Shi, V.; Rose, J.J.; Halverson, D.C.; Fowler, D.H.; Gea-Banacloche, J.C.; Pavletic, S.Z.; Hickstein, D.D.; Lu, T.L.; et al. Allogeneic T Cells That Express an Anti-CD19 Chimeric Antigen Receptor Induce Remissions of B-Cell Malignancies That Progress After Allogeneic Hematopoietic Stem-Cell Transplantation Without Causing Graft-Versus-Host Disease. *J. Clin. Oncol. Off. J. Am. Soc. Clin. Oncol.* **2016**, *34*, 1112–1121. [CrossRef]
10. Yun, H.D.; Waller, E.K. Finding the sweet spot for donor lymphocyte infusions. *Biol. Blood Marrow Transplant. J. Am. Soc. Blood Marrow Transplant.* **2013**, *19*, 507–508. [CrossRef]
11. Alyea, E.P.; DeAngelo, D.J.; Moldrem, J.; Pagel, J.M.; Przepiorka, D.; Sadelin, M.; Young, J.W.; Giralt, S.; Bishop, M.; Riddell, S. NCI First International Workshop on The Biology, Prevention and Treatment of Relapse after Allogeneic Hematopoietic Cell Transplantation: Report from the committee on prevention of relapse following allogeneic cell transplantation for hematologic malignancies. *Biol. Blood Marrow Transplant. J. Am. Soc. Blood Marrow Transplant.* **2010**, *16*, 1037–1069. [CrossRef]
12. Jedlickova, Z.; Schmid, C.; Koenecke, C.; Hertenstein, B.; Baurmann, H.; Schwerdtfeger, R.; Tischer, J.; Kolb, H.J.; Schleuning, M. Long-term results of adjuvant donor lymphocyte transfusion in AML after allogeneic stem cell transplantation. *Bone Marrow Transplant.* **2016**, *51*, 663–667. [CrossRef] [PubMed]
13. Hofmann, S.; Schmitt, M.; Gotz, M.; Dohner, H.; Wiesneth, M.; Bunjes, D.; Greiner, J. Donor lymphocyte infusion leads to diversity of specific T cell responses and reduces regulatory T cell frequency in clinical responders. *Int. J. Cancer J. Int. du Cancer* **2019**, *144*, 1135–1146. [CrossRef] [PubMed]
14. Tanaka, A.; Sakaguchi, S. Regulatory T cells in cancer immunotherapy. *Cell Res.* **2017**, *27*, 109–118. [CrossRef] [PubMed]
15. Gjerdrum, L.M.; Woetmann, A.; Odum, N.; Burton, C.M.; Rossen, K.; Skovgaard, G.L.; Ryder, L.P.; Ralfkiaer, E. FOXP3+ regulatory T cells in cutaneous T-cell lymphomas: Association with disease stage and survival. *Leukemia* **2007**, *21*, 2512–2518. [CrossRef] [PubMed]
16. Yang, W.; Xu, Y. Clinical significance of Treg cell frequency in acute myeloid leukemia. *Int. J. Hematol.* **2013**, *98*, 558–562. [CrossRef]

17. D'Arena, G.; Laurenti, L.; Minervini, M.M.; Deaglio, S.; Bonello, L.; De Martino, L.; De Padua, L.; Savino, L.; Tarnani, M.; De Feo, V.; et al. Regulatory T-cell number is increased in chronic lymphocytic leukemia patients and correlates with progressive disease. *Leuk. Res.* **2011**, *35*, 363–368. [CrossRef]
18. Mailloux, A.W.; Sugimori, C.; Komrokji, R.S.; Yang, L.; Maciejewski, J.P.; Sekeres, M.A.; Paquette, R.; Loughran, T.P., Jr.; List, A.F.; Epling-Burnette, P.K. Expansion of effector memory regulatory T cells represents a novel prognostic factor in lower risk myelodysplastic syndrome. *J. Immunol.* **2012**, *189*, 3198–3208. [CrossRef]
19. Idris, S.Z.; Hassan, N.; Lee, L.J.; Md Noor, S.; Osman, R.; Abdul-Jalil, M.; Nordin, A.J.; Abdullah, M. Increased regulatory T cells in acute lymphoblastic leukaemia patients. *Hematology* **2016**, *21*, 206–212. [CrossRef]
20. Simpson, T.R.; Li, F.; Montalvo-Ortiz, W.; Sepulveda, M.A.; Bergerhoff, K.; Arce, F.; Roddie, C.; Henry, J.Y.; Yagita, H.; Wolchok, J.D.; et al. Fc-dependent depletion of tumor-infiltrating regulatory T cells co-defines the efficacy of anti-CTLA-4 therapy against melanoma. *J. Exp. Med.* **2013**, *210*, 1695–1710. [CrossRef]
21. Hofmann, S.; Gotz, M.; Schneider, V.; Guillaume, P.; Bunjes, D.; Dohner, H.; Wiesneth, M.; Greiner, J. Donor lymphocyte infusion induces polyspecific CD8(+) T-cell responses with concurrent molecular remission in acute myeloid leukemia with NPM1 mutation. *J. Clin. Oncol. Off. J. Am. Soc. Clin. Oncol.* **2013**, *31*, e44–e47. [CrossRef] [PubMed]
22. Greiner, J.; Schneider, V.; Schmitt, M.; Gotz, M.; Dohner, K.; Wiesneth, M.; Dohner, H.; Hofmann, S. Immune responses against the mutated region of cytoplasmatic NPM1 might contribute to the favorable clinical outcome of AML patients with NPM1 mutations (NPM1mut). *Blood* **2013**, *122*, 1087–1088. [CrossRef] [PubMed]
23. Snyder, A.; Makarov, V.; Merghoub, T.; Yuan, J.; Zaretsky, J.M.; Desrichard, A.; Walsh, L.A.; Postow, M.A.; Wong, P.; Ho, T.S.; et al. Genetic basis for clinical response to CTLA-4 blockade in melanoma. *N. Engl. J. Med.* **2014**, *371*, 2189–2199. [CrossRef]
24. McGranahan, N.; Furness, A.J.; Rosenthal, R.; Ramskov, S.; Lyngaa, R.; Saini, S.K.; Jamal-Hanjani, M.; Wilson, G.A.; Birkbak, N.J.; Hiley, C.T.; et al. Clonal neoantigens elicit T cell immunoreactivity and sensitivity to immune checkpoint blockade. *Science* **2016**, *351*, 1463–1469. [CrossRef] [PubMed]
25. Moore, T.; Wagner, C.R.; Scurti, G.M.; Hutchens, K.A.; Godellas, C.; Clark, A.L.; Kolawole, E.M.; Hellman, L.M.; Singh, N.K.; Huyke, F.A.; et al. Clinical and immunologic evaluation of three metastatic melanoma patients treated with autologous melanoma-reactive TCR-transduced T cells. *Cancer Immunol. Immunother. CII* **2018**, *67*, 311–325. [CrossRef]
26. Rambaldi, A.; Biagi, E.; Bonini, C.; Biondi, A.; Introna, M. Cell-based strategies to manage leukemia relapse: Efficacy and feasibility of immunotherapy approaches. *Leukemia* **2015**, *29*, 1–10. [CrossRef]
27. Collins, R.H., Jr.; Shpilberg, O.; Drobyski, W.R.; Porter, D.L.; Giralt, S.; Champlin, R.; Goodman, S.A.; Wolff, S.N.; Hu, W.; Verfaillie, C.; et al. Donor leukocyte infusions in 140 patients with relapsed malignancy after allogeneic bone marrow transplantation. *J. Clin. Oncol. Off. J. Am. Soc. Clin. Oncol.* **1997**, *15*, 433–444. [CrossRef]
28. Posthuma, E.F.M.; Marijt, E.W.A.F.; Barge, R.M.Y.; van Soest, R.A.; Baas, I.O.; Starrenburg, C.W.J.I.; van Zelderen-Bhola, S.L.; Fibbe, W.E.; Smit, W.M.; Willemze, R.; et al. α-Interferon with very-low-dose donor lymphocyte infusion for hematologic or cytogenetic relapse of chronic myeloid leukemia induces rapid and durable complete remissions and is associated with acceptable graft-versus-host disease. *Biol. Blood Marrow Transplant.* **2004**, *10*, 204–212. [CrossRef]
29. Verdonck, L.F.; Petersen, E.J.; Lokhorst, H.M.; Nieuwenhuis, H.K.; Dekker, A.W.; Tilanus, M.G.; de Weger, R.A. Donor leukocyte infusions for recurrent hematologic malignancies after allogeneic bone marrow transplantation: Impact of infused and residual donor T cells. *Bone Marrow Transplant.* **1998**, *22*, 1057–1063. [CrossRef]
30. Bao, H.; Wu, D. Current Status of Leukemia Cytotherapy-Exploitation with Immune Cells. *Curr. Stem Cell Res. Ther.* **2017**, *12*, 188–196. [CrossRef]
31. Kongtim, P.; Lee, D.A.; Cooper, L.J.; Kebriaei, P.; Champlin, R.E.; Ciurea, S.O. Haploidentical Hematopoietic Stem Cell Transplantation as a Platform for Post-Transplantation Cellular Therapy. *Biol. Blood Marrow Transplant. J. Am. Soc. Blood Marrow Transplant.* **2015**, *21*, 1714–1720. [CrossRef] [PubMed]
32. Bleakley, M.; Heimfeld, S.; Loeb, K.R.; Jones, L.A.; Chaney, C.; Seropian, S.; Gooley, T.A.; Sommermeyer, F.; Riddell, S.R.; Shlomchik, W.D. Outcomes of acute leukemia patients transplanted with naive T cell-depleted stem cell grafts. *J. Clin. Investig.* **2015**, *125*, 2677–2689. [CrossRef] [PubMed]

33. De Lima, M.; Porter, D.L.; Battiwalla, M.; Bishop, M.R.; Giralt, S.A.; Hardy, N.M.; Kroger, N.; Wayne, A.S.; Schmid, C. Proceedings from the National Cancer Institute's Second International Workshop on the Biology, Prevention, and Treatment of Relapse After Hematopoietic Stem Cell Transplantation: Part III. Prevention and treatment of relapse after allogeneic transplantation. *Biol. Blood Marrow Transplant. J. Am. Soc. Blood Marrow Transplant.* **2014**, *20*, 4–13. [CrossRef]
34. Kolb, H.J. Hematopoietic stem cell transplantation and cellular therapy. *HLA* **2017**, *89*, 267–277. [CrossRef]
35. Cooper, N.; Rao, K.; Goulden, N.; Amrolia, P.; Veys, P. Alpha interferon augments the graft-versus-leukaemia effect of second stem cell transplants and donor lymphocyte infusions in high-risk paediatric leukaemias. *Br. J. Haematol.* **2012**, *156*, 550–552. [CrossRef] [PubMed]
36. Schmid, C.; Labopin, M.; Nagler, A.; Bornhauser, M.; Finke, J.; Fassas, A.; Volin, L.; Gurman, G.; Maertens, J.; Bordigoni, P.; et al. Donor lymphocyte infusion in the treatment of first hematological relapse after allogeneic stem-cell transplantation in adults with acute myeloid leukemia: A retrospective risk factors analysis and comparison with other strategies by the EBMT Acute Leukemia Working Party. *J. Clin. Oncol. Off. J. Am. Soc. Clin. Oncol.* **2007**, *25*, 4938–4945. [CrossRef]
37. Schmid, C.; Labopin, M.; Nagler, A.; Niederwieser, D.; Castagna, L.; Tabrizi, R.; Stadler, M.; Kuball, J.; Cornelissen, J.; Vorlicek, J.; et al. Treatment, risk factors, and outcome of adults with relapsed AML after reduced intensity conditioning for allogeneic stem cell transplantation. *Blood* **2012**, *119*, 1599–1606. [CrossRef]
38. Zeiser, R.; Vago, L. Mechanisms of immune escape after allogeneic hematopoietic cell transplantation. *Blood* **2019**, *133*, 1290–1297. [CrossRef]
39. Rautenberg, C.; Nachtkamp, K.; Dienst, A.; Schmidt, P.V.; Heyn, C.; Kondakci, M.; Germing, U.; Haas, R.; Kobbe, G.; Schroeder, T. Sorafenib and azacitidine as salvage therapy for relapse of FLT3-ITD mutated AML after allo-SCT. *Eur. J. Haematol.* **2017**, *98*, 348–354. [CrossRef]
40. De Freitas, T.; Marktel, S.; Piemontese, S.; Carrabba, M.G.; Tresoldi, C.; Messina, C.; Lupo Stanghellini, M.T.; Assanelli, A.; Corti, C.; Bernardi, M.; et al. High rate of hematological responses to sorafenib in FLT3-ITD acute myeloid leukemia relapsed after allogeneic hematopoietic stem cell transplantation. *Eur. J. Haematol.* **2016**, *96*, 629–636. [CrossRef]
41. Sommer, S.; Cruijsen, M.; Claus, R.; Bertz, H.; Wasch, R.; Marks, R.; Zeiser, R.; Bogatyreva, L.; Blijlevens, N.M.A.; May, A.; et al. Decitabine in combination with donor lymphocyte infusions can induce remissions in relapsed myeloid malignancies with higher leukemic burden after allogeneic hematopoietic cell transplantation. *Leuk. Res.* **2018**, *72*, 20–26. [CrossRef] [PubMed]
42. Schroeder, T.; Rautenberg, C.; Kruger, W.; Platzbecker, U.; Bug, G.; Steinmann, J.; Klein, S.; Hopfer, O.; Nachtkamp, K.; Kondakci, M.; et al. Treatment of relapsed AML and MDS after allogeneic stem cell transplantation with decitabine and DLI-a retrospective multicenter analysis on behalf of the German Cooperative Transplant Study Group. *Ann. Hematol.* **2018**, *97*, 335–342. [CrossRef] [PubMed]
43. Ghobadi, A.; Choi, J.; Fiala, M.A.; Fletcher, T.; Liu, J.; Eissenberg, L.G.; Abboud, C.; Cashen, A.; Vij, R.; Schroeder, M.A.; et al. Phase I study of azacitidine following donor lymphocyte infusion for relapsed acute myeloid leukemia post allogeneic stem cell transplantation. *Leuk. Res.* **2016**, *49*, 1–6. [CrossRef] [PubMed]
44. Steinmann, J.; Bertz, H.; Wasch, R.; Marks, R.; Zeiser, R.; Bogatyreva, L.; Finke, J.; Lubbert, M. 5-Azacytidine and DLI can induce long-term remissions in AML patients relapsed after allograft. *Bone Marrow Transplant.* **2015**, *50*, 690–695. [CrossRef] [PubMed]
45. Schroeder, T.; Rachlis, E.; Bug, G.; Stelljes, M.; Klein, S.; Steckel, N.K.; Wolf, D.; Ringhoffer, M.; Czibere, A.; Nachtkamp, K.; et al. Treatment of acute myeloid leukemia or myelodysplastic syndrome relapse after allogeneic stem cell transplantation with azacitidine and donor lymphocyte infusions–A retrospective multicenter analysis from the German Cooperative Transplant Study Group. *Biol. Blood Marrow Transplant. J. Am. Soc. Blood Marrow Transplant.* **2015**, *21*, 653–660. [CrossRef] [PubMed]
46. Tessoulin, B.; Delaunay, J.; Chevallier, P.; Loirat, M.; Ayari, S.; Peterlin, P.; Le Gouill, S.; Gastinne, T.; Moreau, P.; Mohty, M.; et al. Azacitidine salvage therapy for relapse of myeloid malignancies following allogeneic hematopoietic SCT. *Bone Marrow Transplant.* **2014**, *49*, 567–571. [CrossRef]
47. Motabi, I.H.; Ghobadi, A.; Liu, J.; Schroeder, M.; Abboud, C.N.; Cashen, A.F.; Stockler-Goldstein, K.E.; Uy, G.L.; Vij, R.; Westervelt, P.; et al. Chemotherapy versus Hypomethylating Agents for the Treatment of Relapsed Acute Myeloid Leukemia and Myelodysplastic Syndrome after Allogeneic Stem Cell Transplant. *Biol. Blood Marrow Transplant. J. Am. Soc. Blood Marrow Transplant.* **2016**, *22*, 1324–1329. [CrossRef]

48. Levine, J.E.; Braun, T.; Penza, S.L.; Beatty, P.; Cornetta, K.; Martino, R.; Drobyski, W.R.; Barrett, A.J.; Porter, D.L.; Giralt, S.; et al. Prospective trial of chemotherapy and donor leukocyte infusions for relapse of advanced myeloid malignancies after allogeneic stem-cell transplantation. *J. Clin. Oncol. Off. J. Am. Soc. Clin. Oncol.* **2002**, *20*, 405–412. [CrossRef]
49. Guieze, R.; Damaj, G.; Pereira, B.; Robin, M.; Chevallier, P.; Michallet, M.; Vigouroux, S.; Beguin, Y.; Blaise, D.; El Cheikh, J.; et al. Management of Myelodysplastic Syndrome Relapsing after Allogeneic Hematopoietic Stem Cell Transplantation: A Study by the French Society of Bone Marrow Transplantation and Cell Therapies. *Biol. Blood Marrow Transplant. J. Am. Soc. Blood Marrow Transplant.* **2016**, *22*, 240–247. [CrossRef]
50. Cornelissen, J.J.; Blaise, D. Hematopoietic stem cell transplantation for patients with AML in first complete remission. *Blood* **2016**, *127*, 62–70. [CrossRef]
51. Dietz, A.C.; Wayne, A.S. Cells to prevent/treat relapse following allogeneic stem cell transplantation. *Hematol. Educ. Program Am. Soc. Hematol. Am. Soc. Hematol. Educ. Program* **2017**, *2017*, 708–715. [CrossRef]
52. Sun, C.; Dotti, G.; Savoldo, B. Utilizing cell-based therapeutics to overcome immune evasion in hematologic malignancies. *Blood* **2016**, *127*, 3350–3359. [CrossRef] [PubMed]
53. Orr, M.T.; Lanier, L.L. Natural killer cell education and tolerance. *Cell* **2010**, *142*, 847–856. [CrossRef] [PubMed]
54. Handgretinger, R.; Schilbach, K. The potential role of gammadelta T cells after allogeneic HCT for leukemia. *Blood* **2018**, *131*, 1063–1072. [CrossRef] [PubMed]
55. Deol, A.; Lum, L.G. Role of donor lymphocyte infusions in relapsed hematological malignancies after stem cell transplantation revisited. *Cancer Treat. Rev.* **2010**, *36*, 528–538. [CrossRef] [PubMed]
56. Tsirigotis, P.; Byrne, M.; Schmid, C.; Baron, F.; Ciceri, F.; Esteve, J.; Gorin, N.C.; Giebel, S.; Mohty, M.; Savani, B.N.; et al. Relapse of AML after hematopoietic stem cell transplantation: Methods of monitoring and preventive strategies. A review from the ALWP of the EBMT. *Bone Marrow Transplant.* **2016**, *51*, 1431–1438. [CrossRef] [PubMed]
57. Schneidawind, C.; Jahnke, S.; Schober-Melms, I.; Schumm, M.; Handgretinger, R.; Faul, C.; Kanz, L.; Bethge, W.; Schneidawind, D. G-CSF administration prior to donor lymphocyte apheresis promotes anti-leukaemic effects in allogeneic HCT patients. *Br. J. Haematol.* **2019**, *186*, 60–71. [CrossRef]
58. Zhao, X.S.; Wang, Y.; Yan, C.H.; Wang, J.Z.; Zhang, X.H.; Xu, L.P.; Liu, K.Y.; Huang, X.J. The cell composition of infused donor lymphocyte has different impact in different types of allogeneic hematopoietic stem cell transplantation. *Clin. Transplant.* **2014**, *28*, 926–934. [CrossRef]
59. Vago, L.; Perna, S.K.; Zanussi, M.; Mazzi, B.; Barlassina, C.; Stanghellini, M.T.; Perrelli, N.F.; Cosentino, C.; Torri, F.; Angius, A.; et al. Loss of mismatched HLA in leukemia after stem-cell transplantation. *N. Engl. J. Med.* **2009**, *361*, 478–488. [CrossRef]
60. Goldsmith, S.R.; Slade, M.; DiPersio, J.F.; Westervelt, P.; Schroeder, M.A.; Gao, F.; Romee, R. Donor-lymphocyte infusion following haploidentical hematopoietic cell transplantation with peripheral blood stem cell grafts and PTCy. *Bone Marrow Transplant.* **2017**, *52*, 1623–1628. [CrossRef]
61. Miyamoto, T.; Fukuda, T.; Nakashima, M.; Henzan, T.; Kusakabe, S.; Kobayashi, N.; Sugita, J.; Mori, T.; Kurokawa, M.; Mori, S.I. Donor Lymphocyte Infusion for Relapsed Hematological Malignancies after Unrelated Allogeneic Bone Marrow Transplantation Facilitated by the Japan Marrow Donor Program. *Biol. Blood Marrow Transplant. J. Am. Soc. Blood Marrow Transplant.* **2017**, *23*, 938–944. [CrossRef] [PubMed]
62. Mo, X.D.; Zhang, X.H.; Xu, L.P.; Wang, Y.; Yan, C.H.; Chen, H.; Chen, Y.H.; Han, W.; Wang, F.R.; Wang, J.Z.; et al. Comparison of outcomes after donor lymphocyte infusion with or without prior chemotherapy for minimal residual disease in acute leukemia/myelodysplastic syndrome after allogeneic hematopoietic stem cell transplantation. *Ann. Hematol.* **2017**, *96*, 829–838. [CrossRef] [PubMed]
63. Schmid, C.; Labopin, M.; Schaap, N.; Veelken, H.; Schleuning, M.; Stadler, M.; Finke, J.; Hurst, E.; Baron, F.; Ringden, O.; et al. Prophylactic donor lymphocyte infusion after allogeneic stem cell transplantation in acute leukaemia-a matched pair analysis by the Acute Leukaemia Working Party of EBMT. *Br. J. Haematol.* **2019**, *184*, 782–787. [CrossRef] [PubMed]
64. Gao, X.N.; Lin, J.; Wang, S.H.; Huang, W.R.; Li, F.; Li, H.H.; Chen, J.; Wang, L.J.; Gao, C.J.; Yu, L.; et al. Donor lymphocyte infusion for prevention of relapse after unmanipulated haploidentical PBSCT for very high-risk hematologic malignancies. *Ann. Hematol.* **2019**, *98*, 185–193. [CrossRef] [PubMed]

65. Cauchois, R.; Castagna, L.; Pagliardini, T.; Harbi, S.; Calmels, B.; Bramanti, S.; Granata, A.; Lemarie, C.; Maisano, V.; Legrand, F.; et al. Prophylactic donor lymphocyte infusions after haploidentical haematopoietic stem cell transplantation for high risk haematological malignancies: A retrospective bicentric analysis of serial infusions of increasing doses of CD3(+) cells. *Br. J. Haematol.* **2018**. [CrossRef] [PubMed]
66. Eefting, M.; Halkes, C.J.; de Wreede, L.C.; van Pelt, C.M.; Kersting, S.; Marijt, E.W.; von dem Borne, P.A.; Willemze, R.; Veelken, H.; Falkenburg, J.H. Myeloablative T cell-depleted alloSCT with early sequential prophylactic donor lymphocyte infusion is an efficient and safe post-remission treatment for adult ALL. *Bone Marrow Transplant.* **2014**, *49*, 287–291. [CrossRef]
67. Ljungman, P.; Brand, R.; Einsele, H.; Frassoni, F.; Niederwieser, D.; Cordonnier, C. Donor CMV serologic status and outcome of CMV-seropositive recipients after unrelated donor stem cell transplantation: An EBMT megafile analysis. *Blood* **2003**, *102*, 4255–4260. [CrossRef]
68. Xuan, L.; Fan, Z.; Zhang, Y.; Zhou, H.; Huang, F.; Dai, M.; Nie, D.; Lin, D.; Xu, N.; Guo, X.; et al. Sequential intensified conditioning followed by prophylactic DLI could reduce relapse of refractory acute leukemia after allo-HSCT. *Oncotarget* **2016**, *7*, 32579–32591. [CrossRef]
69. Michallet, M.; Sobh, M.; Detrait, M.Y.; Labussiere-Wallet, H.; Hayette, S.; Tigaud, I.; Elhamri, M.; Gilis, L.; Lebras, L.L.; Barraco, F.; et al. Flamsa Sequential Chemotherapy Followed By Reduced Intensity Conditioning and Allogeneic Hematopoietic Transplantation for High Risk Acute Myeloid Leukemia Patients. *Blood* **2014**, *124*, 3892. [CrossRef]
70. Yan, C.H.; Liu, D.H.; Liu, K.Y.; Xu, L.P.; Liu, Y.R.; Chen, H.; Han, W.; Wang, Y.; Qin, Y.Z.; Huang, X.J. Risk stratification-directed donor lymphocyte infusion could reduce relapse of standard-risk acute leukemia patients after allogeneic hematopoietic stem cell transplantation. *Blood* **2012**, *119*, 3256–3262. [CrossRef]
71. Chiappinelli, K.B.; Strissel, P.L.; Desrichard, A.; Li, H.; Henke, C.; Akman, B.; Hein, A.; Rote, N.S.; Cope, L.M.; Snyder, A.; et al. Inhibiting DNA Methylation Causes an Interferon Response in Cancer via dsRNA Including Endogenous Retroviruses. *Cell* **2015**, *162*, 974–986. [CrossRef] [PubMed]
72. Platzbecker, U.; Wermke, M.; Radke, J.; Oelschlaegel, U.; Seltmann, F.; Kiani, A.; Klut, I.M.; Knoth, H.; Rollig, C.; Schetelig, J.; et al. Azacitidine for treatment of imminent relapse in MDS or AML patients after allogeneic HSCT: Results of the RELAZA trial. *Leukemia* **2012**, *26*, 381–389. [CrossRef] [PubMed]
73. Platzbecker, U.; Schetelig, J.; Finke, J.; Trenschel, R.; Scott, B.L.; Kobbe, G.; Schaefer-Eckart, K.; Bornhauser, M.; Itzykson, R.; Germing, U.; et al. Allogeneic hematopoietic cell transplantation in patients age 60–70 years with de novo high-risk myelodysplastic syndrome or secondary acute myelogenous leukemia: Comparison with patients lacking donors who received azacitidine. *Biol. Blood Marrow Transplant. J. Am. Soc. Blood Marrow Transplant.* **2012**, *18*, 1415–1421. [CrossRef]
74. Mo, X.D.; Zhang, X.H.; Xu, L.P.; Wang, Y.; Yan, C.H.; Chen, H.; Chen, Y.H.; Han, W.; Wang, F.R.; Wang, J.Z.; et al. Salvage chemotherapy followed by granulocyte colony-stimulating factor-primed donor leukocyte infusion with graft-vs.-host disease control for minimal residual disease in acute leukemia/myelodysplastic syndrome after allogeneic hematopoietic stem cell transplantation: Prognostic factors and clinical outcomes. *Eur. J. Haematol.* **2016**, *96*, 297–308. [CrossRef] [PubMed]
75. Horowitz, M.M.; Gale, R.P.; Sondel, P.M.; Goldman, J.M.; Kersey, J.; Kolb, H.J.; Rimm, A.A.; Ringden, O.; Rozman, C.; Speck, B.; et al. Graft-versus-leukemia reactions after bone marrow transplantation. *Blood* **1990**, *75*, 555–562. [CrossRef] [PubMed]
76. Malard, F.; Labopin, M.; Stuhler, G.; Bittenbring, J.; Ganser, A.; Tischer, J.; Michallet, M.; Kroger, N.; Schmid, C.; Huynh, A.; et al. Sequential Intensified Conditioning Regimen Allogeneic Hematopoietic Stem Cell Transplantation in Adult Patients with Intermediate-or High-Risk Acute Myeloid Leukemia in Complete Remission: A Study from the Acute Leukemia Working Party of the European Group for Blood and Marrow Transplantation. *Biol. Blood Marrow Transplant. J. Am. Soc. Blood Marrow Transplant.* **2017**, *23*, 278–284. [CrossRef]
77. Maury, S.; Lemoine, F.M.; Hicheri, Y.; Rosenzwajg, M.; Badoual, C.; Cherai, M.; Beaumont, J.L.; Azar, N.; Dhedin, N.; Sirvent, A.; et al. CD4+CD25+ regulatory T cell depletion improves the graft-versus-tumor effect of donor lymphocytes after allogeneic hematopoietic stem cell transplantation. *Sci. Transl. Med.* **2010**, *2*, 41ra52. [CrossRef] [PubMed]
78. Peggs, K.S.; Thomson, K.; Hart, D.P.; Geary, J.; Morris, E.C.; Yong, K.; Goldstone, A.H.; Linch, D.C.; Mackinnon, S. Dose-escalated donor lymphocyte infusions following reduced intensity transplantation: Toxicity, chimerism, and disease responses. *Blood* **2004**, *103*, 1548–1556. [CrossRef]

79. Lemieux, J.; Jobin, C.; Simard, C.; Neron, S. A global look into human T cell subsets before and after cryopreservation using multiparametric flow cytometry and two-dimensional visualization analysis. *J. Immunol. Methods* **2016**, *434*, 73–82. [CrossRef]
80. Groger, M.; Gagelmann, N.; Wolschke, C.; von Pein, U.M.; Klyuchnikov, E.; Christopeit, M.; Zander, A.; Ayuk, F.; Kroger, N. Long-Term Results of Prophylactic Donor Lymphocyte Infusions for Patients with Multiple Myeloma after Allogeneic Stem Cell Transplantation. *Biol. Blood Marrow Transplant. J. Am. Soc. Blood Marrow Transplant.* **2018**, *24*, 1399–1405. [CrossRef]
81. Falkenburg, J.H.; Wafelman, A.R.; Joosten, P.; Smit, W.M.; van Bergen, C.A.; Bongaerts, R.; Lurvink, E.; van der Hoorn, M.; Kluck, P.; Landegent, J.E.; et al. Complete remission of accelerated phase chronic myeloid leukemia by treatment with leukemia-reactive cytotoxic T lymphocytes. *Blood* **1999**, *94*, 1201–1208. [CrossRef] [PubMed]
82. Wang, X.; Schmitt, A.; Chen, B.; Xu, X.; Mani, J.; Linnebacher, M.; Freund, M.; Schmitt, M. Streptamer-based selection of WT1-specific CD8+ T cells for specific donor lymphocyte infusions. *Exp. Hematol.* **2010**, *38*, 1066–1073. [CrossRef] [PubMed]
83. Bae, J.; Samur, M.; Richardson, P.; Munshi, N.C.; Anderson, K.C. Selective targeting of multiple myeloma by B cell maturation antigen (BCMA)-specific central memory CD8(+) cytotoxic T lymphocytes: Immunotherapeutic application in vaccination and adoptive immunotherapy. *Leukemia* **2019**. [CrossRef] [PubMed]
84. Tawara, I.; Kageyama, S.; Miyahara, Y.; Fujiwara, H.; Nishida, T.; Akatsuka, Y.; Ikeda, H.; Tanimoto, K.; Terakura, S.; Murata, M.; et al. Safety and persistence of WT1-specific T-cell receptor gene-transduced lymphocytes in patients with AML and MDS. *Blood* **2017**, *130*, 1985–1994. [CrossRef]
85. Boeckh, M.; Murphy, W.J.; Peggs, K.S. Recent advances in cytomegalovirus: An update on pharmacologic and cellular therapies. *Biol. Blood Marrow Transplant. J. Am. Soc. Blood Marrow Transplant.* **2015**, *21*, 24–29. [CrossRef]
86. Ljungman, P.; Boeckh, M.; Hirsch, H.H.; Josephson, F.; Lundgren, J.; Nichols, G.; Pikis, A.; Razonable, R.R.; Miller, V.; Griffiths, P.D.; et al. Definitions of Cytomegalovirus Infection and Disease in Transplant Patients for Use in Clinical Trials. *Clin. Infect. Dis. Off. Publ. Infect. Dis. Soc. Am.* **2017**, *64*, 87–91. [CrossRef]
87. Quinnan, G.V., Jr.; Kirmani, N.; Rook, A.H.; Manischewitz, J.F.; Jackson, L.; Moreschi, G.; Santos, G.W.; Saral, R.; Burns, W.H. Cytotoxic t cells in cytomegalovirus infection: HLA-restricted T-lymphocyte and non-T-lymphocyte cytotoxic responses correlate with recovery from cytomegalovirus infection in bone-marrow-transplant recipients. *N. Engl. J. Med.* **1982**, *307*, 7–13. [CrossRef]
88. Reusser, P.; Riddell, S.R.; Meyers, J.D.; Greenberg, P.D. Cytotoxic T-lymphocyte response to cytomegalovirus after human allogeneic bone marrow transplantation: Pattern of recovery and correlation with cytomegalovirus infection and disease. *Blood* **1991**, *78*, 1373–1380. [CrossRef]
89. Gillespie, G.M.; Wills, M.R.; Appay, V.; O'Callaghan, C.; Murphy, M.; Smith, N.; Sissons, P.; Rowland-Jones, S.; Bell, J.I.; Moss, P.A. Functional heterogeneity and high frequencies of cytomegalovirus-specific CD8(+) T lymphocytes in healthy seropositive donors. *J. Virol.* **2000**, *74*, 8140–8150. [CrossRef]
90. Ma, C.K.K.; Clancy, L.; Simms, R.; Burgess, J.; Deo, S.; Blyth, E.; Micklethwaite, K.P.; Gottlieb, D.J. Adjuvant Peptide Pulsed Dendritic Cell Vaccination in Addition to T Cell Adoptive Immunotherapy for Cytomegalovirus Infection in Allogeneic Hematopoietic Stem Cell Transplantation Recipients. *Biol. Blood Marrow Transplant. J. Am. Soc. Blood Marrow Transplant.* **2018**, *24*, 71–77. [CrossRef]
91. Meyers, J.D.; Flournoy, N.; Thomas, E.D. Risk factors for cytomegalovirus infection after human marrow transplantation. *J. Infect. Dis.* **1986**, *153*, 478–488. [CrossRef] [PubMed]
92. Schmitt, A.; Tonn, T.; Busch, D.H.; Grigoleit, G.U.; Einsele, H.; Odendahl, M.; Germeroth, L.; Ringhoffer, M.; Ringhoffer, S.; Wiesneth, M.; et al. Adoptive transfer and selective reconstitution of streptamer-selected cytomegalovirus-specific CD8+ T cells leads to virus clearance in patients after allogeneic peripheral blood stem cell transplantation. *Transfusion* **2011**, *51*, 591–599. [CrossRef] [PubMed]
93. Papadopoulos, E.B.; Ladanyi, M.; Emanuel, D.; Mackinnon, S.; Boulad, F.; Carabasi, M.H.; Castro-Malaspina, H.; Childs, B.H.; Gillio, A.P.; Small, T.N.; et al. Infusions of donor leukocytes to treat Epstein-Barr virus-associated lymphoproliferative disorders after allogeneic bone marrow transplantation. *N. Engl. J. Med.* **1994**, *330*, 1185–1191. [CrossRef] [PubMed]

94. Einsele, H.; Roosnek, E.; Rufer, N.; Sinzger, C.; Riegler, S.; Loffler, J.; Grigoleit, U.; Moris, A.; Rammensee, H.G.; Kanz, L.; et al. Infusion of cytomegalovirus (CMV)-specific T cells for the treatment of CMV infection not responding to antiviral chemotherapy. *Blood* **2002**, *99*, 3916–3922. [CrossRef]
95. Walter, E.A.; Greenberg, P.D.; Gilbert, M.J.; Finch, R.J.; Watanabe, K.S.; Thomas, E.D.; Riddell, S.R. Reconstitution of cellular immunity against cytomegalovirus in recipients of allogeneic bone marrow by transfer of T-cell clones from the donor. *N. Engl. J. Med.* **1995**, *333*, 1038–1044. [CrossRef]
96. Moosmann, A.; Bigalke, I.; Tischer, J.; Schirrmann, L.; Kasten, J.; Tippmer, S.; Leeping, M.; Prevalsek, D.; Jaeger, G.; Ledderose, G.; et al. Effective and long-term control of EBV PTLD after transfer of peptide-selected T cells. *Blood* **2010**, *115*, 2960–2970. [CrossRef]
97. Styczynski, J.; Einsele, H.; Gil, L.; Ljungman, P. Outcome of treatment of Epstein-Barr virus-related post-transplant lymphoproliferative disorder in hematopoietic stem cell recipients: A comprehensive review of reported cases. *Transpl. Infect. Dis. Off. J. Transplant. Soc.* **2009**, *11*, 383–392. [CrossRef]
98. Tzannou, I.; Papadopoulou, A.; Naik, S.; Leung, K.; Martinez, C.A.; Ramos, C.A.; Carrum, G.; Sasa, G.; Lulla, P.; Watanabe, A.; et al. Off-the-Shelf Virus-Specific T Cells to Treat BK Virus, Human Herpesvirus 6, Cytomegalovirus, Epstein-Barr Virus, and Adenovirus Infections After Allogeneic Hematopoietic Stem-Cell Transplantation. *J. Clin. Oncol. Off. J. Am. Soc. Clin. Oncol.* **2017**, *35*, 3547–3557. [CrossRef]
99. Muranski, P.; Davies, S.I.; Ito, S.; Koklanaris, E.; Superata, J.; Yu, Q.; Highfill, S.L.; Sabatino, M.; Stroncek, D.F.; Battiwalla, M.; et al. Very Early Adoptive Transfer of Ex Vivo Generated Multi-Virus Specific T Cells Is a Safe Strategy for Prevention of Viral Infection after Allogeneic T Cell Depleted Stem Cell Transplantation. *Blood* **2018**, *132*, 812. [CrossRef]
100. Kanate, A.S.; Craig, M.; Cumpston, A.; Saad, A.; Hobbs, G.; Leadmon, S.; Bunner, P.; Watkins, K.; Bulian, D.; Gibson, L.; et al. Higher infused CD34+ cell dose and overall survival in patients undergoing in vivo T-cell depleted, but not t-cell repleted, allogeneic peripheral blood hematopoietic cell transplantation. *Hematol. Oncol. Stem Cell Ther.* **2011**, *4*, 149–156. [CrossRef]
101. Chakrabarti, S.; MacDonald, D.; Hale, G.; Holder, K.; Turner, V.; Czarnecka, H.; Thompson, J.; Fegan, C.; Waldmann, H.; Milligan, D.W. T-cell depletion with Campath-1H "in the bag" for matched related allogeneic peripheral blood stem cell transplantation is associated with reduced graft-versus-host disease, rapid immune constitution and improved survival. *Br. J. Haematol.* **2003**, *121*, 109–118. [CrossRef] [PubMed]
102. Malard, F.; Labopin, M.; Cho, C.; Blaise, D.; Papadopoulos, E.B.; Passweg, J.; O'Reilly, R.; Forcade, E.; Maloy, M.; Volin, L.; et al. Ex Vivo and In Vivo T cell-depleted allogeneic stem cell transplantation in patients with acute myeloid leukemia in first complete remission resulted in similar overall survival: On behalf of the ALWP of the EBMT and the MSKCC. *J. Hematol. Oncol.* **2018**, *11*, 127. [CrossRef] [PubMed]
103. Lee, C.J.; Savani, B.N.; Mohty, M.; Labopin, M.; Ruggeri, A.; Schmid, C.; Baron, F.; Esteve, J.; Gorin, N.C.; Giebel, S.; et al. Haploidentical hematopoietic cell transplantation for adult acute myeloid leukemia: A position statement from the Acute Leukemia Working Party of the European Society for Blood and Marrow Transplantation. *Haematologica* **2017**, *102*, 1810–1822. [CrossRef] [PubMed]
104. Russo, A.; Oliveira, G.; Berglund, S.; Greco, R.; Gambacorta, V.; Cieri, N.; Toffalori, C.; Zito, L.; Lorentino, F.; Piemontese, S.; et al. NK cell recovery after haploidentical HSCT with posttransplant cyclophosphamide: Dynamics and clinical implications. *Blood* **2018**, *131*, 247–262. [CrossRef]
105. Chapuis, A.G.; Ragnarsson, G.B.; Nguyen, H.N.; Chaney, C.N.; Pufnock, J.S.; Schmitt, T.M.; Duerkopp, N.; Roberts, I.M.; Pogosov, G.L.; Ho, W.Y.; et al. Transferred WT1-reactive CD8+ T cells can mediate antileukemic activity and persist in post-transplant patients. *Sci. Transl. Med.* **2013**, *5*, 174ra127. [CrossRef]
106. Van Heijst, J.W.; Ceberio, I.; Lipuma, L.B.; Samilo, D.W.; Wasilewski, G.D.; Gonzales, A.M.; Nieves, J.L.; van den Brink, M.R.; Perales, M.A.; Pamer, E.G. Quantitative assessment of T cell repertoire recovery after hematopoietic stem cell transplantation. *Nat. Med.* **2013**, *19*, 372–377. [CrossRef]
107. Stenger, E.O.; Turnquist, H.R.; Mapara, M.Y.; Thomson, A.W. Dendritic cells and regulation of graft-versus-host disease and graft-versus-leukemia activity. *Blood* **2012**, *119*, 5088–5103. [CrossRef]
108. Boelens, J.J.; Admiraal, R.; Kuball, J.; Nierkens, S. Fine-Tuning Antithymocyte Globulin Dosing and Harmonizing Clinical Trial Design. *J. Clin. Oncol. Off. J. Am. Soc. Clin. Oncol.* **2018**, *36*, 1175–1176. [CrossRef]
109. Admiraal, R.; Nierkens, S.; de Witte, M.A.; Petersen, E.J.; Fleurke, G.J.; Verrest, L.; Belitser, S.V.; Bredius, R.G.M.; Raymakers, R.A.P.; Knibbe, C.A.J.; et al. Association between anti-thymocyte globulin exposure and survival outcomes in adult unrelated haemopoietic cell transplantation: A multicentre, retrospective, pharmacodynamic cohort analysis. *Lancet Haematol.* **2017**, *4*, e183–e191. [CrossRef]

110. Pasquini, M.C.; Devine, S.; Mendizabal, A.; Baden, L.R.; Wingard, J.R.; Lazarus, H.M.; Appelbaum, F.R.; Keever-Taylor, C.A.; Horowitz, M.M.; Carter, S.; et al. Comparative outcomes of donor graft CD34+ selection and immune suppressive therapy as graft-versus-host disease prophylaxis for patients with acute myeloid leukemia in complete remission undergoing HLA-matched sibling allogeneic hematopoietic cell transplantation. *J. Clin. Oncol. Off. J. Am. Soc. Clin. Oncol.* **2012**, *30*, 3194–3201. [CrossRef]
111. Mielcarek, M.; Furlong, T.; O'Donnell, P.V.; Storer, B.E.; McCune, J.S.; Storb, R.; Carpenter, P.A.; Flowers, M.E.; Appelbaum, F.R.; Martin, P.J. Posttransplantation cyclophosphamide for prevention of graft-versus-host disease after HLA-matched mobilized blood cell transplantation. *Blood* **2016**, *127*, 1502–1508. [CrossRef] [PubMed]
112. Locatelli, F.; Merli, P.; Pagliara, D.; Li Pira, G.; Falco, M.; Pende, D.; Rondelli, R.; Lucarelli, B.; Brescia, L.P.; Masetti, R.; et al. Outcome of children with acute leukemia given HLA-haploidentical HSCT after alphabeta T-cell and B-cell depletion. *Blood* **2017**, *130*, 677–685. [CrossRef] [PubMed]
113. Kanakry, C.G.; Coffey, D.G.; Towlerton, A.M.; Vulic, A.; Storer, B.E.; Chou, J.; Yeung, C.C.; Gocke, C.D.; Robins, H.S.; O'Donnell, P.V.; et al. Origin and evolution of the T cell repertoire after posttransplantation cyclophosphamide. *JCI Insight* **2016**, *1*. [CrossRef] [PubMed]
114. Yew, P.Y.; Alachkar, H.; Yamaguchi, R.; Kiyotani, K.; Fang, H.; Yap, K.L.; Liu, H.T.; Wickrema, A.; Artz, A.; van Besien, K.; et al. Quantitative characterization of T-cell repertoire in allogeneic hematopoietic stem cell transplant recipients. *Bone Marrow Transplant.* **2015**, *50*, 1227–1234. [CrossRef]
115. Van Bergen, C.A.; van Luxemburg-Heijs, S.A.; de Wreede, L.C.; Eefting, M.; von dem Borne, P.A.; van Balen, P.; Heemskerk, M.H.; Mulder, A.; Claas, F.H.; Navarrete, M.A.; et al. Selective graft-versus-leukemia depends on magnitude and diversity of the alloreactive T cell response. *J. Clin. Investig.* **2017**. [CrossRef]
116. Ravens, S.; Schultze-Florey, C.; Raha, S.; Sandrock, I.; Drenker, M.; Oberdorfer, L.; Reinhardt, A.; Ravens, I.; Beck, M.; Geffers, R.; et al. Publisher Correction: Human gammadelta T cells are quickly reconstituted after stem-cell transplantation and show adaptive clonal expansion in response to viral infection. *Nat. Immunol.* **2018**, *19*, 1037. [CrossRef]

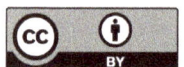

© 2019 by the authors. Licensee MDPI, Basel, Switzerland. This article is an open access article distributed under the terms and conditions of the Creative Commons Attribution (CC BY) license (http://creativecommons.org/licenses/by/4.0/).

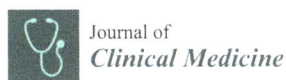

Review

FLAMSA-RIC for Stem Cell Transplantation in Patients with Acute Myeloid Leukemia and Myelodysplastic Syndromes: A Systematic Review and Meta-Analysis

Weerapat Owattanapanich [1,*], Patompong Ungprasert [2], Verena Wais [3], Smith Kungwankiattichai [1], Donald Bunjes [3] and Florian Kuchenbauer [4,5,*]

1. Division of Hematology, Department of Medicine, Faculty of Medicine Siriraj Hospital, Mahidol University, Bangkok 10700, Thailand
2. Clinical Epidemiology Unit, Department of Research and Development, Faculty of Medicine Siriraj Hospital, Mahidol University, Bangkok 10700, Thailand
3. Department of Internal Medicine III, University Hospital of Ulm, 89081 Ulm, Germany
4. Vancouver General Hospital, L/BMT Program of British Columbia, Vancouver, BC V5Z 1M9, Canada
5. Terry Fox Laboratory, British Columbia Research Centre, Vancouver, BC V5Z 1L3, Canada
* Correspondence: weerapato36733@gmail.com (W.O.); fkuchenbauer@bccrc.ca (F.K.)

Received: 2 July 2019; Accepted: 3 September 2019; Published: 11 September 2019

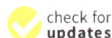

Abstract: Reduced-intensity conditioning (RIC) regimens are established options for hematopoietic stem cell transplantation (HSCT) for patients with acute myeloid leukemia (AML) and myelodysplastic syndrome (MDS). However, the efficacy of RIC regimens for patients with high-risk disease is limited. The addition of a fludarabine, amsacrine, and cytarabine (FLAMSA)-sequential conditioning regimen was introduced for patients with high-risk MDS and AML to combine a high anti-leukemic activity with the advantages of RIC. The current systematic literature review and meta-analysis was conducted with the aim of identifying all cohort studies of patients with AML and/or MDS who received FLAMSA-RIC to determine its efficacy and toxicity. Out of 3044 retrieved articles, 12 published studies with 2395 overall patients (18.1–76.0 years; 96.8% AML and 3.2% MDS; follow-up duration of 0.7–145 months; 50.3% had active AML disease before HSCT) met the eligibility criteria and were included in the meta-analysis. In the pooled analysis, the 1- and 3-year overall survival (OS) rates were 59.6% (95% confidence interval (CI), 47.9–70.2%) and 40.2% (95% CI, 28.0–53.7%), respectively. The pooled 3-year OS rate of the patients who achieved CR1 or CR2 prior to HSCT was 60.1% (95% CI, 55.1–64.8%) and the percentage of those with relapse or refractory disease was 27.8% (95% CI, 23.3–32.8%). The pooled 3-year leukemia-free survival (LFS) rate was 39.3% (95% CI, 26.4–53.9%). Approximately 29% of the patients suffered from grades 2–4 acute graft-versus-host disease (GVHD), while 35.6% had chronic GVHD. The pooled 1- and 3-year non-relapse mortality (NRM) rates were 17.9% (95% CI, 16.1–19.8%) and 21.1% (95% CI, 18.8–23.7%), respectively. Our data indicates that the FLAMSA-RIC regimen is an effective and well-tolerated regimen for HSCT in patients with high-risk AML and MDS.

Keywords: FLAMSA; reduced-intensity; acute myeloid leukemia; myelodysplastic syndrome

---

1. Introduction

Reduced-intensity conditioning (RIC) regimens were initially introduced to reduce the adverse effects associated with myeloablative conditioning (MAC) and to improve the chance of successful hematopoietic stem cell transplantation (HSCT), especially in elderly and frail patients [1]. However, the efficacy of RIC regimens for patients who do not achieve a complete remission (CR) is limited [2]. The combination of fludarabine, amsacrine, and cytarabine (FLAMSA)-polychemotherapy with RIC was initially adopted by Schmid et al. for patients with high-risk myelodysplastic syndrome (MDS) and acute myeloid leukemia (AML) [3–5] to combine high anti-leukemic activity with the advantages of RIC. Although several variations have been published [6–16], the 'classic' FLAMSA-RIC regimen consists of fludarabine, amsacrine, and cytarabine, followed by RIC with 4-Gy total body irradiation (TBI), high-dose cyclophosphamide (Cy), antithymocyte globulin (ATG), and prophylactic donor lymphocyte infusions (DLI) if indicated. Because of initially promising data, especially in poor prognosis AML patients, FLAMSA-RIC was adopted by many transplantation centers, and variations that included busulfan (Bu) or treosulfan were established. The current systematic review and meta-analysis was conducted with the aim of identifying all cohort studies that have investigated the efficacy and toxicity of the FLAMSA-RIC regimen and summarize their results.

2. Materials and Methods

2.1. Data Sources and Searches

Three investigators (W.O., P.U. and S.K.) independently searched for published articles indexed in MEDLINE and EMBASE databases from their inception to May 2019. The search strategy is available as Supplementary Data 1. The references of the included studies were also manually reviewed for additional eligible studies. This study was undertaken in accordance with the Preferred Reporting Items for Systematic Reviews and Meta-Analyses (PRISMA) statement, which is available as Supplementary Data 2 [17].

2.2. Selection Criteria and Data Extraction

Studies included in this meta-analysis were cohort studies (either prospective or retrospective) of patients with AML and/or MDS who received FLAMSA-RIC regimens, which reported our primary outcomes of interest (overall survival (OS) and/or leukemic-free survival (LFS) rates). The secondary outcomes of interest, which included non-relapse mortality (NRM) rate, relapse rate (RR), full chimerism rate, grades 2–4 acute GVHD (aGVHD) rate, and chronic GVHD (cGVHD) rate were also collected for analysis but were not part of the inclusion criteria. Assessment of the eligibility of each study was independently conducted by three investigators. In the event of opposing decisions regarding a study's eligibility, the study in question was reviewed by the three investigators together and the final determination was reached by mutual consensus.

2.3. Definition of Treatment Response and Outcome

Complete remission (CR) was defined as bone marrow blasts of < 5%, the absence of circulating blasts and blasts with Auer rods, the absence of an extramedullary disease, an absolute neutrophil count (ANC) of $\geq 1.0 \times 10^9$/L and a platelet count of $\geq 100 \times 10^9$/L [8]. Refractory AML was defined as failure to achieve CR following induction or salvage chemotherapy. Relapse AML was defined as recurrence of disease after CR. Overall survival (OS) rate was defined as the percentage of patients who were still alive at the time of interest (such as at 1 year after transplantation). Leukemia-free survival (LFS) rate was defined as the percentage of patients who were still alive and did not have leukemia at the time of interest. Non-relapse mortality (NRM) was defined as any death without previous relapse or progression.

2.4. Statistical Analysis

All data analyses were performed using the Comprehensive Meta-Analysis program, version 2.2 (Biostat, Englewood, NJ, USA). Using a standardized data extraction algorithm, two authors (W.O. and P.U.) extracted and tabulated all data from each study. The pooled rates and 95% confidence interval of OS rate, LFS rate, NRM rate, relapse rate, full chimerism rate, aGVHD rate, and cGVHD rate were calculated using the DerSimonian-Laird random-effect model with double arcsine transformation [18]. A random-effect model, rather than fixed-effect, was used because of the high likelihood of between-study heterogeneity. Cochran's Q test and I^2 statistic were used to determine the between-study heterogeneity. I^2 statistic quantified the proportion of total variation across studies that is due to heterogeneity rather than chance. An I^2 value of 0% to 25% represents insignificant heterogeneity, greater than 25% but less than or equal to 50% represents low heterogeneity, greater than 50% but less than or equal to 75% represents moderate heterogeneity, and greater than 75% represents high heterogeneity [19].

3. Results

The search strategy yielded 3044 potentially relevant articles (504 articles from MEDLINE and 2540 from EMBASE). After exclusion of 416 duplicated articles using the EndNote X8 software, 2628 articles underwent title and abstract review. A total of 2607 articles were excluded at this stage as they did not meet the inclusion criteria based on type of article, study design, subjects and interventions used. A total of eighteen articles underwent full-text review and 9 of them were excluded because they did not report the primary outcomes of interest. Finally, 12 studies fulfilled the eligibility criteria and were included in the meta-analysis [3,6–16]. A manual review of the bibliography of the included studies, and some selected review articles, did not yield any additional eligible studies. Figure 1 summarizes the literature review and identification process. The main characteristics of the included studies are described in Table 1.

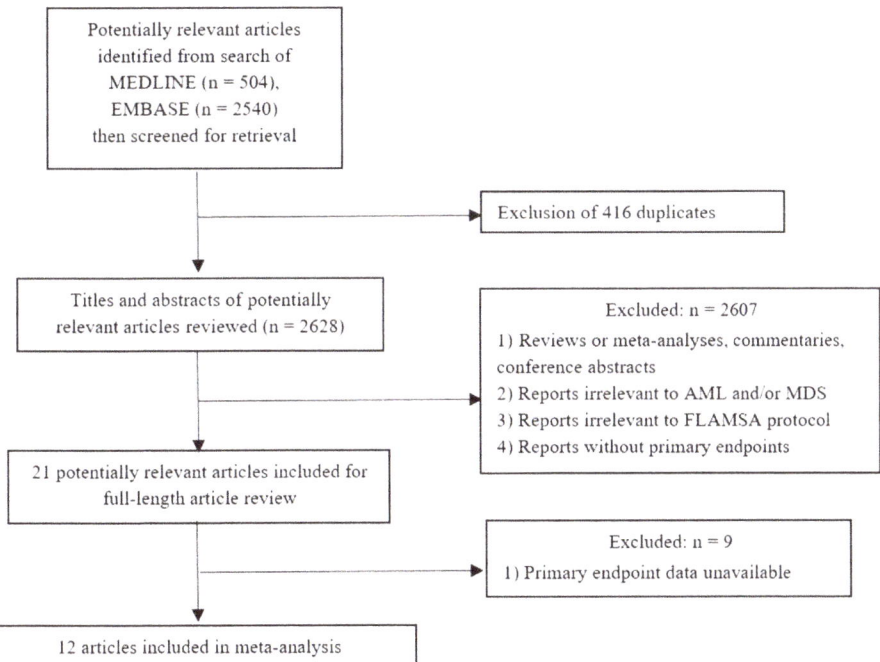

Figure 1. Flowchart of literature review process.

Table 1. Baseline patient characteristics of each included article.

References	No.	Sex (M/F)	Median Age (Years, Range)	Diseases	Disease Status	Stem Cell Source	Donor Source	CD34+ (×10^6 cells/kg)	Study Period	Median Follow Up (Months, Range)	Type
Schmid et al. (2005) [4]	75	42/33	52.3 (18.5–65.8)	50 dAML, 15 sAML, 10 MDS	8 CR1, 8 CR2, 49 R/R, 10 MDS	61 PBSC, 14 BM	31 MRD, 30 MUD 6 MMRD, 8 MMUD	9.6	1999–2002	31.5 (13.6–47.6)	P
Saure et al. (2012) [5]	30	20/10	49 (36–66)	10 sAML, 20 MDS	10 untreated AML, 20 MDS	30 PBSC	13 MRD, 13 MUD 4 MMUD	7.7	2003–2010	28 (7–81)	P
Krejci et al. (2013) [7]	60	28/32	52 (20–63)	50 dAML, 10 sAML	34 CR1, 26 R/R	56 PBSC, 4 BM	15 MRD, 29 MUD, 16 MMUD	6.3	2006–2011	37 (10–69)	P
Schneidawind et al. (2013) [10]	62	34/28	55 (20–72)	35 dAML, 27 sAML	62 R/R	62 PBSC	11 MRD, 22 MUD 4 MMRD, 25 MMUD	5.4	2005–2012	17.5 (2.2–77.6)	R
Bohl et al. (2016) [8]	84	46/38	48.7	67 dAML, 17 sAML	13 CR1, 12 CR2, 59 R/R	NR	NR	NR	2000–2012	NR	R
Holtick et al. (2016) [9]	130	59/71	50.9 (19–73)	NR	47 CR1, 26 CR2, 57 R/R	127 PBSC, 3 BM	42 MRD, 64 MUD 1 MMRD, 23 MMUD	7.07	2004–2015	37 (10–125)	R
Pfrepper et al. (2016) [11]	44	25/19	52 (21–65)	NR	44 R/R	44 PBSC	3 MRD, 27 MUD, 14 MMUD	NR	2006–2013	34 (6–71)	R
Ringden et al. (2016) [12]	267	131/136	51.7 (19.4–72.5)	NR	267 R/R	256 PBSC, 11 BM	77 MRD, 190 MUD	NR	NR	68.2 (2–157)	R
Malard et al. (2017) [13]	265	143/122	55 (19–76)	156 dAML, 109 sAML	216 CR1, 49 CR2	251 PBSC, 14 BM	74 MRD, 191 MUD	NR	2002–2014	46 (1–145)	R
Heinicke et al. (2018) [14]	399	206/193	(18–74.4)	NR	305 CR1, 94 CR2	379 PBSC, 20 BM	139 MRD, 198 MUD, 62 MMUD	NR	2005–2016	(0.7–121.5)	R
Sheth et al. (2019) [15]	348	179/169	(40.1–65)	294 dAML, 54 sAML	264 CR1, 84 CR2	330 PBSC, 18 BM	113 MRD, 182 MUD, 53 MMUD	NR	2007–2016	NR	R
Saraceni et al. (2019) [16]	631	336/295	51.5 (18.1–76)	NR	631 RR	616 PBSC, 15 BM	252 MRD, 268 MUD, 111 MMUD	NR	2005–2016	53 (4–35)	R

Abbreviations: BM bone marrow; CR1 complete remission after first induction therapy; CR2 complete remission after relapse; dAML denovo acute myeloid leukemia; F Female; M Male; MDS myelodysplastic syndromes; MRD match related donor; MMRD mismatch related donor; MUD match unrelated donor; MMUD mismatch unrelated donor; NR not reported; P prospectively; PBSC peripheral blood stem cell; R retrospectively; R/R relapse and/or refractory diseases; sAML secondary acute myeloid leukemia.

3.1. Baseline Patient Characteristics

A total of 12 studies with 2395 patients receiving FLAMSA-RIC regimen were included in this meta-analysis. 52.2% were male, age ranged from 18.1 to 76.0 years (46% were age 55 years or older). AML was by far the most common underlying hematological disease (70.6% de novo AML and 26.2% secondary AML). Only 3.2% of the analyzed patients had high-risk MDS. Thirty-seven per cent of the patients were in CR1, 11.4% of the patients were in CR2, and 50.3% of the patients had active AML prior to HSCT (49.9% relapse and/or refractory disease and 0.4% untreated AML). Baseline clinical characteristics of those patients are summarized in Table 2.

Table 2. Clinical characteristics of the patients from the included studies.

		Number of Patients (N = 2395)	Percent (%) or Range
Sex	Male	1249	52.2
	Female	1146	47.8
Age range in years		-	18.1–6.0
Diseases (n = 924)	dAML	652	70.6
	sAML	242	26.2
	MDS	30	3.2
Disease status (n = 2395)	CR1	887	37.0
	CR2	273	11.4
	R/R	1195	49.9
	Untreated AML	10	0.4
	High-risk MDS	30	1.3
Stem cell source (n = 2311)	PBSC	2212	95.7
	BM	99	4.3
Donor source (n = 2311)	MRD	770	33.3
	MUD	1214	52.5
	MMRD	11	0.5
	MMUD	316	13.7
CD 34+ in 10^6 cells/kg (n = 357)		-	1.2–23.1
Follow up duration in months (n = 933)		-	0.7–145

Abbreviations; BM bone marrow; CR1 complete remission after first induction therapy; CR2 complete remission after relapse; dAML denovo acute myeloid leukemia; MDS myelodysplastic syndromes; MRD match related donor; MMRD mismatch related donor; MMUD mismatch unrelated donor; MUD match unrelated donor; PBSC peripheral blood stem cell; R/R relapse and/or refractory diseases; sAML secondary acute myeloid leukemia.

3.2. FLAMSA Variations, Stem Sources, and GVHD Prophylaxis

The FLAMSA regimen consists of fludarabine (30 mg/m^2; total dose 120 mg/m^2), amsacrine (100 mg/m^2; total dose 400 mg/m^2), and cytarabine (2 g/m^2; total dose 8 g/m^2) therapy from days minus 12 to minus 9, followed by a three-day interval without therapy and RIC. Several RIC protocols were included in this meta-analysis: (1) 4 Gy TBI plus Cy, (2) Bu/Cy, (3) treosulfan/Cy, (4) melphalan (Mel), (5) fludarabine (Flu)/Bu, (6) Bu alone, or (7) Mel/thiotepa. Almost all patients received rabbit anti-thymocyte globulin (rATG; 10–20 mg/kg from day minus 4 to day minus 2, according to donor type). Details of all included FLAMSA-RIC regimens, GvHD prophylaxis, and prophylactic donor lymphocyte transfusions are summarized in Supplementary Table S1.

Donors were investigated for human leukocyte antigen (HLA)-A, HLA-B, HLA-C, HLA-DRB1, and HLA-DQB1. In this study, 10/10 HLA-matched related (MRD), unrelated donors (MUD), 1–2 antigen/allele mismatched related (MMRD) and unrelated donors (MMUD) were included. The most frequent donors were MUD (52.5%), followed by MRD (33.3%), MMUD (13.7%) and MMRD (0.5%). The most frequent stem cell source (95.7%) were stem cells collected from peripheral blood. CD 34$^+$ cell infusions ranged from 1.2 to 23.1 × 10^6 cells/kg.

GVHD prophylaxis was available for 720 patients, most of them received cyclosporine A (CyA) plus mycophenolate mofetil (MMF; n = 573), followed by tacrolimus plus MMF (n = 112), CyA alone (n = 28), and CyA plus methotrexate (n = 7). Prophylactic donor lymphocyte transfusions were given if patients did not show any evidence for GVHD either at day 120 or 30 days after discontinuation of the immunosuppression [3,7,10–12].

3.3. Survival Outcome

The follow-up period ranged from 0.7 to 145 months. The pooled 1-, 2- and 3-year OS rates were 59.6% (95% CI, 47.9–70.2%; I^2 94%; Figure 2A) [6–8,14–16], 48.4% (95% CI, 37.3–59.6%; I^2 96%; Figure 2B [3,6,8,10,13–16], and 40.2% (95% CI, 28.0–53.7%; I^2 96%; Figure 2C) [6,7,11,12,14–16], respectively. The pooled 1-, 2- and 3-year LFS were 57.4% (95% CI, 38.6–74.2%; I^2 98%; Figure 2D) [6, 14–16], 49.4% (95% CI, 38.1–60.8%; I^2 95%; Figure 2E [3,6,9,13–16], and 39.3% (95% CI, 26.4–53.9%; I^2 97%; Figure 2F) [6,7,12,14–16], respectively. The pooled 2- and 3-year RR were 31.3% (95% CI, 21.1–43.8%; I^2 96%; Figure 3A) [3,6,10,13–16] and 41.9% (95% CI, 30.9–53.8%; I^2 95%; Figure 3B) [6,7,11, 12,14–16], respectively.

A total of 4 studies [3,6,9,11] reported the rate of full chimerism at day +28 (defined as the presence of > 98% of HLA belonging to the donor) and the pooled rate across the 4 studies was 82.9% (95% CI, 69.7–91.1%; I^2 77%) (Figure 3C).

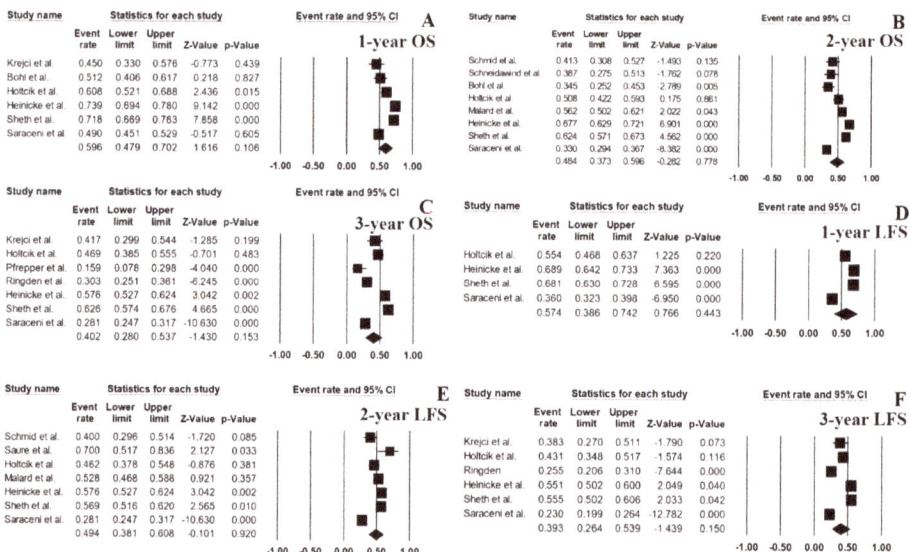

Figure 2. Forest plots of pooled estimates (95% confidence interval (CI)) for overall survival (OS) and leukemia-free survival (LFS) after hematopoietic stem cell transplantation (HSCT); (**A**): 1-year OS; (**B**): 2-year OS; (**C**): 3-year OS; (**D**): 1-year LFS; (**E**): 2-year LFS; (**F**): 3-year LFS.

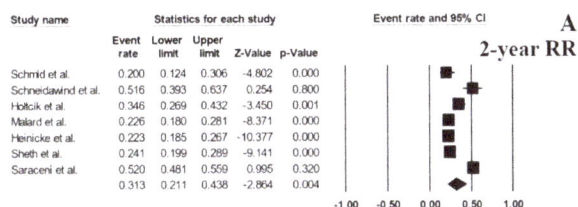

Figure 3. Forest plots of pooled estimates (95% CI) for relapse rate (RR) and outcome after HSCT; (**A**): 2-year RR; (**B**): 3-year RR; (**C**): full chimerism at 4 weeks after HSCT.

3.4. Complications of HSCT

A total of 9 studies reported the rate of Grade 2–4 aGVHD. The pooled rate across those studies was 29.0% (95% CI, 25.5–32.7%; I^2 63%; Figure 4A) [3,9–16], whereas the pooled rate of cGVHD was 35.6% (95% CI, 30.0–41.6%; I^2 84%; Figure 4B), which was derived from 9 studies [3,7,9,10,12–16]. There was a slight increase in the rate of NRM for each year of follow-up with the pooled 1-year NRM rate of 17.9% (95% CI, 16.1–19.8%; I^2 0%; Figure 4C) [3,6,7,14–16], and the pooled 3-year NRM rate of 21.1% (95% CI, 18.8–23.7%; I^2 30%; Figure 4D) [6,7,9,11,12,14–16].

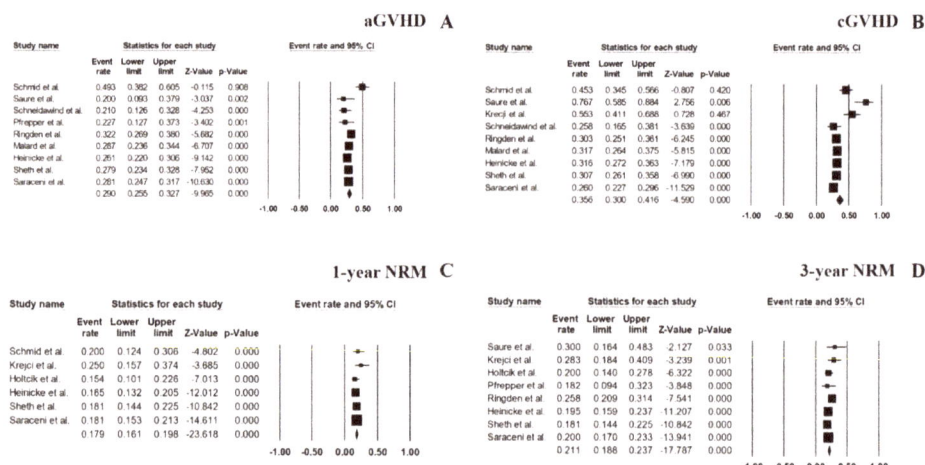

Figure 4. Forest plots of pooled estimates (95% CI) for complications after HSCT; (**A**): Acute graft-versus-host disease (aGVHD); (**B**): Chronic graft-versus-host disease (cGVHD); (**C**): 1-year non-relapse mortality (NRM); (**D**): 3-year NRM.

3.5. Subgroup Analysis

The pooled 3-year OS rate of the patients who achieved CR1 or CR2 prior to HSCT was 60.1% (95% CI, 55.1–64.8%; I^2 48%; Figure 5A) [14,15] and 3-year LFS was 55.2% (95% CI, 51.6–58.7%; I^2 0%; Figure 5B) [14,15]. As for the patients with relapse or refractory disease, the pooled 3-year OS and LFS rates were 27.8% (95% CI, 23.3–32.8%; I^2 47%; Figure 5C) [11,12,16] and 23.7% (95% CI, 21.1–26.6%; I^2 0%; Figure 5D) [12,16], respectively.

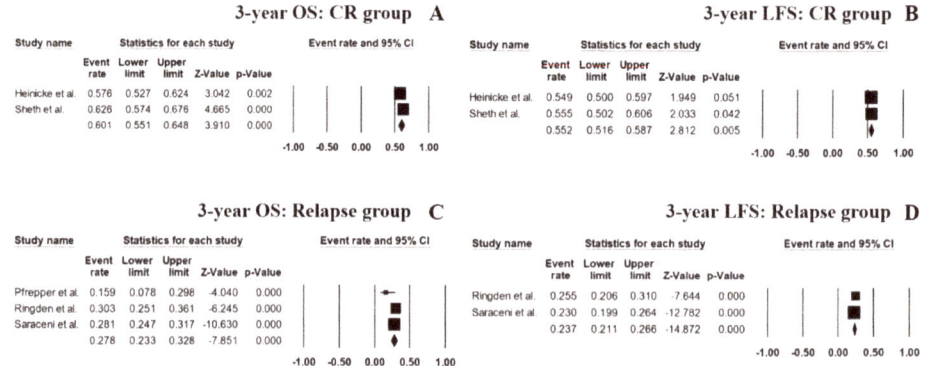

Figure 5. Forest plots of pooled estimates (95% CI) for outcomes of the patient's subgroups; (**A**): 3-year OS of CR1 or CR2 patients; (**B**): 3-year LFS of CR1 or CR2 patients; (**C**): 3-year OS of acute myeloid leukemia (AML) patients with relapse and/or refractory disease; (**D**): 3-year LFS of high risk AML patients with relapse and/or refractory disease.

A subgroup analysis based on the reported conditioning regimens showed that the patients receiving a TBI-based regimen had a pooled 3-year OS rate of 58.5% (95% CI, 47.2–68.9%; I^2 82%; Figure 6A) [7,14,15] and a pooled 3-year LFS of 54.0% (95% CI, 43.6–64.1%; I^2 80%; Figure 6B) [7,14,15]. With regard to the patients receiving Bu-based regimens, the pooled 3-year OS rate was 52.8% (95%

CI, 39.8–65.3%; I^2 80%; Figure 6C) [14,15] and the 3-year LFS was 48.2% (95% CI, 41.4–51.1%; I^2 29%; Figure 6D) [14,15].

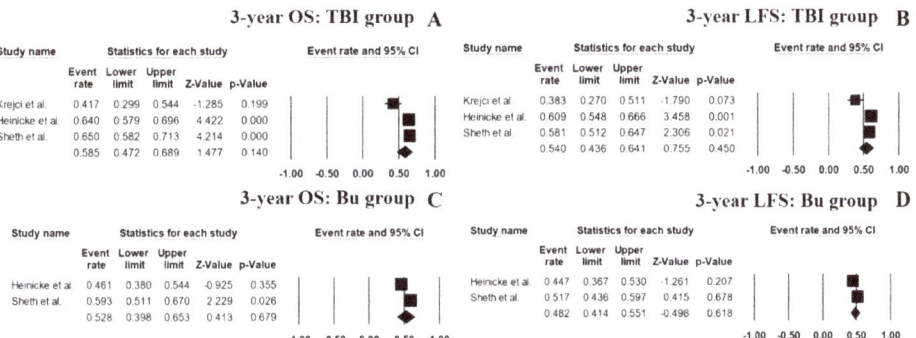

Figure 6. Forest plots of pooled estimates (95% CI) for outcome outcomes of the patient's subgroups; (**A**): 3-year OS of patients receiving total body irradiation (TBI)-based conditioning regimen; (**B**): 3-year LFS of patients receiving TBI-based conditioning regimen; (**C**): 3-year OS of patients receiving busulfan-based conditioning regimen; (**D**): 3-year LFS of patients receiving busulfan-based conditioning regimen.

3.6. Sensitivity Analysis

A sensitivity analysis was performed by excluding five studies by Ringden et al. [12], Malard et al. [13], Heinicke et al. [14], Sheth et al. [15] and Saraceni et al. [16] from the pooled analyses based on a concern over double-counting of patients. These five studies collected and reported data of patients who were treated at several medical centers and some centers also reported their own data separately (including the studies by Schmid et al. [3], Holtick et al. [6], Krejci et al. [7], Saure et al. [9], Schneidawind et al. [10], and Pfrepper et al. [11], which were included in this meta-analysis). The pooled 3-year OS, 3-year RR, and 3-year LFS were 34.9%, 47.2% and 41.6%, respectively. The new pooled results, after exclusion of the aforementioned studies, were fairly similar to the results of the original analysis as demonstrated in Supplementary Data 3.

4. Discussion

Although HSCT remains the most effective treatment option for AML, data from the National Cancer Data Base on patients with AML aged ≥ 61 years who were diagnosed between 2003 and 2012 found that only about 6% of older patients (n = 17,555) underwent HSCT [20]. RIC regimens were subsequently introduced with the aim of reducing adverse effects and making HSCT feasible for elderly and fragile patients. However, RIC regimens alone may not be sufficient for patients with high-risk features, such as persisting disease [21]. To overcome this limitation, FLAMSA-RIC was introduced in 2005 and has been adopted in many countries [3]. The current study is the first systematic review and meta-analysis to examine the efficacy and toxicity of the FLAMSA-RIC regimen for patients with AML and MDS. Recently published trials comparing MAC vs. RIC showed controversial results. For example, in the study of Scott et al., RIC led to significantly lower TRM but higher relapse rates compared with MAC, suggesting the use of MAC as the standard of care for fit patients with AML and MDS in CR [22]. In contrast, Bornhäuser et al. did not observe any difference between RIC and MAC with regards to relapse rate, OS and TRM for intermediate and high-risk AML patients [23]. We found a pooled 2-year OS rate of approximately 50%, which is lower than the reported results of Scott et al. (18-month OS: 76.4% MAC and 63.4% RIC) and Bornhäuser et al. (3-year OS: 61% vs. 58%), but similar or lower RR (FLAMSA: 2-year RR: 31.3%) compared to Scott et al. (18-month RR: 65.2%: MAC and 45.3%: RIC) and Bornhäuser et al. (3-year RR: 28% MAC and 26% RIC). In a retrospective analysis, Eapen et al. analyzed the impact of conditioning regimes with varying intensity on outcome in 2209

AML and MDS patients transplanted in complete remission [24]. The authors reported a higher 3-year RR with 46% with Flu/Bu2 and 56% with Flu/Bu2+ATG. In line with this finding, a recent retrospective EBMT analysis demonstrated a lower RR for FLAMSA-RIC compared to Flu/Bu2 in AML patients in CR1 and CR2 [14], suggesting that this patient group could benefit from FLAMSA-RIC. The clinical outcome was similar using either a TBI or Bu-based FLAMSA regimen. Considering the side-effects of TBI, FLAMSA-Bu appears to be an effective alternative to FLAMSA-TBI.

With regard to patients with active disease in this meta-analysis, the 3-year OS and LFS rates were 27.8% and 23.7%, respectively. Given, that only 46% of AML patients with induction failure respond to chemotherapy and that 52% with refractory disease die within 90 days [25], FLAMSA-RIC is a reasonable treatment option for this otherwise difficult to treat patient cohort. Interestingly, Bohl et al. recently showed a correlation between tumor load and outcome for FLAMSA-RIC, underscoring the relevance of a high tumor burden as one of the strongest negative predictors for treatment outcome after HSCT especially in relapsed or refractory AML patients [8]. Although Goyal et al. showed that the exclusive presence of extramedullary disease did not impact on outcome after HSCT [26], Bohl et al. noted that that FLAMSA-RIC followed by HSCT is not effective in patients with concurrent active bone marrow and extramedullary disease [8], which led to a change of practice in our institution.

The results may also suggest that the addition of FLAMSA to RIC may help to alleviate the aggressive behavior of the disease, which will ultimately help to improve survival outcome. Furthermore, the FLAMSA-RIC regimen did not appear to increase the risk of serious toxicity with the comparable 1-year NRM rate to those who received RIC regimens alone (17.9% versus 28% [27], respectively), as well as the comparable rate of grade 2–4 aGVHD events (29% versus 35% [27], respectively).

The limitations of this study are mainly due to the observational nature of the included primary studies. Varying event rates such as OS, LFS and RR among the included studies could attributed to differences in the analyzed patient cohorts and treatment protocols in each study. Furthermore, without a direct prospective head-to-head comparison, a conclusion on whether the FLAMSA-RIC regimen offers a superior survival benefit compared with RIC regimens alone among patients who do not achieve CR cannot be made. Randomized controlled trials comparing the FLAMSA-RIC regimen with RIC regimens alone are still needed. Ongoing randomized trials such as NCT01423175 and NCT00606723 comparing FLAMSA-RIC with alternative conditioning regimes will eventually prove its efficacy and toxicity as a standard conditioning protocol for high risk AML.

5. Conclusions

A FLAMSA-RIC regimen is an effective and well-tolerated regimen for HSCT in patients with AML and MDS, even among those who do not achieve complete remission.

Supplementary Materials: The following are available online at http://www.mdpi.com/2077-0383/8/9/1437/s1, Supplementary data 1: Search strategy, Supplementary data 2: The Preferred Reporting Items for Systematic Reviews and Meta-Analyses statement, Supplementary data 3: Sensitivity analysis of the odds of outcomes after HSCT; A: 3-year OS; B: 2-year relapse rate; C: 3-year relapse rate; D: 3-year LFS; E: aGVHD; F: cGVHD; G: 3-year NRM., Table S1: FLAMSA-RIC regimen, GvHD prophylaxis, and prophylactic donor lymphocyte transfusions in each study.

Author Contributions: All authors designed the study. W.O., P.U., S.K. designed the study, collected the data, and performed the statistical analyses. W.O. and F.K. drafted the manuscript. V.W., D.B. and F.K. made critical revisions to the manuscript. W.O. and F.K. revised the final manuscript. All authors read and approved the final manuscript.

Funding: This research received no external funding.

Conflicts of Interest: The authors declare no conflict of interest.

Abbreviation

Abbreviation	Full Name
aGVHD	acute graft-versus-host disease;
AML	acute myeloid leukemia
Bu	busulfan
CI	confidence interval
cGVHD	chronic graft-versus-host disease
CR	complete remission
Cy	cyclophosphamide
CyA	cyclosporine A
Flu	fludarabine
GVHD	graft-versus-host disease
HLA	human leukocyte antigen
HSCT	hematopoietic stem cell transplantation
LFS	leukemia-free survival
MAC	myeloablative conditioning
MDS	MMUD mismatched unrelated donors
MRD	matched related donor
MUD	matched unrelated donors
NRM	non-relapse mortality
OS	overall survival
rATG	rabbit anti-thymocyte globulin
RIC	reduced-intensity conditioning
RR	relapse rate
TBI	total body irradiation

References

1. Slavin, S.; Nagler, A.; Naparstek, E.; Kapelushnik, Y.; Aker, M.; Cividalli, G.; Varadi, G.; Kirschbaum, M.; Ackerstein, A.; Samuel, S.; et al. Non-MA stem cell transplantation and cell therapy as an alternative to conventional bone marrow transplantation with lethal cytoreduction for the treatment of malignant and nonmalignant hematologic diseases. *Blood* **1998**, *91*, 756–763. [PubMed]
2. Wais, V.; Kundgen, L.; Bohl, S.R.; von Harsdorf, S.; Schlenk, R.F.; Dohner, K.; Teleanu, V.; Bullinger, L.; Nguyen, T.M.; Drognitz, K.; et al. Reduced-toxicity conditioning for allogeneic hematopoietic cell transplantation in elderly or comorbid patients with AML using fludarabine, BCNU and melphalan: Disease stage at transplant determines outcome. *Bone Marrow Transplant.* **2018**, *53*, 94–96. [CrossRef] [PubMed]
3. Schmid, C.; Schleuning, M.; Ledderose, G.; Tischer, J.; Kolb, H.-J. Sequential Regimen of Chemotherapy, Reduced-Intensity Conditioning for Allogeneic Stem-Cell Transplantation, and Prophylactic Donor Lymphocyte Transfusion in High-Risk Acute Myeloid Leukemia and Myelodysplastic Syndrome. *J. Clin. Oncol.* **2005**, *23*, 5675–5687. [CrossRef] [PubMed]
4. Schmid, C.; Schleuning, M.; Schwerdtfeger, R.; Hertenstein, B.; Mischak-Weissinger, E.; Bunjes, D.; Harsdorf, S.V.; Scheid, C.; Holtick, U.; Greinix, H.; et al. Long-term survival in refractory acute myeloid leukemia after sequential treatment with chemotherapy and reduced-intensity conditioning for allogeneic stem cell transplantation. *Blood* **2006**, *108*, 1092–1099. [CrossRef] [PubMed]
5. Schmid, C.; Schleuning, M.; Hentrich, M.; Markl, G.E.; Gerbitz, A.; Tischer, J.; Ledderose, G.; Oruzio, D.; Hiddemann, W.; Kolb, H.-J. High antileukemic efficacy of an intermediate intensity conditioning regimen for allogeneic stem cell transplantation in patients with high-risk acute myeloid leukemia in first complete remission. *Bone Marrow Transplant.* **2008**, *41*, 721–727. [CrossRef] [PubMed]
6. Holtick, U.; Shimabukuro-Vornhagen, A.; Chakupurakal, G.; Theurich, S.; Leitzke, S.; Burst, A.; Hallek, M.; von Bergwelt-Baildon, M.; Scheid, C.; Chemnitz, J.M. FLAMSA reduced-intensity conditioning is equally effective in AML patients with primary induction failure as well as in first or second complete remission. *Eur. J. Haematol.* **2016**, *96*, 475–482. [CrossRef] [PubMed]

7. Krejci, M.; Doubek, M.; Dušek, J.; Brychtova, Y.; Racil, Z.; Navrátil, M.; Tomiska, M.; Horky, O.; Pospisilova, S.; Mayer, J. Combination of fludarabine, amsacrine, and cytarabine followed by reduced-intensity conditioning and allogeneic hematopoietic stem cell transplantation in patients with high-risk acute myeloid leukemia. *Ann. Hematol.* **2013**, *92*, 1397–1403. [CrossRef] [PubMed]
8. Bohl, S.; Von Harsdorf, S.; Mulaw, M.; Hofmann, S.; Babiak, A.; Maier, C.P.; Schnell, J.; Hütter-Krönke, L.-M.; Scholl, K.; Wais, V.; et al. Strong impact of extramedullary involvement in high-risk AML patients with active disease receiving the FLAMSA conditioning regimen for HSCT. *Bone Marrow Transplant.* **2016**, *51*, 994–996. [CrossRef] [PubMed]
9. Saure, C.; Schroeder, T.; Zohren, F.; Groten, A.; Bruns, I.; Czibere, A.; Galonska, L.; Kondakci, M.; Weigelt, C.; Fenk, R.; et al. Upfront Allogeneic Blood Stem Cell Transplantation for Patients with High-Risk Myelodysplastic Syndrome or Secondary Acute Myeloid Leukemia Using a FLAMSA-Based High-Dose Sequential Conditioning Regimen. *Biol. Blood Marrow Transplant.* **2012**, *18*, 466–472. [CrossRef]
10. Schneidawind, D.; Federmann, B.; Faul, C.; Vogel, W.; Kanz, L.; Bethge, W.A. Allogeneic hematopoietic cell transplantation with reduced-intensity conditioning following FLAMSA for primary refractory or relapsed acute myeloid leukemia. *Ann. Hematol.* **2013**, *92*, 1389–1395. [CrossRef]
11. Pfrepper, C.; Klink, A.; Behre, G.; Schenk, T.; Franke, G.N.; Jentzsch, M.; Schwind, S.; Al-Ali, H.K.; Hochhaus, A.; Niederwieser, D.; et al. Risk factors for outcome in refractory acute myeloid leukemia patients treated with a combination of fludarabine, cytarabine, and amsacrine followed by a reduced-intensity conditioning and allogeneic stem cell transplantation. *J. Cancer Res. Clin. Oncol.* **2016**, *142*, 317–324. [CrossRef] [PubMed]
12. Ringdén, O.; Labopin, M.; Schmid, C.; Sadeghi, B.; Polge, E.; Tischer, J.; Ganser, A.; Michallet, M.; Kanz, L.; Schwerdtfeger, R.; et al. Sequential chemotherapy followed by reduced-intensity conditioning and allogeneic haematopoietic stem cell transplantation in adult patients with relapse or refractory acute myeloid leukaemia: A survey from the Acute Leukaemia Working Party of EBMT. *Br. J. Haematol.* **2017**, *176*, 431–439. [CrossRef] [PubMed]
13. Malard, F.; Labopin, M.; Stuhler, G.; Bittenbring, J.; Ganser, A.; Tischer, J.; Michallet, M.; Kröger, N.; Schmid, C.; Huynh, A.; et al. Sequential Intensified Conditioning Regimen Allogeneic Hematopoietic Stem Cell Transplantation in Adult Patients with Intermediate- or High-Risk Acute Myeloid Leukemia in Complete Remission: A Study from the Acute Leukemia Working Party of the European Group for Blood and Marrow Transplantation. *Biol. Blood Marrow Transplant.* **2017**, *23*, 278–284. [PubMed]
14. Heinicke, T.; Labopin, M.; Schmid, C.; Polge, E.; Socié, G.; Blaise, D.; Mufti, G.J.; Huynh, A.; Brecht, A.; LeDoux, M.-P.; et al. Reduced Relapse Incidence with FLAMSA–RIC Compared with Busulfan/Fludarabine for Acute Myelogenous Leukemia Patients in First or Second Complete Remission: A Study from the Acute Leukemia Working Party of the European Society for Blood and Marrow Transplantation. *Biol. Blood Marrow Transplant.* **2018**, *24*, 2224–2232. [PubMed]
15. Sheth, V.; Labopin, M.; Canaani, J.; Volin, L.; Brecht, A.; Ganser, A.; Mayer, J.; Labussière-Wallet, H.; Bittenbring, J.; Shouval, R.; et al. Comparison of FLAMSA-based reduced intensity conditioning with treosulfan/fludarabine conditioning for patients with acute myeloid leukemia: An ALWP/EBMT analysis. *Bone Marrow Transplant.* **2019**, *54*, 531–539. [CrossRef] [PubMed]
16. Saraceni, F.; Labopin, M.; Brecht, A.; Kröger, N.; Eder, M.; Tischer, J.; Labussière-Wallet, H.; Einsele, H.; Beelen, D.; Bunjes, D.; et al. Fludarabine-treosulfan compared to thiotepa-busulfan-fludarabine or FLAMSA as conditioning regimen for patients with primary refractory or relapsed acute myeloid leukemia: A study from the Acute Leukemia Working Party of the European Society for Blood and Marrow Transplantation (EBMT). *J. Hematol. Oncol.* **2019**, *12*, 44.
17. Moher, D.; Liberati, A.; Tetzlaff, J.; Altman, D.G. Preferred Reporting Items for Systematic Reviews and Meta-Analyses: The PRISMA Statement. *J. Clin. Epidemiol.* **2009**, *62*, 1006–1012. [CrossRef]
18. Mathes, T.; Kuss, O. A comparison of methods for meta-analysis of a small number of studies with binary outcomes. *Res. Synth. Methods* **2018**, *9*, 366–381. [CrossRef]
19. Higgins, J.P.T.; Thompson, S.G.; Deeks, J.J.; Altman, D.G. Measuring inconsistency in meta-analyses. *BMJ* **2003**, *327*, 557–560. [CrossRef]
20. Bhatt, V.R.; Chen, B.; Gyawali, B.; Lee, S.J. Socioeconomic and health system factors associated with lower utilization of hematopoietic cell transplantation in older patients with acute myeloid leukemia. *Bone Marrow Transplant.* **2018**, *53*, 1288–1294. [CrossRef]

21. De Lima, M.; Anagnostopoulos, A.; Munsell, M.; Shahjahan, M.; Ueno, N.; Ippoliti, C.; Andersson, B.S.; Gajewski, J.; Couriel, D.; Cortes, J.; et al. Nonablative versus reduced-intensity conditioning regimens in the treatment of acute myeloid leukemia and high-risk myelodysplastic syndrome: Dose is relevant for long-term disease control after allogeneic hematopoietic stem cell transplantation. *Blood* **2004**, *104*, 865–872. [CrossRef] [PubMed]
22. Scott, B.L.; Pasquini, M.C.; Logan, B.R.; Wu, J.; Devine, S.M.; Porter, D.L.; Maziarz, R.T.; Warlick, E.D.; Fernandez, H.F.; Alyea, E.P.; et al. Myeloablative Versus Reduced-Intensity Hematopoietic Cell Transplantation for Acute Myeloid Leukemia and Myelodysplastic Syndromes. *J. Clin. Oncol.* **2017**, *35*, 1154–1161. [CrossRef] [PubMed]
23. Bornhäuser, M.; Kienast, J.; Trenschel, R.; Burchert, A.; Hegenbart, U.; Stadler, M.; Baurmann, H.; Schäfer-Eckart, K.; Holler, E.; Kröger, N.; et al. Reduced-intensity conditioning versus standard conditioning before allogeneic haemopoietic cell transplantation in patients with acute myeloid leukaemia in first complete remission: A prospective, open-label randomised phase 3 trial. *Lancet Oncol.* **2012**, *13*, 1035–1044. [CrossRef]
24. Eapen, M.; Brazauskas, R.; Hemmer, M.; Perez, W.S.; Steinert, P.; Horowitz, M.M.; Deeg, H.J. Hematopoietic cell transplant for acute myeloid leukemia and myelodysplastic syndrome: Conditioning regimen intensity. *Blood Adv.* **2018**, *2*, 2095–2103. [CrossRef] [PubMed]
25. Wattad, M.; Amlsg, F.T.G.-A.; Weber, D.; Döhner, K.; Krauter, J.; Gaidzik, V.I.; Paschka, P.; Heuser, M.; Thol, F.; Kindler, T.; et al. Impact of salvage regimens on response and overall survival in acute myeloid leukemia with induction failure. *Leukemia* **2017**, *31*, 1306–1313. [CrossRef] [PubMed]
26. Goyal, S.D.; Zhang, M.J.; Wang, H.L.; Akpek, G.; Copelan, E.A.; Freytes, C.; Gale, R.P.; Hamadani, M.; Inamoto, Y.; Kamble, R.T.; et al. Allogeneic hematopoietic cell transplant for AML: No impact of pre-transplant extramedullary disease on outcome. *Bone Marrow Transplant.* **2015**, *50*, 1057–1062. [CrossRef] [PubMed]
27. Zhang, Z.-H.; Lian, X.-Y.; Yao, D.-M.; He, P.-F.; Ma, J.-C.; Xu, Z.-J.; Guo, H.; Zhang, W.; Lin, J.; Qian, J. Reduced intensity conditioning of allogeneic hematopoietic stem cell transplantation for myelodysplastic syndrome and acute myeloid leukemia in patients older than 50 years of age: A systematic review and meta-analysis. *J. Cancer Res. Clin. Oncol.* **2017**, *143*, 1853–1864. [CrossRef] [PubMed]

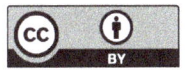

© 2019 by the authors. Licensee MDPI, Basel, Switzerland. This article is an open access article distributed under the terms and conditions of the Creative Commons Attribution (CC BY) license (http://creativecommons.org/licenses/by/4.0/).

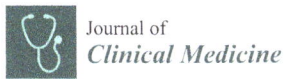

Review

Antibody Therapies for Acute Myeloid Leukemia: Unconjugated, Toxin-Conjugated, Radio-Conjugated and Multivalent Formats

Brent A. Williams [1,*], Arjun Law [2], Judit Hunyadkurti [3], Stephanie Desilets [4], Jeffrey V. Leyton [3,5,6] and Armand Keating [1]

[1] Cell Therapy Program, Princess Margaret Cancer Centre, Toronto, ON M5G 2C1, Canada
[2] Hans Messner Allogeneic Blood and Marrow Transplant Program, Princess Margaret Cancer Centre, Toronto, ON M5G 2C1, Canada
[3] Département de Medécine Nucléaire et Radiobiology, Faculté de Medécine et des Sciences de la Santé, Centre Hospitalier Universitaire de Sherbrooke (CHUS), Université de Sherbrooke, Sherbrooke, QC J1H 5N4, Canada
[4] Service de Hemato-Oncologie, CHUS, Sherbrooke, QC J1H 5N4, Canada
[5] Sherbrooke Molecular Imaging Centre, Centre de Recherche du CHUS, Sherbrooke, QC J1H 5N4, Canada
[6] Institute de Pharmacologie de Sherbrooke, Université de Sherbrooke, Sherbrooke, QC J1H 5N4, Canada
* Correspondence: brentwilliams.brent@gmail.com

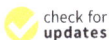

Received: 1 July 2019; Accepted: 16 August 2019; Published: 20 August 2019

Abstract: In recent decades, therapy for acute myeloid leukemia (AML) has remained relatively unchanged, with chemotherapy regimens primarily consisting of an induction regimen based on a daunorubicin and cytarabine backbone, followed by consolidation chemotherapy. Patients who are relapsed or refractory can be treated with allogeneic hematopoietic stem-cell transplantation with modest benefits to event-free and overall survival. Other modalities of immunotherapy include antibody therapies, which hold considerable promise and can be categorized into unconjugated classical antibodies, multivalent recombinant antibodies (bi-, tri- and quad-specific), toxin-conjugated antibodies and radio-conjugated antibodies. While unconjugated antibodies can facilitate Natural Killer (NK) cell antibody-dependent cell-mediated cytotoxicity (ADCC), bi- and tri-specific antibodies can engage either NK cells or T-cells to redirect cytotoxicity against AML targets in a highly efficient manner, similarly to classic ADCC. Finally, toxin-conjugated and radio-conjugated antibodies can increase the potency of antibody therapies. Several AML tumour-associated antigens are at the forefront of targeted therapy development, which include CD33, CD123, CD13, CLL-1 and CD38 and which may be present on both AML blasts and leukemic stem cells. This review focused on antibody therapies for AML, including pre-clinical studies of these agents and those that are either entering or have been tested in early phase clinical trials. Antibodies for checkpoint inhibition and microenvironment targeting in AML were excluded from this review.

Keywords: acute myeloid leukemia; AML; antibody; bi-specific antibody; therapy

1. Introduction

The discovery of a means to generate murine monoclonal antibodies by George Köhler and César Milstein garnered the 1984 Nobel Prize in Medicine and paved the way for a new class of therapeutics [1]. Monoclonal antibodies (mAbs) have transformed therapy for numerous diseases, including cancer. Rituximab (anti-CD20 chimeric antibody) was the first monoclonal antibody approved for use in cancer and tested experimentally in a clinical trial for lymphoma in 1998 [2]. The approach to the antibody therapy of cancer has developed rapidly, leading to several general therapeutic approaches: (1) unconjugated classical antibodies (e.g., rituximab/Rituxan), (2) toxin-conjugated antibodies (e.g., gemtuzumab ozogamicin (GO)/Mylotarg), (3) bi- and tri-specific recombinant antibodies (e.g., blinatumomab/Blincyto), and 4) radio-conjugated antibodies (e.g., ^{131}I-BC8/Iomab-B). Acute myeloid leukemia (AML) represents a challenging malignancy to treat, particularly in the situation of relapsed and refractory AML (R/R AML), and antibody therapeutics have not, in general, become a standard of care for most patients. In this review, we will discuss basic aspects of AML biology, which inform the strategies that have been used in developing targeted antibody therapies to complement, enhance or replace existing standards of care. We highlighted four major approaches to antibody therapy, emphasizing mechanisms of cytotoxicity and data from both pre-clinical and clinical studies of specific agents. We will not cover checkpoint inhibitors that facilitate T-cell anti-tumour responses (e.g., ipilimumab/Yervoy; anti-CTLA-4), or similar approaches to facilitate macrophage anti-tumour responses (i.e., Hu5F9-G4; anti-CD47), or antibodies not directed at cancer cells specifically, such as those that target stroma (BMS-936564/MDX1338/ulocuplumab; anti-CXCR4).

1.1. Current Standard of Care for AML

The core of most AML chemotherapy regimens consists of continuously infused cytarabine with anthracyclines such as daunorubicin [3]. The most frequently used regimen, referred to as "3 + 7", consists of continuous infusion of cytarabine at 100 mg/m^2 for seven days and rapid intravenous injection of daunorubicin on the first three days of the treatment cycle [4]. Another subsequent trial showed improved complete response (CR) rates, with 45 mg/m^2 of daunorubicin over lower doses, particularly in younger patients [5]. Dose intensification of cytarabine and daunorubicin at 45 or 90 mg/m^2 for 3 days was assessed in a large prospective trial showing that adverse events were similar in both arms and a significantly higher complete remission rate was achieved with higher dosing of daunorubicin (67.6% vs. 57.2%). However, in this study, OS was only significantly improved in patients with favorable or intermediate risk cytogenetics [6]. Further studies also confirmed the improved efficacy of high dose daunorubicin (90 mg/m^2), including subgroup analysis that showed superior outcomes in patients with mutations in *DNMT3A*, *NPM1*, and *MLL* [7–9]. The UK National Cancer Research Institute AML17 trial compared an intermediate 60 mg/m^2 dose to 90 mg/m^2 and found no differences in CR rate but a higher dose arm was associated with greater mortality at day 60 [10]. Current recommendations suggest that daunorubicin doses should be ≥60 mg/m^2 in all cases [11].

Several attempts have been made to improve upon the success of induction chemotherapy by adding other agents, but none have shown significant improvements in outcomes without increasing toxicity. The topoisomerase II inhibitor, etoposide, has single agent activity against AML and has been incorporated into induction or consolidation protocols depending on the risk category, age, and cardiac status of the patient [12]. However, there are no data to suggest that adding etoposide or 6-thioguanine to 3 + 7 improves outcomes [13,14]. More intense combination regimens, such as FLAG-Ida (Fludarabine, Cytarabine, Idarubicin, and Filgrastim), have higher rates of CR but are associated with increased toxicity, resulting in no improvement in overall survival [15,16].

A risk-adapted approach may be beneficial in certain situations. AML with *FLT3*-ITD mutations may benefit from the addition of targeted therapy with tyrosine kinase inhibitors (TKIs) like midostaurin [17]. Similarly, the addition of GO has improved outcomes in patients with favourable risk of AML with core binding factor mutations [18]. More recently, a specialized liposomal formulation containing cytarabine and daunorubicin (CPX-351/Vyxeos) was evaluated in patients with R/R-AML, and later, in patients with de novo high-risk or secondary AML, with improvements in survival in both settings [19–21]. This drug is now approved for use in therapy-related AML and AML with myelodysplasia-related changes [22,23].

Furthermore, patients unable to tolerate standard chemotherapy have benefited from venetoclax, an oral B-cell leukemia/lymphoma-2 (BCL-2) inhibitor with a 19% overall response rate and an additional 19% demonstrating partial anti-leukemic activity [24]. A subsequent phase 1b study of venetoclax in patients ≥65 years of age with treatment-naive AML ineligible for standard chemotherapy who received oral venetoclax in combination with the hypomethylating agents decitabine or azacytidine resulted in a 67% CR or Cri, maintained with a median duration of 11.3 months [25].

Virtually all patients who achieve CR relapse without post-remission therapy [26]. Consolidation chemotherapy with high-dose cytarabine (HiDAC) was found to be effective in preventing relapse in up to 44% of patients who did not receive allogeneic hematopoietic stem-cell transplantation (HSCT) [27]. While there are significant variations in doses between centers, a dose of 3 g/m^2 administered on days 1, 3, and 5 of each course was considered optimal [28]. Finally, it has been well established that allogeneic HSCT is the post-remission treatment of choice in eligible patients with intermediate or high-risk AML [29].

However, despite these therapies, five-year survival for AML patients was approximately 40% in adults [30] and 60% in children [31], with high-risk groups faring much worse (<10%) [32]. Survival outcomes remained particularly poor for patients over the age of 60 [33]. To improve outcomes, novel therapeutics are needed and antibody-based therapeutics have the potential to integrate with currently used standard-of-care regimens. However, selecting the right antibody-based treatment strategy in combination with complementary AML biological aspects, such as target antigens and leukemogenic stem cells, is key to providing patients with long-term leukemic-free survival.

1.2. AML Cell Surface Antigens

AML cells typically express antigens found on normal myeloid progenitor and differentiated cells, such as macrophages and monocytes, with aberrant expression of other lineage markers. AML expresses the pan-leukocyte marker CD45 and other myeloid markers such as CD11b, CD13 and CD33. A review of 106 adult AML cases was conducted to assess immunophenotypic variation based on the French-American-British (FAB) classification using a 22-antibody panel [34]. The most commonly expressed antigens were CD45 (97.2%), CD33 (95.3%), and CD13 (94.3%). Lymphoid-associated antigens were expressed in approximately half of cases, with the following descending order of frequency: CD20 (17%), CD7 (16%), CD19 (9.8%), CD2 (7.5%), CD3 (6.7%), CD5 (4.8%), and CD10 (2.9%). CD56, typically found on NK cells, can also be found on AML cells, but not on normal myeloid cells. CD56 expression in t(8;21) AML was associated with a higher rate of relapse [35]. These markers provide potential therapeutic targets to exploit.

1.3. Cancer Stem Cell Hypothesis and Optimal Antigen Targets in AML

Normal hematopoietic stem cells were first discovered by Till and McCulloch [36], which led them to explore the underlying process that determined cell fate decision to self-renew or differentiate based on stochastic or deterministic models. Ultimately, hematopoietic stem cells (HSCs) were identified as being enriched in the CD34 + CD38- fraction of bone marrow cells and cord blood [37] and capable of recapitulating an entire hematopoietic system in both animal and human models. The concept of a cancer stem cell in leukemia was proposed by Bruce et al. [38] and provided an alternative to the stochastic model to explain rare tumour-initiating cells. One additional feature of this theory was that cancer cells could differentiate along a hierarchy somewhat analogous to normal HSCs. Leukemia stem cells (LSCs) in AML were the first identified cancer stem-cell population, which were shown to be enriched in the CD34 + CD38- fraction of whole blasts, as measured by the ability to engraft in the bone marrow of immunodeficient mice [39,40]. Most subsequent studies of leukemic stem cells (LSCs) have focused on the CD34 + CD38- definition with or without addition of CD123 or CLL-1 [41–43], and these have informed the majority of therapeutic strategies to date that target LSCs. Other markers that are expressed on LSCs and have utility in further discriminating them from HSCs include CD7, CD32, CD45RA, CD96, CD99, CD157, CD244, IL-1 receptor accessory protein (IL-1RAP) [44], and T cell immunoglobulin mucin-3 (TIM-3), which are discussed briefly below. However, some of these antigens are expressed on normal tissues and might pose challenges to target therapeutically. CD7 and CD96 were both found on T and NK cells populations [45,46], CD32 on myeloid cells and B-cells [47], CD45RA on naïve T-cells [48], CD99 on all leukocytes [49], CD244 on NK and T cells [50], CD157 on all myeloid progenitors, neutrophils and macrophage [51], IL-1RAP on neutrophils, monocytes and lymphocytes [52] and TIM-3 on T, NK, macrophage and dendritic cells [53]. CD96 has been shown to be expressed on the majority of AML LSCs, with minimal expression on HSCs making it a potential target [54]. TIM-3 is expressed on LSCs in most types of AML, but is absent on HSCs and can be therapeutically targeted in AML xenograft models with TIM-3 specific antibodies [55]. CD157 has been shown to be present on 97% of primary AML blasts, with some expression on LSC sub-populations and a novel humanized antibody has been generated with in vitro activity in combination with NK cells [56]. CD244 has been implicated in maintaining and driving LSCs and represents an emerging target [57].

Finally, several lines of evidence support the clinical relevance of what is commonly referred to in the field as the leukemic stem cell (LSC) hypothesis: (1) a higher engraftment capacity in the bone marrow of murine recipients correlates with worse survival [58], (2) patients whose whole AML samples had a gene expression profile similar to LSCs or HSCs had worse survival and could risk stratify patients independent of known prognostic factors [59], and (3) patients with a high burden of CD34 + CD38- AML cells at diagnosis correlated with poor survival [41,42]. These findings support the notion that an optimal target would include a LSC population in the whole cell leukemic population. In this review, we focused primarily on LSC- and leukemic blast-associated cell-surface antigens for the various targeting strategies, as these are optimal targets for achieving curative therapy.

1.4. Optimal Targets in AML Therapy (CD33, CD123, CD13, CLL-1 and CD38)

CD33 is a 67 kDa immunoglobulin superfamily glycoprotein that is classified as a sialic acid-binding immunoglobulin-like lectin (Siglec) which has two immunoreceptor tyrosine-based inhibitor motifs (ITIMs). Phosphorylation events lead to distal activation of SHP1 and SHP2. CD33 appears on early myelomonocytic lineage-committed cells in normal hematopoiesis. It is expressed on 99% of AML blasts and LSCs.

CD123 is the interleukin (IL)-3 receptor alpha chain and is a type I transmembrane glycoprotein [60]. The beta chain (CDw131) for the IL-3 receptor is common to the IL-5 and granulocyte monocyte-colony stimulating factor (GM-CSF) receptors [61]. When CD123 is coupled to CDw131, the binding infinity for IL-3 increases dramatically, facilitating signal transduction from low concentrations of IL-3 [62]. IL-3 is important in driving myeloid differentiation and can activate STAT5. CD123 is present on ~99% of CD34 + CD38- LSCs [63] and on the majority of leukemic blasts. Importantly, CD123 is not highly expressed on normal hematopoietic stem cells [64], making it a potential therapeutic target. CD123 is expressed on committed hematopoietic progenitor cells and mediates differentiation and proliferation. CD123 is also expressed on cells of the hematopoietic system (monocytes, neutrophils, basophils, eosinophils, megakaryocytes and erythroid precursors, mast cells, macrophages, some B lymphocytes) and non-hematopoietic tissue (Leyding cells of the testis, placenta, and brain) [60].

CD13 is a zinc-dependent metalloprotease with enzymatic activity of N-terminal amino acid cleavage from peptides [65]. It is present on normal myeloid cells and is involved in several cellular functions, including adhesion, differentiation, proliferation, apoptosis, and phagocytosis, and is overexpressed on AML cells [66]. It is expressed on both blasts and LSCs. Antibodies which can bind to CD13 can not only facilitate ADCC, but also inhibit proliferation and trigger apoptosis of AML cells, but not against normal CD13-expressing blood cells [67].

C-type lectin-like receptor 1 (CLL-1) belongs to group V of the C-type lectin-like receptor family, which is calcium independent [68,69]. Based on the structure, C-type lectin and C-type-like lectin receptors are categorized into type I and type II receptor. CLL-1 is not expressed on HSCs, but is expressed on myeloid committed progenitors and on differentiated myeloid cells, such as peripheral blood monocytes, dendritic cells, and granulocytes [68]. However, it is expressed on LSCs [70], making it a potentially relevant target for antibody therapeutics.

CD38 is made up of a single chain of 300 amino acids with a molecular weight of 45 kDa and is expressed by hematopoietic and non-hematopoietic cells, including NK cells and monocytes (reviewed in [71]). Other CD38+ cells include smooth and striated muscle cells, renal tubules, retinal ganglion cells, and cornea (reviewed in [72]). CD38 is involved in lymphocyte signal transduction [73] and adhesion [74]. The binding of CD38 to the ligand CD31 (PECAM-1) initiates a signaling cascade that includes the phosphorylation of sequential intracellular targets and increases cytoplasmic Ca^{2+} levels, mediating different biological events, depending on the cell type (e.g., activation, proliferation, apoptosis, cytokine secretion and homing). While the absence of CD38 was used to establish classic LSC definitions [39], subsequent work demonstrated that LSCs can exist in the CD34+CD38+ compartment of a significant number of primary AML samples [75]. Interestingly, CD38, a well-studied target for multiple myeloma [76], has been less focused on as a target for AML. This target is of potential interest for AML, given that 75% of AML samples express CD38 and there are anti-CD38 mAbs approved for multiple myeloma with established safety profiles.

1.5. Additional Targets in AML (WT-1, CD15, CD25, CD30, CD45)

Several other AML target candidates that have greater limitations than the previously listed antigens have been studied and are briefly summarized here. WT1 is a zinc finger transcription factor and an oncogene in AML progression and detectable in the majority of AML samples [77], but is an intracellular protein not expressed on the cell surface. However, mutations can be detected by T-cells through the presentation of mutant peptides in the context of HLA class I. This antigen presentation has been exploited by a novel BiTE construct specific for CD3 and a WT1 epitope presented in the context of HLA-A*02:01 [78]. However, this approach is limited compared with targeting tumour-associated antigens (TAAs) and may be complicated by cross-reactivity with other antigens presented with this HLA subtype [79]. CD15 is another antigen expressed on AML cells, but is only expressed on AML blasts and not LSCs, and is also present on many normal myeloid cells, making it a suboptimal target. CD25 (IL-2R alpha chain), another target selected by some investigators, is present on blasts and LSCs, but is not as widely expressed as other AML antigens, and is present on other IL-2-dependent cell types such as regulatory T-cells (Tregs), which could lead to undesirable side-effects.

CD45 is a type 1 transmembrane glycoprotein present on all hematopoietic cells [80]. It has tyrosine phosphatase activity and is involved in signal transduction with several isoforms (E3_8, CD45RO, CD45RB, CD45 RABC) derived from alternative splicing [81,82]. While CD45 is not an ideal target, as it is expressed on all hematopoietic cells, it can be used for myeloablative conditioning prior to HSCT, which is covered in the section on radio-immunotherapy.

2. Unconjugated Antibody Therapies

Unconjugated antibody therapy relies on important structural regions, each of which have a specific function. The basic structure of a mAb involves two identical heavy chains each with variable regions (V_H) and two identical light chains each with variable regions (V_L). These are joined by disulphide bonds to create the classical antibody Y structure. The fragment crystallizable (Fc) portion has regions that allow for cells of the innate immune system to bind by Fcγ receptors (FcγRs) or for complement binding. The V_L and V_H contain the complementarity determining regions which provide mAbs with a high antigen binding affinity and specificity.

The major mechanism of action of many classical therapeutic mAbs is NK cell antibody-dependent cell-mediated cytotoxicity (ADCC), which involves exocytosis of granules containing perforin and granzymes onto target cells (Figure 1G) [83]. Following an encounter with another cell, an NK cell forms an immunological synapse (IS) [84]. If there are sufficient activation signals on the potential target cell and also a lack of inhibitory signals, a cytolytic response will be triggered. Antibody-coated targets may bind Fcγ receptor III (CD16) on NK cells and induce cytotoxicity, which can over-ride inhibitory signals. This requires cytoskeletal rearrangement and re-orientation of the granules to the IS, followed by fusion into the synapse, and subsequent contact of granule contents with the plasma membrane of the target cell. Granules contain perforin, which can create pores in the membranes of target cells following cytolytic effector degranulation [85,86]. Serine proteases termed granzymes are also contained within granules. Granzyme A was the first characterized family member in T cell granules [87,88]. Granzymes are facilitated entry by perforin, where they are able to initiate apoptosis by both caspase-dependent and independent pathways. Perforin is a 70-Kda protein that requires free calcium and neutral pH to optimally integrate into the target membrane. Granzyme B induces DNA damage through the activation of caspase activity and has been shown to partially process procaspase 3, which requires the release of other proapoptotic factors from the mitochondria to complete apoptosis [89]. By contrast, granzyme A is unable to activate caspases, but instead targets nuclear proteins directly to induce DNA single-stranded DNA breaks and fragmentation by a caspase-independent pathway [90].

Furthermore, antibodies may also bind to activating receptors on NK cells and engage FcγR on AML cells in the reverse position to classical ADCC, in a process termed reverse-ADCC (R-ADCC) (Figure 1J) first demonstrated by Saxena et al. [91]. R-ADDC can stimulate granule exocytosis with similar potency to ADCC at concentrations as low as 0.001 µg/mL by bridging an FcγR positive target with an NK cell [92]. Pre-treatment of NK cell lines with mAbs to the natural cytotoxicity receptors (NCRs), NKp30 and NKp44, can facilitate a several-fold enhancement of cytotoxicity against leukemia cell lines and primary AML blasts which express FcγRs [93]. Although no humanized anti-NKp30 antibody has been developed yet, this approach could be used to target FcγR-positive cancers, which includes approximately two thirds of the primary AML samples [94].

Antibodies can facilitate antibody-dependent phagocytosis (ADCP) by macrophage and neutrophils owing to their expression of all classes of FcγRs, in contrast to NK cells, which express only FcγRIIIA (CD16) (reviewed in [95]). Antibody-coated cancer cells may become engulfed by macrophages or neutrophils, leading to their destruction and also to antigen presentation that could result in an adaptive anti-tumour immune response. Elotuzumab (anti-SLAMF7) has been approved for treatment of multiple myeloma and has demonstrated ADCP as a mechanism [96] in addition to ADDC and NK-cell activation.

Antibodies can also mediate cytotoxicity against cancer cells by complement dependent cytotoxicity (CDC) via the classical pathway (reviewed in [97]). Briefly, CDC involves initial binding of C1 via its C1q subcomponent to two adjacent cell-bound antibodies, leading to the recruitment of other components (C4, C2) and ultimately forming a C3 and C5 convertase. This leads to another cascade involving components C5-C9 with the final formation of the membrane attack complex, which results in pore formation in the target cell, and ultimately, osmotic lysis.

2.1. CSL360/CSL362 (Talacotuzumab)

The murine anti-human CD123 mAb 7G3 has been modified into two versions: chimeric CSL360 and humanized CSL362 (talcotuzumab). CSL360 has the variable region of 7G3 and is fused with the backbone of a human IgG1 through genetic engineering. Unfortunately, in a phase I clinical trial of 40 relapsed and refractory AML patients, CSL360 was unable to provide therapeutic benefit in all but two cases [98]. As a consequence, CSL360 was not pursued for further clinical development. A second-generation version of this antibody, CSL362, was Fc optimized to bind CD16A on NK cells with better affinity, as well as affinity matured to better bind to CD123 by its variable region (Figure 1G). CSL362 was tested in a Phase 1 clinical trial of AML patients in first or second CR as consolidation therapy which, at interim report, had 25 patients and was generally well tolerated, with three severe adverse events reported and no deaths from toxicity [99]. Ten patients maintained a CR for greater than or equal to 6 months (median 34 weeks) and of six MRD-positive patients, three converted to MRD-negative. While a further Phase II study of talocotuzumab and decitabine for AML (NCT02472145) was completed by Janssen, this trial did not meet the endpoint criterion to justify the further development of CSL362. However, these clinical results indicate that targeting CD123 has some anti-leukemic effect, when the mAb is engineered to provide more potent ADCC activation.

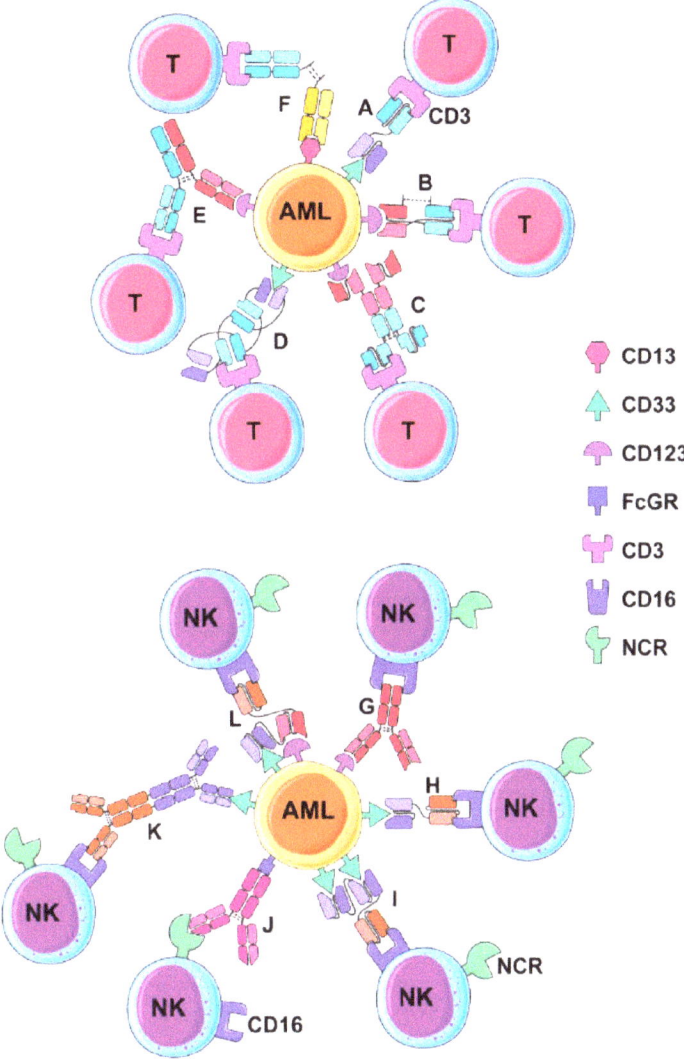

Figure 1. Antibody facilitated T and natural killer (NK) cell cytolysis of leukemia cells. T-cells and NK cells can be redirected to kill acute myeloid leukemia (AML) targets using a variety of antibody formats derived from the natively occurring IgG immunoglobulin molecule. Various approaches are diagrammed with key examples of each antibody format that has been developed. T-cell redirecting antibodies include (**A**) Bispecific tandem fragment variable format (BiTE, scBsTaFv), of which AMG 330 is an example (CD33 × CD3); (**B**) Dual Affinity Re-targeting Antibody (DART) (CD123 × CD3); (**C**) Bispecific single-chain Fv (scFv) immunofusion (Bif) (CD123 × CD3); (**D**) Bispecific tandem diabodies (TandAb) (AMV-564) (CD33 × CD3); (**E**) Duobody (CD123 × CD3); (**F**) Chemically conjugated Fab (CD3 × CD13). NK cell redirecting antibodies include (**G**) native IgG via antibody-dependent cell-mediated cytotoxicity (ADCC) (e.g., anti-CD123 mAb) CSL362); (**H**) Bi-specific Killer cell Engager (BiKE) (CD16 × CD33); (**I**) Tandem triple scfv (sctb); (CD33 × CD33 × CD16); (**J**) native IgG via reverse-ADCC; antibody directed against a natural cytotoxicity receptor (e.g., anti-NKp30); (**K**) Chemically conjugated antibodies (CD16 × CD33); (**L**) Tandem triple scfv (sctb); (CD33 × CD123 × CD16).

2.2. Lintuzimab and BI 835858

Lintuzumab (SGN-33, HuM195) is an unconjugated anti-CD33 mAb which has been tested in several clinical trials for AML (NCT00002609, NCT00002800, NCT00006084, NCT00016159, NCT00283114, NCT00502112, NCT00528333, and NCT00997243) in combination with standard induction chemotherapy and a maintenance monotherapy in R/R AML (reviewed in [100]). Both a phase 2b randomized trial [101] and a phase 3 randomized trial [102] of lintuzumab did not demonstrate survival benefit and the agent was not pursued further but has been applied for the delivery of radionuclides and described in a subsequent section. Another unconjugated anti-CD33 mAb, BI 836858, is Fc optimized through engineering, leading to improved NK cell-mediated ADCC relative to native antibody Fc [103]. Several clinical trials of BI 836,858 are currently underway for R/R AML (NCT02632721 NCT01690624) and AML relapsing post HSCT (NCT03207191).

2.3. Daratumumab (Darzalex), Isatuximab

Daratumumab is a fully human IgG1 kappa mAb that targets CD38 and was generated using the HuMAb platform with human antibody transgenic mice [104]. Daratumumab was originally evaluated in and approved for use in multiple myeloma (MM) in 2015 [105]. Daratumumab has been tested against primary AML targets in vitro, demonstrating apoptosis induction, ADCC and CDC as mechanisms of cytotoxicity, as well as being shown to reduce leukemic burden in the spleen and peripheral blood, but not in bone marrow in primary AML xenograft models [106]. Its mechanism of action includes (CDC), ADCC [107] and (ADCP). Investigators at MD Anderson Cancer Center are currently evaluating the efficacy of daratumumab as a stand-alone treatment for R/R AML (NCT 03067571), while Ohio State University is evaluating its effectiveness in combination with donor leukocyte infusions (DLI) for AML patients who have relapsed after allogeneic HSCT (NCT 03537599).

Another anti-CD38 antibody, isatuximab, has also been tested in MM, NHL, and CLL patients in a phase 1 trial [108] and a phase 3 trial in patients with MM, which showed improvement in progression-free survival. One advantage of isatuximab versus daratumumab is the need for less frequent dosing, though no head-to-head comparison of efficacy has been performed. A study of isatumximab recently opened a phase I/II trial for pediatric patients with R/R AML and ALL for use with combination chemotherapy (NCT 03860844).

3. Multivalent Antibody Therapies

Multivalent antibodies with, bi-, tri- and quadri-specific binding domains are engineered constructs which combine specificities of two or more antibodies into one molecular product that is designed to bind to both a TAA and an activating receptor on the effector cells, typically a T cell or natural-killer (NK) cell. There are several different structural variants of bispecific antibodies, which, in turn, can be utilized to target various combinations of effector and tumour targets antigens [109]. The first FDA-approved dual-binding antibody was blinatumomab, a bispecific T-cell engager (BiTE) developed by Amgen with specificities for CD3 and CD19 for treatment of acute lymphoblastic leukemia (ALL). BiTE format antibodies (tandem di-scFv) are engineered products involving combining the V_L and V_H domains of a monoclonal antibody into a single chain fragment variable (scFv) specific to an activating receptor (e.g., CD3) and further linked to the scFv of an antibody specific to a target antigen (e.g., CD19). The CD19 × CD3 BiTE was able to induce remissions in relapsed and refractory ALL that had failed other therapies [110,111] and was recently approved by the FDA for ALL patients with minimal residual disease (MRD) [112]. Because of the low molecular weight of blinatumomab, it is rapidly cleared by the kidneys and excreted through the urine, requiring administration by continuous infusion for up to several weeks [110]. Hence, for clinical use, there are challenges in cost and practical applications. Nonetheless, this technology is powerful, as it can be used as a general approach to redirect T-cells toward any antigen of interest. It can also be applied to engineered antibody fragments with different formats than the BiTE, such as DART and Duobody, also increasing valency, such as with tri-specific antibodies.

In general, most bi- and tri-specific engineered antibodies lack an Fc region and therefore, do not have the ability to mediate CDC and ADCC. Moreover, the engagement of NK cells to targets by bi- or tri-specific antibodies can result in immediate degranulation, owing to their preformed granules [113,114], whereas only a subset of primed T-cells can optimally be redirected to mediated cytotoxicity against against cancer-cell targets [115]. Only three bi-specific antibodies have been entered into clinical trials for AML, which are registered on ClinicalTrials.gov (Table 1) and are discussed in more detail with other bi-, tri- and quadri-specific formats in the pre-clinical stage of development.

Table 1. Clinical trials of bispecific antibody therapy for AML.

NCI Clinical Trial and Phase	Target	Agent(s)	Inclusion Criteria	Estimated Start and End Dates	Outcomes	Status
NCT02715011 Phase 1	CD123	JNJ-63709178 CD123 × CD3 Duobody	≥18 years of age with R/R AML	June 2016 October 2021	MTD, ORR, 1.5 year EFS and RFS	Suspended
NCT02520427 Phase 1	CD33	AMG330 CD33 × CD3 Tandem scFv (BiTE)	≥18 years of age with R/R AML	August 2015 January 2020	MTD and ORR duration at 3 years	Suspended
NCT02152956 Phase 1	CD123	MGD006 CD123 × CD3 DART flotetuzumab	≥18 years of age with R/R AML	May 2014 April 2020	MTD and OS at 2 years	Recruiting

AML: acute myeloid leukemia; R/R: relapsed/refractory; MTD: maximum tolerated dose; ORR: overall response rate (CR + CRi); OS: overall survival; RFS: relapse free survival.

3.1. Bispecific Tandem Fragment Variable Format (BiTE, scBsTaFv)

Given the success of blinatumomab for ALL, Amgen subsequently developed AMG 330, which is a CD33 × CD3 specific BiTE for treatment of AML (Figure 1A). The CD33 × CD3 BiTE can facilitate T-cell activation, expansion and in vitro lysis of primary AML cells [116,117]. Furthermore, AMG 330, in combination with infusions of activated human T cells, could suppress the growth of AML cells in a MOLM-13 cell line xenograft model, leading to improved survival [118]. Furthermore, AMG 330 could facilitate the cytotoxicity of both autologous and healthy donor allogenic T-cells against primary AML [119]. Recently, preliminary data for AMG330 was presented at the American Society for Hematology (ASH) meeting for patients with relapsed and refractory AML (NCT02520427) [120]. This was a phase 1 dose escalation study with 35 patients (enrolment to 40 in progress) to evaluate the safety, pharmacokinetics and tolerance. Four patients (10%) achieved a CR or a CR with incomplete blood count recovery treated with 120 or 240 ug/day. However, these CRs were not sustained beyond one cycle of treatment and the majority of patients discontinued treatment because of disease progression. Adverse events included cytokine release syndrome (CRS), febrile neutropenia, pneumonia, leukopenia, pyrexia, thrombocytopenia and subdural hematoma. Although this study established a tolerable dose, there was a low frequency of remission induction and short durations of remission in the four responders.

Another bispecific antibody format termed single-chain bispecific tandem fragment variable (scBsTaFv) provides an alternative to tandem scFv fragments in the BiTE format. This approach attaches the V_H of an anti-CD3 mAb to the V_L of an anti-CD33 mAb with the two tandem scFv joined by a glycine-serine linker. Further optimization of this format was resolved by rearranging the variable regions. A CD33 × CD3 scBsTaFv construct was able to facilitate the cytotoxicity of allogeneic mononuclear cells (PBMC) against CD33-expressing target cells [121]. This CD33 × CD3 scBsTaFv bispecific antibody was further humanized, reducing the probability of the patient mounting an immune response against the agent and was effective in picomolar concentrations, was independent of CD33 antigen density and did not redirect cytotoxicity to HSCs, as measured by a clonogenic assay [122]. An additional modification was to add 4-1BB ligand (4-1BBL), a co-stimulatory molecule which further enhanced T cell cytotoxicity against AML cells, against $CD33_{low}$ targets, relative to the parental construct [123].

3.2. Dual-Affinity Retargeting (DART)

Dual-affinity retargeting (DART) molecules are generated from a V_H and V_L taken from two distinct mAbs in a format distinct from BiTE to target two distinct antigens (Figure 1B). Specifically, a CD123 × CD3 DART was developed by Macrogenics (flotetuzumab), which can redirect T cells to target and kill AML cells, as well as stimulate T-cell proliferation [124]. The CD123 × CD3 DART was able to suppress leukemia progression in a CD123 + GFP + CBRLuc K562 murine xenograft model as measured by bioluminescence. The preliminary results of a phase 1 clinical trial of flotetuzumab demonstrated that it had anti-leukemic activity in 57% of a cohort of 45 patients with R/R AML/MDS (89% AML). Toxicity was reported and included infusion-related fever, chills, tachycardia, and hypotension, which were not severe. Importantly, the overall response rate (ORR) was 43%. Thus, the preliminary results are encouraging for DART as a potential effective targeted therapeutic for R/R AML.

3.3. Bispecific scFv Immunofusion or BIf

A novel and interesting bi-specific antibody format is the Bispecific scFv Immunofusion (BIf) with an scFv fused at the N-terminus of human IgG1 hinge region with a second scFv at the C-terminus (Figure 1C). The first described BIf was an CD123 × CD3 construct which would form pairs as a homodimer with a tumour target binding Kd of 1.0×10^{-10} molar which is superior to other bispecific antibody formats and can facilitate T-cell mediated cytotoxicity in vitro at low effector:target ratios [125]. Due to an intact Fc, it has a longer half-life than the lower molecular weight classical BiTE molecules and, hence, a longer therapeutic exposure to AML cells.

3.4. Bispecific Tandem Diabodies (TandAb)

Bispecific tandem diabodies (TandAb), also termed bispecific tetravalent antibodies, have a unique structure with two homologous immunoglobulin chains running counter to each other $(V_HA-V_LB-V_HB-V_LA)_2$ (Figure 1D) [126]. A CD30 × CD3 TandAb (AFM13) is being tested in clinical trials for cutaneous lymphoma (NCT 03192202—recruiting), R/R Hodgkin lymphoma (NCT 02321592 (recruiting and NCT 02665650—completed). A CD33 × CD3 TandAb has been generated (AMV-564) which, in the presence of T cells, can mediate dose-dependent cytotoxicity against primary AML targets from newly diagnosed and refractory or relapsed patients in vitro. AMV-564 had efficacy in treating a murine AML xenograft model [127]. A trial of AMV-564 has been initiated for R/R AML (NCT 03144245) and is sponsored by this platform's developer, Affimed Therapeutics Inc. (Heidelberg, Germany).

3.5. Chemically Conjugated Bispecific Antibodies

An early approach to dual target antigens was to chemically conjugate two different antibodies. A chemical conjugate of anti-CD16 and anti-CD33 monoclonal antibodies was developed which could redirect the cytotoxicity of NK cells toward AML blasts (Figure 1K) [128]. Another variant of this approach was to develop a bispecific $(Fab')_2$ fragment derived from two different antibodies [129,130]. Specifically, antibodies underwent cleavage and separation of $(Fab')_2$ fragments with dithiothreitol to create Fab'-SH fragments which could be recombined using a thiol-disulfide interchain reagent, ultimately producing a bispecific hybrid $F(ab')_2$. This approach was used to combine an anti-CD3 (OKT3) and anti-CD13 mAb (Figure 1F) [131]. These anti-CD3 and anti-CD13 Fab' fragments were mixed and reduced to form a bispecific $F(ab')_2$. This CD13 × CD3 Fab was able to enhance lysis of AML blasts by PMBCs. Also, this CD13 × CD3 antibody construct had some inhibition of AML colony-forming units (CFU), and had a lesser effect on granulocyte/macrophage CFU from normal bone marrow [131].

3.6. Bispecific Full-Length Antibodies (Duobody and Biclonics)

Genmab developed the DuoBody platform to develop bispecific human IgG1 antibodies. Two mAbs of different specificity, each containing single matched mutations in the third constant (C_H3) domain, were produced using mammalian recombinant cell lines and are then in a bispecific antibody. A CD123 × CD3 duobody was developed from an IgG4 backbone with a silenced Fc function and termed JNA-63709178 (Figure 1E) [132]. A phase 1 trial of a CD123 × CD3 Duobody (JNJ-63709178) sponsored by Janssen is in active recruitment of R/R AML patients (NCT 02715011). A full-length bispecific CLL-1 × CD3 antibody was developed by Merus using their proprietary Biclonics platform with preclinical activity demonstrated against AML [133], with an ongoing Phase 1/2 clinical trial ongoing for R/R AML in adults and newly diagnosed elderly patients with complex cytogenetics (NCT 03038230).

3.7. BiKEs and TriKEs

A CD33 × CD16 bispecific scfv was designed to activate NK cells and redirect them to lyse CD33+ AML targets and also secrete cytokines (IFNγ and TNFα) [134]. This construct is structurally similar to BiTE and was termed a bispecific killer-cell engager (BiKE) (Figure 1H). The observation that CD16 can be shed from NK cells by cleavage with ADAM17 limited this approach, but this was overcome with an ADAM17 inhibitor that could enhance NK cell cytotoxicity and cytokine secretion in the presence of the CD33 × CD16 BiKE. The BiKE platform was also functional using NK cells from patients with myelodysplastic syndrome, facilitating cytotoxicity against both AML targets and myeloid-derived suppressor cells [135].

Further modification of BiKEs was carried out to incorporate a third functional domain, specifically, to incorporate the IL-15 cytokine, and accordingly named a trispecific killer cell engager (TriKE) [136]. This approach facilitated additional expansion and activation capacity of NK cells, and when compared to the BiKE, yielded superior anti-leukemic results in mouse models of human AML. Three scFv components can be inserted to create a (scFv)$_3$ construct termed a single-chain Fv triplebody (sctb). One such construct linked two anti-CD33 scFv fragments to a single anti-CD16 scFv and was compared with a bispecific format (bsscFv) that consisted of only a single anti-CD33 scFv (Figure 1I). The CD33 × CD33 × CD16 sctb had a greater binding affinity for CD33 compared to the affinity obtained with the CD33 × CD16 bsscFv. More importantly, the sctb had increased by ≥2-logs the NK cell cytotoxic potency against AML cells relative to bsscFv [137]. Another approach using the triple scFv involves targeting two different antigens on a single target cell (Figure 1L). Using this approach, a CD33 × CD123 × CD16 was developed and shown to facilitate superior leukemic cell killing by NK cells relative to the dual targeting of the same antigen (CD123) [138]. A clinical trial of TriKE therapy is underway for patients with CD33 + R/R AML (NC T03214666).

4. Toxin-Conjugated Antibody Therapy for AML

Conceptually, the combination of highly potent anti-neoplastic agents and targeted antibodies in a single antibody-drug conjugate is not a recent development [139]. The principle of attaching a targeted antibody to a cytotoxic drug or radioactive isotope (referred to as 'payload' or 'warhead') through covalent linkage has led to a number of antibody-drug conjugates (ADCs) approved for use in the management of hematological malignancies. Although several warheads are being tested in cancer, the warheads that will be described have been used in AML.

Structurally, there are three components of equal importance in the design of an ADC, namely the mAb itself, the cytotoxic agent, and the conjugation linker [140]. The mAbs can be human, humanized, or chimeric, and may be engineered to target the antigen of choice with high specificity. For optimal drug delivery, the linker must bind with sufficient integrity to prevent premature de-conjugation, yet must release the drug once the antibody has bound to the target [141]. Linkers may be cleavable or non-cleavable. Typically, ADCs are reliant on efficient degradation in lysosomes to release the payload inside the target tumour cell [140]. Each approach is associated with its unique advantages and drawbacks and should be engineered with the target cell and the payload in mind. Finally, the drug itself must be sufficiently potent to ensure tumour killing with minimal off-target toxicity.

Calicheamicin is an anti-tumour antibiotic synthesized from *Micromonospora echinospora* that induces double-stranded DNA breaks, leading to cell death [142]. This is used in conjugation with antibodies targeting CD33 (gemtuzumab ozogamicin/Mylotarg) in AML, or CD22 (inotuzumab ozogamicin) in B-cell acute lymphoblastic leukemia (ALL). Monomethyl auristatin E (MMAE) is conjugated to an anti-CD30 antibody in brentuximab vedotin, an ADC that is FDA-approved for Hodgkin lymphoma [143]. Most recently, an investigational agent was developed using a pyrrolobenzodiazepine (PBD) dimer to induce DNA damage in tumour cells [144]. Vadastuximab talirine (SGN-CD33A) is a third generation ADC construct whereby an anti-CD33 antibody is conjugated to two molecules of a pyrrolobenzodiazepine (PBD) dimer via a maleimidocaproyl valine-alanine dipeptide connecting segment [145]. The PBD dimer is released after protease cleavage and induces DNA cross-linking, leading to target-cell apoptosis [146]. Several ADCs for AML have been tested in publish clinical trials and are discussed below, while other novel ADC trials for AML are ongoing.

4.1. Gemtuzumab Ozogamicin (GO)

The first clinically viable ADC to be approved in hematological malignancies was gemtuzumab ozogamicin (GO; Mylotarg), which targets CD33 [147]. In phase III studies of GO as monotherapy in patients over the age of 60 with relapsed AML, an overall response rate of 30% was reported. Based on these data, GO received accelerated FDA approval in 2000 [148]. However, a subsequent multicenter phase 3 randomized clinical trial comparing GO 6 mg/m^2 on day 4 of a daunorubicin and cytarabine induction chemotherapy protocol failed to demonstrate differences in survival. In fact, the patients receiving GO had a higher rate of mortality during induction due to Veno-Occlusive Disease (VOD) (5.5% death rate in the combination arm versus 1.4% in the chemotherapy alone arm) [149]. As a result, the drug was voluntarily withdrawn from the market in 2010. However, subsequent randomized trials evaluating lower doses of GO in combination with chemotherapy demonstrated improved overall survival without increased toxicities such as VOD. For example, The MRC AML15 trial combined GO at a dose of 3 mg/m^2 on day 1 of conventional induction chemotherapy in 1113 patients with previously untreated AML and reported a significant survival benefit without increased toxicity in younger patients with favorable cytogenetics, particularly core binding factor leukemias [150]. Another trial of a similar dosage regimen in older patients showed no difference in CR rates but significantly improved the three-year OS and relapse-free survival (RFS) with no appreciable increase in toxicity [151]. This demonstrated that lower doses of GO are effective in AML. As a result, GO was reapproved by the FDA for the treatment of newly-diagnosed CD33-positive acute myeloid leukemia (AML) in adults and for treatment of relapsed or refractory CD33-positive AML in adults and in pediatric patients 2 years and older.

4.2. Vadastuximab Talirine (SGN33A) and IMGN779

Other ADCs that target CD33 have been developed and are being actively investigated for AML therapy. Early in vitro experiments and animal studies showed that SGN33A was active even in multi-drug resistant and p53 mutated AML cell lines [152]. A phase 1 trial of SGN-CD33A in 27 older (median age 74 years) treatment naïve AML patients reported responses in 54%, with 14 patients achieving CR/CRi and five achieving a morphological leukemia-free state [153]. MRD negativity by flow cytometry was noted in six of 13 patients for whom data were available. VOD was not reported with this drug. Current trials are focused on evaluating SGN-CD33A in combination with standard induction chemotherapy. For example, a trial of SGN-CD33A in combination with decitabine or azacitidine in 24 patients with AML unfit or unwilling for conventional chemotherapy had a response rate (CR + CRi) of 73% amongst 49 evaluable patients [154]. In addition, 47% of the responding patients achieved MRD negativity by flow cytometry. Noteworthily, the combinations were well tolerated, with a 30-day mortality rate of 2%. Another CD33-directed antibody-drug conjugate IMGN779 in which the mAb is bound to a novel alkylating agent DGN462 was active in preclinical models [155] and a phase 1 clinical trial is currently underway in R/R AML (NCT 02674763).

4.3. Current Clinical Trials

There are many current clinical trials evaluating ADCs for AML which are registered on ClinicalTrials.gov (Table 2). GO is under investigation as a single agent for R/R AML in a phase 2 trial (NCT 03374332). Given that treatment of R/R AML is challenging and would not address its role in treating minimal residual disease (MRD), a phase 2 trial of GO is being examined after standard induction chemotherapy in patients achieving a CR who remain MRD + (NCT 03737955). Finally, another phase 1/2 study is aiming to evaluate the efficacy of GO in combination with chemotherapy in the up-front setting (NCT 03531918). Another CD33-directed antibody-drug conjugate IMGN779, in which the mAb is bound to a novel alkylating agent DGN462, was active in preclinical models [155], and a phase 1 clinical trial of this agent is currently underway in R/R AML (NCT 02674763). Other currently active clinical trials are examining the role of ADCs targeting CD30, CD123, CD71, and *FLT3* in patients with AML and other hematological malignancies expressing these antigens.

Table 2. Clinical trials of toxin-conjugated antibodies for AML.

NCI Clinical Trial and Phase	Target	Agent(s)	Inclusion Criteria	Estimated Start and End Dates	Status
NCT03374332 Phase 2	CD33	gemtuzmab ozogamicin	≥18 years of age with R/R AML	June 2019 March 2021	Not yet recruiting
NCT03737955 Phase 2	CD33	gemtuzmab ozogamicin	≥2 years of age with AML in CR with MRD after induction chemotherapy	November 2018 August 2021	Recruiting
NCT03531918 Phase 1/2	CD33	gemtuzmab ozogamicin in combination with GCLAM	≥18 years of age with untreated "high-grade" myeloid neoplasm (≥10% Blasts in blood or BM) or AML, exluding APL	September 2018 July 2025	Recruiting
NCT02674763 Phase 1	CD33	IMGN779	≥18 years of age with R/R AML	March 2016 December 2019	Recruiting
NCT03386513 Phase 1	CD123	IMGN632	≥18 years of age with R/R CD123 + AML and other CD123 + malignancies	January 2018 February 2021	Recruiting
NCT02864290 Phase 1	FLT3	ASP1235 (AGS62P1)	≥18 years of age with R/R AML	November 2016 January 2024	Recruiting
NCT03957915 Phase 1	CD71	INA03	≥18 years of age R/R AML, ALL, or MPAL with ≥ 20% CD71 positive blasts	September 2019 November 2021	Active, not recruiting
NCT01830777 Phase 1	CD30	Brentuximab vedotin in combination with Mitoxantrone, Etoposide, and Cytarabine	≥18 years of age with CD30 + relapsed AML	May 2013 December 2019	Active, not recruiting

NCI: National Cancer Institute; AML: Acute Myeloid Leukemia; R/R: Relapsed/Refractory; MRD: Measurable Residual Disease; BM: Bone Marrow; GCLAM: Granulocyte-Colony Stimulating Factor, Cladribine, Cytarabine and Mitoxantrone.

5. Radioimmunotherapy of AML

Radioimmunotherapy (RIT) for R/R AML is a scientifically sound approach that is translatable to clinical practice and can improve treatment outcome in patients. RIT utilizes mAbs labeled with radionuclides, providing continuous ionizing particle-based radiation exposure to cells expressing target antigens. RIT for AML has been investigated for the past three decades, demonstrating its ability to kill leukemic cells and deliver radiation specifically to sites harboring AML disease.

Although clinical testing is in place, important aspects such as target antigens on AML (or also on normal hematopoietic) cells and the properties of the payload radionuclides are still being optimized. Therefore, in this section, we put into context how RIT works and demonstrated the unique properties of select radionuclides and what has been learned from several clinical trials. Here, we identified clinical trials that are currently recruiting patients or are in preparation.

Due to exquisite affinity and specificity for target antigens preferentially expressed on diseased cells by mAbs and because radiolabeled mAbs have an increasingly well-understood pharmacokinetic profile, they target tumours with high target-to-nonspecific organ ratios [156]. Hence, radiolabeled mAbs are able to deliver ionizing radiation to disease sites more specifically than traditional total body irradiation (TBI). Ionizing radiation is then delivered with increased precision to AML cells and induces cell-death by two main mechanisms—apoptosis and necrosis—as a result of unrepaired DNA strand breaks [157]. Although RIT efficiency depends on many additional factors, this is beyond the scope of this summary and was reviewed in Desouky et al. [158].

A key RIT property is the type of radionuclide that is attached to the mAb. The nature of radiation emitted from radioisotopes that radioactively decay via α-particle or β-particle emission is different (Table 3). For example, the most relevant radionuclides for AML ^{225}Ac and ^{211}At decay by the emission of α-particles, whereas ^{131}I and ^{90}Y decay by the emission of β-particles. These radionuclides have different energies and another unique important property called linear energy transfer (LET). LET is the amount of energy that an ionizing particle transfers to material traversed per unit distance. Typically, α-particles have a range in tissue of 50–80 μm, which results in an LET of 50–230 keV/μm (Table 1). In contrast, β-particles have a considerably reduced LET of 0.1–1 keV/μm as they have a range of 0.5–12 mm in tissue. This signifies that α-particles provide an increased relative biological effectiveness (RBE) relative to β-particles. RBE is a measure of the extent of damage (e.g., DNA double strand breaks) to the cell an emitted particle produces. The RBE for α-particles is 3–7-fold increased relative to β-particles [159].

Table 3. Radionuclides used in active clinical trials for AML.

Radionuclide	T ½	Emission	Emax (keV)	Range (μm)
β-Emitting Radionuclides (LET = 0.1–1.0 keV/μm)				
Iodine-131	8.02 days	β and γ	610/362	2300
Yttrium-90	2.67 days	β	2250	11,300
α-Emitting Radionuclides (LET = 50–230 keV/μm)				
Astatine-211	7.2 h	α and X	5870 and 7450/ 77–92	80
Actinium-225	9.92 days	4α, 2β and γ	6000–8000/ 198–659/218–444	90
Bismuth-213	45.59 min	α and γ	8400/440	17

In general, ^{131}I and ^{90}Y have been employed in >95% of clinical RIT trials and represent the current standard to which all other radionuclides are compared [160]. Both isotopes have distinct favorable properties. ^{131}I emits a second ionizing particle, the γ-ray and can thus be utilized for both imaging and therapy. However, ^{131}I-mAbs degrades rapidly if the receptor internalizes upon mAb binding. This results in the release of ^{131}I-tyrosine in the bloodstream. In addition, the γ-rays emitted by ^{131}I increases the absorbed radiation dose to tissues and pose a risk to family members and healthcare professionals and, hence, require patient isolation. Both of these properties increase the absorbed radiation to healthy organs. Alternatively, ^{90}Y is an almost exclusive β-particle emitter (Table 3). Since the travel distance of β-particles is short compared to γ-rays and does not leave the patient's body,

^{90}Y is safer and more practical to work with for healthcare professionals. ^{90}Y also emits β-particles that are more energetic by 5-fold compared to the β-particles emitted by ^{131}I. In addition, if ^{90}Y-mAbs are internalized, the isotope is retained in the cell and is not released into the bloodstream. With either case, it is vital to have knowledge that the radionuclide targets tissue harboring the leukemic cells several fold higher than the liver, kidney, and lung—the dose limiting normal tissues. Since ^{90}Y cannot be imaged, dosimetry relies on utilizing another isotope labeled on the mAb, typically 111-indium (^{111}In).

A caveat for β-particle-based RIT is that the emitted β-particles often overshoot single AML cells and ablate surrounding normal hematopoietic cells residing in the bone marrow [161] (Figure 2A,B). This often results in dose-limiting toxicity (DLT) to the bone marrow, as normal hematopoietic cells are also highly sensitive to irradiation [162]. In contrast, the short range of emitted α-particles in theory makes them ideal for eradicating individual leukemic cells (Figure 2A,C). However, the energy of α-particles is several-fold higher than β-particles and thus, can also cause unwanted toxicities.

Although this is not a focus in this brief summary, short-ranged and high LET Auger electrons may provide an approach to eradicate AML cells. Recent preclinical studies have shown that the Auger-emitter ^{111}In labeled to mAbs targeting CD33 and CD123 and conjugated to short peptides harboring a nuclear localization signal sequence could kill AML cell lines and primary AML cell engrafted into mice. In addition, single-photon emission computed tomography (SPECT) imaging could be used as a companion to evaluate the targeting of AML cells in the bone marrow and extramedullary sites in these preclinical models to the γ-ray emissions by ^{111}In [163–166].

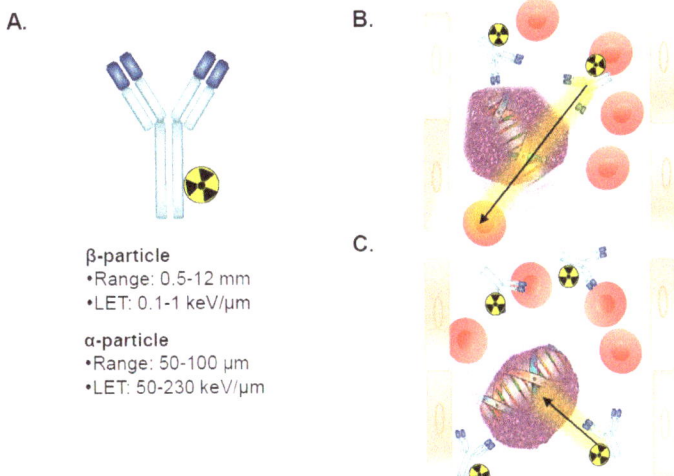

Figure 2. Radioimmunotherapy for acute myeloid leukemia. Illustration of (**A**) a mAb radiolabeled with either a (**B**) β-particle or (**C**) α-particle-emitting radionuclide and the track of the particles perfusing the bone marrow to target AML cells. Note that the path length of β-particles is greater than for α-particles leading to β-particle-based RIT used primarily in preparative regimens to myeloablate the bone marrow prior to hematopoietic cell transplantation.

5.1. β-Particle RIT for AML

Because of the properties of β-particles and the need to overcome the limitation of normal organ tolerance with current preparative regimens HSCT, The Fred Hutchinson Cancer Research Center (FHCRC) made an important breakthrough for developing an effective niche for RIT utilization. As detailed in a review by Gyurkocza and Sandmaier, successful HCT relies on the effectiveness of the preparative or conditioning regimen administered to patients prior to transplantation [167]. The goals of the regimen are to provide sufficient immunoablation to prevent the graft rejection of the donor cells and to reduce the leukemic burden [167].

In general, myeloablative regimens consist of alkylating agents with or without TBI that ablate marrow hematopoiesis to the point where autologous hematologic recovery does not occur. The greater part of regimens combines 12- to 16-Gy TBI, typically fractionated, with chemotherapy, and includes cyclophosphamide, cytarabine, etoposide, melphelan, and busulphan [167]. These chemotherapeutic agents have shown the ability to simultaneously exert cytotoxic and cytostatic effects on leukemic cells and to suppress the patient's own immune system to reduce graft rejection. While increased doses of TBI reduce the risk of AML relapse, this also increases treatment-related mortality (TRM), often due to toxicity in the gastrointestinal system, the liver, and the lungs. Hence, HSCT is not an option for many older and medically infirm patients. In addition, TBI-induced malignancies and development impairment in children are significant concerns.

As an alternative, non-myeloablative regimens have been developed for patients with AML that provide more favorable toxicity profiles yet are sufficiently immunosuppressive. There is a considerable range in intensity of these regimens. However, the approach developed at FHCRC is relevant since most RIT trials have occurred there. In particular, in older patients, conventional conditioning regimens prior to HCT often leads to a high TRM [168]. A low-dose 2-Gy TBI-based preparative regimen is administered to patients at FHCRC with the addition of 90 mg/m^2 of fludarabine to prevent graft rejection and increase pre-transplantation host T-cell immunosuppression [169]. Cyclosporine and mycophenolate mofetil is also administered to increase immunosuppression.

Although high-intensity TBI doses reduce relapse rates, this is offset by increased conditioning regimen-related death [170,171]. Conversely, reducing the TBI allows for increased utilization of HCT for patients with AML, however AML relapse rates increase [172,173]. Hence, there is a dilemma to find an ideal regimen that allows for low toxicity yet potent myeloablation/myelosuppression before transplantation that improves patient survival. Thus, targeted radiation is an alternative.

The mAb BC8 is specific for CD45 and radiolabeled with ^{131}I was developed as means to myeloablate since the antigen is expressed on the surface of almost all hematopoietic cells, except mature red blood cells and platelets and is also present on AML blasts [174]. CD45 is an attractive target because it is expressed by most AML samples at relatively high levels (~200,000 receptors per cell), and the antigen does not internalize, which is important for ^{131}I. Because CD45 is expressed on both normal and leukemic cells, it can be used to target the bone marrow. The strategy is to reduce the radiation dose and, hence, the overall toxicity to the patient by delivering radiation specifically to sites harboring leukemia cells.

An early clinical trial evaluating RIT for AML combined escalating doses of radiation delivered by the ^{131}I-BC8 with cyclophosphamide and 12-Gy TBI in patients with advanced AML [175]. Patients received a "tracer" infusion of the radiolabeled mAb weeks before HCT to allow for the mAb to penetrate the hematopoietic tissues harboring the leukemic cells and for sufficient washout from the blood and normal organs. At ~72 h post-injection, patients were imaged with a focus on region-of-interests such as the bone marrow (acetabulum and sacrum), spleen, liver, lungs, kidneys, and spleen. The study showed that 84% of patients contained radiation in the bone marrow and spleen 2.3- and 4.8-fold higher than the liver, the normal organ receiving the highest dose due to normal mAb metabolism. The ratios of radiation delivered to the bone marrow and spleen relative to the lung and kidneys were even greater than the liver. More importantly, this procedure could be safely performed with a conventional HCT preparative regimen.

The effectiveness of targeting radiation to specific hematopoietic/AML sites was then expanded to patients with AML in a first remission with a human leukocyte antigens (HLA)-identical family donor [176]. In addition to ^{131}I-BC8, patients underwent a preparative regimen consisting of busulfan and cyclophosphamide without TBI. The three-year survival among the patients in this study was 63% and the TRM was 21%. In patients with unfavorable cytogenetics, the percentages of survival and TRM were 26% and 27%, respectively. This study demonstrated that ^{131}I-BC8 could be used to intensify the amount of radiation delivered to leukemic cells to a greater extent than that delivered to normal organs, which provided increased survival benefit without excessive TRM. As a result, the effectiveness of ^{131}I-BC8 is now being evaluated to validate its use for AML as part of preparative conditioning prior to HSCT. Distinct evaluations are currently active, such as testing ^{131}I-BC8 in combination with fludarabine and 2-Gy TBI for allogeneic HCT, specifically in patients ≥50 years old (NCT 00008177). This trial reported outcomes in 58 patients with R/R-AML or myelodysplastic syndrome (MDS) [177]. Treatment resulted in the MTD of ^{131}I-BC8 delivered to the liver was 24-Gy. At day 28 post-transplantation, all the patients had a complete remission and donor-cell engraftment. Seven patients ultimately succumbed to TRM by day 100. The one-year survival estimate was 41%. Another phase 1 trial is evaluating ^{131}I-BC8 with fludarabine and 2-Gy TBI in 15 R/R-AML patients that were ≥16–50 years of age (NCT 00119366) [178]. This study capped the maximum dose delivered to the liver at 43-Gy as was carried out in the trial with older AML patients out of concern for causing stromal damage and marrow failure. In these younger patients, no cases of DLTs or TRM were observed. At ~12 months since treatment, 11 of the 15 patients survived and at five years, there were six surviving patients. This study suggested that increased doses from ^{131}I-BC8 are tolerable and provide even more survival benefit to younger adults with R/R AML. The results from these completed and active trials show the feasibility of using ^{131}I-BC8 to enhance the efficacy of allogeneic HCT in both young and older patients in a reduced conditioning setting.

One area in need of progress to extend RIT is for patients who do not have closely HLA-matched allogeneic donors and instead are reliant on haploidentical donor engraftment, especially patients from ethnic minority groups. Orozco et al. demonstrated that ^{90}Y-anti-CD45 RIT and cyclophosphamide without TBI or fludarabine before haploidentical HCT resulted in a high rate of engraftment, which remained stable for six months after transplantation in a murine mouse model [179]. An ongoing phase 2 trial is evaluating the use of ^{131}I-BC8 in R/R AML patients receiving haploidentical donor HCT (NCT00589316). Thus far, six of eight patients have been reported to achieve complete remission by day 28 post-HSCT and all patient had 100% donor chimerism [180].

As previously described, a significant barrier to expanding ^{131}I-BC8 as a mainstream approach to treat patients with AML is that many Nuclear Medicine Departments have difficulty properly handling large quantities of ^{131}I. Thus, a phase 1 study was undertaken to establish the safety, feasibility and optimized dose of ^{90}Y-BC8 in patients undergoing reduced-intensity regimen before allogeneic HCT (NCT01300572). Favorable outcome measures were reported with ^{90}Y-BC8 for multiple myeloma and lymphoma [181,182]. A previous Phase 1 clinical trial studying ^{90}Y conjugated to rat mAb YAML568 that recognizes CD45 was evaluated in eight patients [183]. No significant administration-related side effects were observed. However, in order for ^{90}Y-YAML568 to deliver preferentially increased radiation doses to the bone marrow and spleen, the patients were required to be preloaded with cold antibody. This indicates that patients may have produced an anti-YAML immune response that causes clearance of the mAb. Patient outcome was not reported.

^{90}Y has also been conjugated to the mAb lintuzumab that targets CD33. CD33 is exclusively expressed on myeloid cells and lymphocytes and not on all hematopoietic cells, such as CD45. Importantly, as CD33 is frequently expressed on AML cells it is an attractive target for RIT. Lintuzumab is a humanized mAb and binds CD33 with a very high affinity, as previously discussed. Two completed trials (NCT 00002890 and NCT 00006040) have investigated the MTD of ^{90}Y-BC8 in patients with R/R AML with and without HCT, respectively. No findings have yet been published.

5.2. α-Particle RIT for AML

The relative increased energy of α-particles, relative to β-particles, coupled with a range of only a few cell diameters and high LET in theory makes this RIT approach ideal for the treatment of small-volume disease or MRD. Hence, there has been high clinical activity to test α-particle-based RIT in AML. A Phase 1 study from the 1990s evaluating ^{213}Bi-lintuzumab administered at escalating doses in patients with R/R AML revealed that the absorbed dose was preferential to the bone marrow and spleen and was calculated to be 1000-fold higher than for β-particle-emitting radionuclides [184,185]. A subsequent phase I/II trial of ^{213}Bi-lintuzumab produced remissions in patients after partial leukemic cell reductions were achieved due to patients receiving cytarabine (NCT 00014495). The MTD of ^{213}Bi-lintuzumab in combination with cytarabine was 37 MBq/kg. Partial or complete remissions were observed in 34% of patients. However, no responses were achieved for patients receiving reduced doses of ^{213}Bi-lintuzumab. These studies provided proof-of-concept for α-particle RIT, however the 45.6 min half-life of ^{213}Bi and the requirement of an on-site generator makes its application challenging.

A phase 1 trial of ^{225}Ac-lintuzumab was evaluated in 18 patients with R/R AML (NCT 00672165). Patients tolerated doses of ^{225}Ac-lintuzumab up to 111 kBq/kg and peripheral AML blasts were eliminated in 63% of patients at doses starting at 37 kBq/kg. Importantly, extramedullary toxicities were limited to transient grade-3 liver-function abnormalities in three patients. No evidence of radiation-induced nephrotoxicity was observed [186]. ^{225}Ac-lintuzumab was then tested in 40 older patients. Objective responses were observed in nine and six patients receiving doses of 2.0 µCi/kg and 1.5 µCi/kg, respectively. Although myelosuppression was observed in all patients, the study has thus far concluded that fractionated-dosing of ^{225}Ac-lintuzumab can be combined safely with cytarabine and has antileukemic activity [187].

5.3. Ongoing Clinical Trials of RIT in AML

A number of ongoing clinical trials of RIT for AML are at various stages (Table 4). The SIERRA trial (NCT 02665065) is the first randomized Phase III study comparing a conventional myeloablative conditioning regimen plus allogeneic HCT versus ^{131}I-BC8 plus HCT. The trial was specifically designed to enroll an estimated 150 patients >55 years old with R/R AML. Because the SIERRA trial is randomized, if patients in the conventional treatment arm do not respond to conventional treatment, the trial allows for crossover for patients to receive ^{131}I-BC8 as well. Findings from the first 25% ($n = 38$) of patients enrolled demonstrated the feasibility of the trial. [181] At randomization, the median ranges for bone marrow blasts in the investigational and control arms were 30% (range, 4–74%) and 26% (range, 6–97%). Eighteen of 19 patients treated with ^{131}I-BC8 successfully engrafted with a median of 13 days (range, 9–22). Fifteen patients (79%) receiving conventional therapy did not achieve complete remission, and of these, 10 crossed over to receive ^{131}I-BC8 and were able to undergo HSCT. Thus far, hematologic and nonhematologic toxicities have been similar between arms. However, NRM was observed in patients who were randomized to the ^{131}I-BC8 arm. Further updates are planned for 50% and 75% of enrolled patients.

For α-particle RIT, a multicenter phase 1/2 trial (NCT 03867682) is in the planning stages to recruit patients ≥18 years of age with R/R AML. The trial will determine the MTD and the overall response of ^{225}Ac-lintuzumab when combined with the drugs venetoclax. Recently, the B-cell lymphoma 2 (BCL-2) protein was demonstrated to play a central role in the survival of AML cells [188]. Venetoclax, an inhibitor of BCL-2, has recently been demonstrated in a Phase Ib dose-escalation study in ≥65 years of age with naive AML and ineligible for conventional treatment had favorable outcomes [189]. In November 2018, the U.S. Food and Drug Administration granted an accelerated approval to venetoclax for use in newly diagnosed AML who are 75 years or older or who have comorbidities that preclude use of intensive chemotherapy.

A Phase 1 trial (NCT 03441048) is currently recruiting patients ≥18 years of age with naive/secondary and R/R-AML to evaluate the therapeutic effectiveness of ^{225}Ac-lintuzumab when combined with cladribine, cytarabine, granulocyte colony stimulating factor, and mitoxantrone (CLAG-M). Because CLAG-M has been shown to have impressive anti-leukemic activity and acceptable toxicity in young and older patients with R/R AML, it is rapidly becoming a valuable addition to chemotherapeutic options available to patients [190,191]. The primary outcomes will be to determine the MTD and the toxicities from the therapeutic combination.

Table 4. Clinical trials of RIT for AML.

NCI Clinical Trial and Phase	Target	Agent(s)	Inclusion Criteria	Estimated Start and End Dates	Outcomes	Status
NCT02665065 (SIERRA) Phase 3	CD45	^{131}I-BC8 Fludarabine 2-Gy TBI	≥55 years of age with R/R AML patients	June 2015 June 2020	Durable CR and OS at 1 year	Recruiting
NCT03867682 Phase 1/2	CD33	^{225}Ac-lintuzumab Venetoclax Spironolactone	≥18 years of age with refractory R/R AML.	May 2019 November 2022	MTD and complete and partial remission status at 6, 12, and 24 months	Not yet recruiting
NCT03670966 Phase 1/2	CD45	^{211}At-BC8 Fludarabine Cyclophosphamide 2-Gy TBI Haplotype transplant	≥18 years of age with R/RAML who have an available haploindentical donor for a haplo HSCT.	March 2019 September 2024	Toxicity (GVHD, and NRM), donor chimerism, rate of engraftment, and OS up to 100 days and maintenance of remission at 2 years	Recruiting
NCT03128034 Phase 1/2	CD45	^{211}At-BC8 Fludarabine 2-3-Gy TBI Haplotype transplant	≥18 years of age with R/R AML who have an available haploindentical donor for a haplo HSCT.	October 2017 March 2023	Toxicity (GVHD, and NRM), donor chimerism, rate of engraftment, and OS up to 100, remission at 2 years	Recruiting
NCT03441048 Phase 1	CD45	^{211}At-BC8 CLAG-M (cladribine, cytarabine, G-CSF, mitoxantrone)	≥18 years of age with R/R AML	May 2018 October 2020	MTD and toxicity	Recruiting

AML: acute myeloid leukemia; R/R: relapsed/refractory; MTD: maximum tolerated dose; OS: overall survival; GVHD: graft versus host disease; NRM: non-relapse mortality.

FHCRC is currently recruiting patients with advanced or R/R AML who can receive ^{211}At-BC8 combined with fludarabine and 2–3-Gy TBI as a preparative regimen for HLA-matched (NCT 03128034) or related haplo-identical (NCT 03670966) allogeneic HCT. Thirty participants are estimated for recruitment in each trial. The objectives will be to determine the MTD of ^{211}At-BC8 and AML response.

5.4. Future of RIT for AML

Future optimization of RIT will require better quantitative methods to estimate the dose of radiation absorbed in critical tissues which will allow for individualizing patient treatment and further reducing toxicity. This concept has matured in recent years and is widely known as "theranostics". As previously described, AML patients treated with ^{131}I-BC8 were first imaged to visualize the distribution and estimate the absorbed radiation dose in various organs in humans. These patients were administered the same reagent, which served as both a diagnostic and therapeutic purpose. Currently, dose-escalation with radiolabeled mAbs determines the MTD based on several toxicity parameters. Despite being in the era of precision medicine, which RIT conforms with, current protocols still implement a "one-dose-fits-all" approach. As the distribution of radiolabeled mAbs is variable among patients with AML, it is vital that the accuracy for individualized organ doses be improved by being able to monitor and adjust dosages [192]. The development of more precise and streamlined methods for individualized patient dosimetric determination will increase the effectiveness of RIT for R/R AML.

It is important to note that radiolabeled mAbs undergo extensive preclinical development prior to clinical testing—a drug maturation process the National Cancer Institute (NCI) supports [193]. Kunos and colleagues [193] recently summarized the launch of the NCI Cancer Therapy Evaluation Program, which has determined that radioactive drugs are an important strategic experimental therapeutic approach for AML for patients with R/R AML. The NCI is developing organizational plans for scientific review, oversight, medical monitoring, and further infrastructure elements essential for full radioactive drug development. Commercial partners, such as Actinium Pharmaceuticals, Inc., also realize the commercialization impact with radiolabeled antibodies and further benefit the development of these agents by providing funding for clinical trials. With governmental and industrial support and with the radiolabeled mAbs ^{131}I-BC8, ^{225}Ac-lintuzumab, and ^{211}At-BC8 currently being tested in clinical trials, RIT is on the cusp of becoming a realistic alternative for patients with R/R AML. Certainly, there is a need for further development and optimization, such as broader availability of α-emitters and delivering appropriate radiation dose to circumvent radioresistance while sparing radiosensitive tissues. Thus, we eagerly await the outcome of the active and recruiting trials to provide guidance on future directions for more effective clinical implementation.

6. Conclusions

In this study, we outlined the four major approaches to treat AML with antibody therapeutics. The initial development of unconjugated antibody therapy was not successful for AML possibly owing to limitations of patients' innate immune systems to be activated by ADCC.

However, the subsequent development of Mylotarg demonstrated that antibody potency could be enhanced by conjugation to a toxin and impact clinical outcomes in subsets of patients. Another similar approach would be to add a radiolabeled molecule capable of emitting alpha or beta particles to enhance antibody potency. As more infrastructure and support for RIT becomes widespread, this modality will provide patients with relapsed or refractory AML with additional options. Finally, molecular recombination techniques have allowed numerous antibody format variations with the possibly of multivalency increasing the binding affinity, specificity or activation properties over native antibodies. It is also conceivable that some or all of the four major pathways of antibody therapeutics be combined to take advantage of the higher binding affinity that dual targeting mAbs possess and co-label them with toxins or potent radioisotopes. Furthermore, a combination of novel antibody formats with adoptive cell therapy approaches such as CAR-T cells and NK cells presents an attractive means to develop a multimodal therapy with the potential for better therapeutic efficacy.

Author Contributions: B.A.W. designed the review outline, wrote the sections on unconjugated antibody therapy and multivalent antibody therapy, developed and edited figures, wrote the conclusion and reviewed and edited the entire manuscript. A.L. wrote the sections on AML standard of care and toxin-conjugated antibody therapy, and reviewed the entire manuscript. J.H. wrote and contributed to the section on radioimmunotherapy. S.D. wrote and contributed to the section on radioimmunotherapy and developed and edited figures. J.V.L. wrote and contributed to the section on radioimmunotherapy and reviewed and edited the entire manuscript. A.K. contributed to review outline, figure development and reviewed and edited the entire manuscript.

Conflicts of Interest: The authors declare no conflict of interest.

References

1. Kohler, G.; Milstein, C. Continuous cultures of fused cells secreting antibody of predefined specificity. *Nature* **1975**, *256*, 495–497. [CrossRef] [PubMed]
2. McLaughlin, P.; Grillo-López, A.J.; Link, B.K.; Levy, R.; Czuczman, M.S.; Williams, M.E.; Heyman, M.R.; Bence-Bruckler, I.; White, C.A.; Cabanillas, F.; et al. Rituximab chimeric anti-CD20 monoclonal antibody therapy for relapsed indolent lymphoma: Half of patients respond to a four-dose treatment program. *J. Clin. Oncol.* **1998**, *16*, 2825–2833. [CrossRef] [PubMed]
3. Yates, J.W. Cytosine arabinoside (NSC-63878) and daunorubicin (NSC-83142) therapy in acute nonlymphocytic leukemia. *Cancer Chemother. Rep.* **1973**, *57*, 485–488. [PubMed]
4. Rai, K.R.; Holland, J.F.; Glidewell, O.J.; Weinberg, V.; Brunner, K.; Obrecht, J.P.; Preisler, H.D.; Nawabi, I.W.; Prager, D.; Carey, R.W.; et al. Treatment of acute myelocytic leukemia: A study by cancer and leukemia group B. *Blood* **1981**, *58*, 1203–1212. [PubMed]
5. Yates, J.; Glidewell, O.; Wiernik, P.; Cooper, M.R.; Steinberg, D.; Dosik, H.; Levy, R.; Hoagland, C.; Henry, P.; Gottlieb, A.; et al. Cytosine arabinoside with daunorubicin or adriamycin for therapy of acute myelocytic leukemia: A CALGB study. *Blood* **1982**, *60*, 454–462. [PubMed]
6. Fernandez, H.F.; Sun, Z.; Yao, X.; Litzow, M.R.; Luger, S.M.; Paietta, E.M.; Racevskis, J.; Dewald, G.W.; Ketterling, R.P.; Bennett, J.M.; et al. Anthracycline dose intensification in acute myeloid leukemia. *N. Engl. J. Med.* **2009**, *361*, 1249–1259. [CrossRef] [PubMed]

7. Löwenberg, B.; Ossenkoppele, G.J.; van Putten, W.; Schouten, H.C.; Graux, C.; Ferrant, A.; Sonneveld, P.; Maertens, J.; Jongen-Lavrencic, M.; von Lilienfeld-Toal, M.; et al. High-dose daunorubicin in older patients with acute myeloid leukemia. *N. Engl. J. Med.* **2009**, *361*, 1235–1248.
8. Lee, J.H.; Joo, Y.D.; Kim, H.; Bae, S.H.; Kim, M.K.; Zang, D.Y.; Lee, J.L.; Lee, G.W.; Lee, J.H.; Park, J.H.; et al. A randomized trial comparing standard versus high-dose daunorubicin induction in patients with acute myeloid leukemia. *Blood* **2011**, *118*, 3832–3841. [CrossRef] [PubMed]
9. Patel, J.P.; Gönen, M.; Figueroa, M.E.; Fernandez, H.; Sun, Z.; Racevskis, J.; Van Vlierberghe, P.; Dolgalev, I.; Thomas, S.; Aminova, O.; et al. Prognostic relevance of integrated genetic profiling in acute myeloid leukemia. *N. Engl. J. Med.* **2012**, *366*, 1079–1089. [CrossRef] [PubMed]
10. Burnett, A.K.; Russell, N.H.; Hills, R.K.; Kell, J.; Cavenagh, J.; Kjeldsen, L.; McMullin, M.F.; Cahalin, P.; Dennis, M.; Friis, L.; et al. A randomized comparison of daunorubicin 90 mg/m2 vs. 60 mg/m2 in AML induction: Results from the UK NCRI AML17 trial in 1206 patients. *Blood* **2015**, *125*, 3878–3885. [CrossRef] [PubMed]
11. Murphy, T.; Yee, K.W.L. Cytarabine and daunorubicin for the treatment of acute myeloid leukemia. *Expert Opin Pharm.* **2017**, *18*, 1765–1780. [CrossRef] [PubMed]
12. Ho, A.D.; Brado, B.; Haas, R.; Hunstein, W. Etoposide in acute leukemia. Past experience and future perspectives. *Cancer* **1991**, *67* (Suppl. 1), 281–284. [CrossRef]
13. Preisler, H.; Davis, R.B.; Kirshner, J.; Dupre, E.; Hoagland, H.C.; Kopel, S.; Levy, R.N.; Carey, R.; Schulman, P. Comparison of three remission induction regimens and two postinduction strategies for the treatment of acute nonlymphocytic leukemia: A cancer and leukemia group B study. *Blood* **1987**, *69*, 1441–1449. [PubMed]
14. Bishop, J.F.; Lowenthal, R.M.; Joshua, D.; Matthews, J.P.; Todd, D.; Cobcroft, R.; Whiteside, M.G.; Kronenberg, H.; Ma, D.; Dodds, A. Etoposide in acute nonlymphocytic leukemia. Australian Leukemia Study Group. *Blood* **1990**, *75*, 27–32. [PubMed]
15. Clavio, M.; Gatto, S.; Beltrami, G.; Quintino, S.; Canepa, L.; Pierri, I.; Galbusera, V.; Carrara, P.; Miglino, M.; Varaldo, R.; et al. Fludarabine, ARA-C, idarubicin and G-CSF (FLAG-Ida), high dose ARA-C and early stem cell transplant. A feasable and effective therapeutic strategy for de novo AML patients. *J. Exp. Clin. Cancer Res.* **2002**, *21*, 481–487. [PubMed]
16. Burnett, A.K.; Russell, N.H.; Hills, R.K.; Hunter, A.E.; Kjeldsen, L.; Yin, J.; Gibson, B.E.; Wheatley, K.; Milligan, D. Optimization of chemotherapy for younger patients with acute myeloid leukemia: Results of the medical research council AML15 trial. *J. Clin. Oncol.* **2013**, *31*, 3360–3368. [CrossRef]
17. Stone, R.M.; Mandrekar, S.J.; Sanford, B.L.; Laumann, K.; Geyer, S.; Bloomfield, C.D.; Thiede, C.; Prior, T.W.; Döhner, K.; Marcucci, G.; et al. Midostaurin plus Chemotherapy for Acute Myeloid Leukemia with a FLT3 Mutation. *N. Engl. J. Med.* **2017**, *377*, 454–464. [CrossRef]
18. Lambert, J.; Pautas, C.; Terré, C.; Raffoux, E.; Turlure, P.; Caillot, D.; Legrand, O.; Thomas, X.; Gardin, C.; Gogat-Marchant, K.; et al. Gemtuzumab ozogamicin for de novo acute myeloid leukemia: Final efficacy and safety updates from the open-label, phase III ALFA-0701 trial. *Haematologica* **2019**, *104*, 113–119. [CrossRef]
19. Lancet, J.E.; Cortes, J.E.; Hogge, D.E.; Tallman, M.S.; Kovacsovics, T.J.; Damon, L.E.; Komrokji, R.; Solomon, S.R.; Kolitz, J.E.; Cooper, M.; et al. Phase 2 trial of CPX-351, a fixed 5:1 molar ratio of cytarabine/daunorubicin, vs. cytarabine/daunorubicin in older adults with untreated AML. *Blood* **2014**, *123*, 3239–3246. [CrossRef]
20. Cortes, J.E.; Goldberg, S.L.; Feldman, E.J.; Rizzeri, D.A.; Hogge, D.E.; Larson, M.; Pigneux, A.; Recher, C.; Schiller, G.; Warzocha, K.; et al. Phase II, multicenter, randomized trial of CPX-351 (cytarabine:daunorubicin) liposome injection versus intensive salvage therapy in adults with first relapse AML. *Cancer* **2015**, *121*, 234–242. [CrossRef]
21. Lancet, J.E.; Uy, G.L.; Cortes, J.E.; Newell, L.F.; Lin, T.L.; Ritchie, E.K.; Stuart, R.K.; Strickland, S.A.; Hogge, D.; Solomon, S.R.; et al. CPX-351 (cytarabine and daunorubicin) Liposome for Injection Versus Conventional Cytarabine Plus Daunorubicin in Older Patients with Newly Diagnosed Secondary Acute Myeloid Leukemia. *J. Clin. Oncol.* **2018**, *36*, 2684–2692. [CrossRef] [PubMed]
22. Wei, A.H.; Tiong, I.S. Midostaurin, enasidenib, CPX-351, gemtuzumab ozogamicin, and venetoclax bring new hope to AML. *Blood* **2017**, *130*, 2469–2474. [CrossRef] [PubMed]

23. Krauss, A.C.; Gao, X.; Li, L.; Manning, M.L.; Patel, P.; Fu, W.; Janoria, K.G.; Gieser, G.; Bateman, D.A.; Przepiorka, D.; et al. FDA Approval Summary: (Daunorubicin and Cytarabine) Liposome for Injection for the Treatment of Adults with High-Risk Acute Myeloid Leukemia. *Clin. Cancer Res.* **2019**, *25*, 2685–2690. [CrossRef] [PubMed]
24. Konopleva, M.; Pollyea, D.A.; Potluri, J.; Chyla, B.; Hogdal, L.; Busman, T.; McKeegan, E.; Salem, A.H.; Zhu, M.; Ricker, J.L.; et al. Efficacy and Biological Correlates of Response in a Phase II Study of Venetoclax Monotherapy in Patients with Acute Myelogenous Leukemia. *Cancer Discov.* **2016**, *6*, 1106–1117. [CrossRef] [PubMed]
25. DiNardo, C.D.; Pratz, K.; Pullarkat, V.; Jonas, B.A.; Arellano, M.; Becker, P.S.; Frankfurt, O.; Konopleva, M.; Wei, A.H.; Kantarjian, H.M.; et al. Venetoclax combined with decitabine or azacitidine in treatment-naive, elderly patients with acute myeloid leukemia. *Blood* **2019**, *133*, 7–17. [CrossRef] [PubMed]
26. Cassileth, P.A.; Harrington, D.P.; Hines, J.D.; Oken, M.M.; Mazza, J.J.; McGlave, P.; Bennett, J.M.; O'Connell, M.J. Maintenance chemotherapy prolongs remission duration in adult acute nonlymphocytic leukemia. *J. Clin. Oncol.* **1988**, *6*, 583–587. [CrossRef] [PubMed]
27. Mayer, R.J.; Davis, R.B.; Schiffer, C.A.; Berg, D.T.; Powell, B.L.; Schulman, P.; Omura, G.A.; Moore, J.O.; McIntyre, O.R.; Frei, E. Intensive postremission chemotherapy in adults with acute myeloid leukemia. Cancer and Leukemia Group B. *N. Engl. J. Med.* **1994**, *331*, 896–903. [CrossRef] [PubMed]
28. Magina, K.N.; Pregartner, G.; Zebisch, A.; Wölfler, A.; Neumeister, P.; Greinix, H.T.; Berghold, A.; Sill, H. Cytarabine dose in the consolidation treatment of AML: A systematic review and meta-analysis. *Blood* **2017**, *130*, 946–948. [CrossRef]
29. Döhner, H.; Estey, E.; Grimwade, D.; Amadori, S.; Appelbaum, F.R.; Büchner, T.; Dombret, H.; Ebert, B.L.; Fenaux, P.; Larson, R.A.; et al. Diagnosis and management of AML in adults: 2017 ELN recommendations from an international expert panel. *Blood* **2017**, *129*, 424–447. [CrossRef]
30. Lowenberg, B.; Downing, J.R.; Burnett, A. Acute myeloid leukemia. *N. Engl. J. Med.* **1999**, *341*, 1051–1062. [CrossRef]
31. Rubnitz, J.E. How I treat pediatric acute myeloid leukemia. *Blood* **2012**, *119*, 5980–5988. [CrossRef] [PubMed]
32. Grimwade, D.; Hills, R.K.; Moorman, A.V.; Walker, H.; Chatters, S.; Goldstone, A.H.; Wheatley, K.; Harrison, C.J.; Burnett, A.K. Refinement of cytogenetic classification in acute myeloid leukemia: Determination of prognostic significance of rare recurring chromosomal abnormalities among 5876 younger adult patients treated in the United Kingdom Medical Research Council trials. *Blood* **2010**, *116*, 354–365. [CrossRef] [PubMed]
33. Laubach, J.; Rao, A.V. Current and emerging strategies for the management of acute myeloid leukemia in the elderly. *Oncologist* **2008**, *13*, 1097–1108. [CrossRef] [PubMed]
34. Khalidi, H.S.; Medeiros, L.J.; Chang, K.L.; Brynes, R.K.; Slovak, M.L.; Arber, D.A. The immunophenotype of adult acute myeloid leukemia: High frequency of lymphoid antigen expression and comparison of immunophenotype, French-American-British classification, and karyotypic abnormalities. *Am. J. Clin. Pathol.* **1998**, *109*, 211–220. [CrossRef] [PubMed]
35. Iriyama, N.; Hatta, Y.; Takeuchi, J.; Ogawa, Y.; Ohtake, S.; Sakura, T.; Mitani, K.; Ishida, F.; Takahashi, M.; Maeda, T.; et al. CD56 expression is an independent prognostic factor for relapse in acute myeloid leukemia with t(8;21). *Leuk. Res.* **2013**, *37*, 1021–1026. [CrossRef] [PubMed]
36. McCulloch, E.A.; Till, J.E. The radiation sensitivity of normal mouse bone marrow cells, determined by quantitative marrow transplantation into irradiated mice. *Radiat. Res.* **1960**, *13*, 115–125. [CrossRef] [PubMed]
37. Hao, Q.L.; Shah, A.J.; Thiemann, F.T.; Smogorzewska, E.M.; Crooks, G.M. A functional comparison of CD34 + CD38- cells in cord blood and bone marrow. *Blood* **1995**, *86*, 3745–3753. [PubMed]
38. Bruce, W.R.; Ash, C.L. Survival of Patients Treated for Cancer of the Breast, Cervix, Lung, and Upper Respiratory Tract at the Ontario Cancer Institute (Toronto) from 1930 to 1957. *Radiology* **1963**, *81*, 861–870. [CrossRef]
39. Lapidot, T.; Sirard, C.; Vormoor, J.; Murdoch, B.; Hoang, T.; Caceres-Cortes, J.; Minden, M.; Paterson, B.; Caligiuri, M.A.; Dick, J.E. A cell initiating human acute myeloid leukaemia after transplantation into SCID mice. *Nature* **1994**, *367*, 645–648. [CrossRef]
40. Bonnet, D.; Dick, J.E. Human acute myeloid leukemia is organized as a hierarchy that originates from a primitive hematopoietic cell. *Nat. Med.* **1997**, *3*, 730–737. [CrossRef]

41. Van Rhenen, A.; Feller, N.; Kelder, A.; Westra, A.H.; Rombouts, E.; Zweegman, S.; Van Der Pol, M.A.; Waisfisz, Q.; Ossenkoppele, G.J.; Schuurhuis, G.J. High stem cell frequency in acute myeloid leukemia at diagnosis predicts high minimal residual disease and poor survival. *Clin. Cancer Res.* **2005**, *11*, 6520–6527. [CrossRef] [PubMed]
42. Witte, K.E.; Ahlers, J.; Schäfer, I.; André, M.; Kerst, G.; Scheel-Walter, H.G.; Schwarze, C.P.; Pfeiffer, M.; Lang, P.; Handgretinger, R.; et al. High proportion of leukemic stem cells at diagnosis is correlated with unfavorable prognosis in childhood acute myeloid leukemia. *Pediatr. Hematol. Oncol.* **2011**, *28*, 91–99. [CrossRef] [PubMed]
43. Van Rhenen, A.; Moshaver, B.; Kelder, A.; Feller, N.; Nieuwint, A.W.; Zweegman, S.; Ossenkoppele, G.J.; Schuurhuis, G.J. Aberrant marker expression patterns on the CD34 + CD38- stem cell compartment in acute myeloid leukemia allows to distinguish the malignant from the normal stem cell compartment both at diagnosis and in remission. *Leukemia* **2007**, *21*, 1700–1707. [CrossRef] [PubMed]
44. Ho, T.C.; Jordan, C.T.; LaMere, M.W.; Ashton, J.M.; O'Dwyer, K.; Mendler, J.H.; Liesveld, J.L.; Wang, E.S.; Guzman, M.L.; Calvi, L.M.; et al. A Role for IL1RAP in Acute Myelogenous Leukemia Stem Cells Following Treatment and Progression. *Blood* **2015**, *126*, 4266.
45. Rabinowich, H.; Pricop, L.; Herberman, R.B.; Whiteside, T.L. Expression and function of CD7 molecule on human natural killer cells. *J. Immunol.* **1994**, *152*, 517–526. [PubMed]
46. Blake, S.J.; Dougall, W.C.; Miles, J.J.; Teng, M.W.; Smyth, M.J. Molecular Pathways: Targeting CD96 and TIGIT for Cancer Immunotherapy. *Clin. Cancer Res.* **2016**, *22*, 5183–5188. [CrossRef] [PubMed]
47. Anania, J.C.; Chenoweth, A.M.; Wines, B.D.; Hogarth, P.M. The Human FcγRII (CD32) Family of Leukocyte FcR in Health and Disease. *Front. Immunol.* **2019**, *10*, 464. [CrossRef]
48. Seddiki, N.; Santner-Nanan, B.; Tangye, S.G.; Alexander, S.I.; Solomon, M.; Lee, S.; Nanan, R.; de Saint Groth, B.F. Persistence of naive CD45RA+ regulatory T cells in adult life. *Blood* **2006**, *107*, 2830–2838. [CrossRef]
49. Pasello, M.; Manara, M.C.; Scotlandi, K. CD99 at the crossroads of physiology and pathology. *J. Cell Commun. Signal.* **2018**, *12*, 55–68. [CrossRef]
50. Yang, B.; Wang, X.; Jiang, J.; Cheng, X. Involvement of CD244 in regulating CD4+ T cell immunity in patients with active tuberculosis. *PLoS ONE* **2013**, *8*, e63261. [CrossRef]
51. Ortolan, E.; Augeri, S.; Fissolo, G.; Musso, I.; Funaro, A. CD157: From immunoregulatory protein to potential therapeutic target. *Immunol. Lett.* **2019**, *205*, 59–64. [CrossRef] [PubMed]
52. Peters, V.A.; Joesting, J.J.; Freund, G.G. IL-1 receptor 2 (IL-1R2) and its role in immune regulation. *Brain Behav. Immun.* **2013**, *32*, 1–8. [CrossRef] [PubMed]
53. Banerjee, H.; Kane, L.P. Immune regulation by Tim-3. *F1000Research* **2018**, *7*, 316. [CrossRef] [PubMed]
54. Hosen, N.; Park, C.Y.; Tatsumi, N.; Oji, Y.; Sugiyama, H.; Gramatzki, M.; Krensky, A.M.; Weissman, I.L. CD96 is a leukemic stem cell-specific marker in human acute myeloid leukemia. *Proc. Natl. Acad. Sci. USA* **2007**, *104*, 11008–11013. [CrossRef] [PubMed]
55. Kikushige, Y.; Shima, T.; Takayanagi, S.I.; Urata, S.; Miyamoto, T.; Iwasaki, H.; Takenaka, K.; Teshima, T.; Tanaka, T.; Inagaki, Y.; et al. TIM-3 is a promising target to selectively kill acute myeloid leukemia stem cells. *Cell Stem Cell* **2010**, *7*, 708–717. [CrossRef] [PubMed]
56. Krupka, C.; Lichtenegger, F.S.; Köhnke, T.; Bögeholz, J.; Bücklein, V.; Roiss, M.; Altmann, T.; Do, T.U.; Dusek, R.; Wilson, K.; et al. Targeting CD157 in AML using a novel, Fc-engineered antibody construct. *Oncotarget* **2017**, *8*, 35707–35717. [CrossRef] [PubMed]
57. Zhang, F.; Liu, X.; Chen, C.; Zhu, J.; Yu, Z.; Xie, J.; Xie, L.; Bai, H.; Zhang, Y.; Fang, X.; et al. CD244 maintains the proliferation ability of leukemia initiating cells through SHP-2/p27(kip1) signaling. *Haematologica* **2017**, *102*, 707–718. [CrossRef]
58. Pearce, D.J.; Taussig, D.; Zibara, K.; Smith, L.L.; Ridler, C.M.; Preudhomme, C.; Young, B.D.; Rohatiner, A.Z.; Lister, T.A.; Bonnet, D. AML engraftment in the NOD/SCID assay reflects the outcome of AML: Implications for our understanding of the heterogeneity of AML. *Blood* **2006**, *107*, 1166–1173. [CrossRef]
59. Eppert, K.; Takenaka, K.; Lechman, E.R.; Waldron, L.; Nilsson, B.; Van Galen, P.; Metzeler, K.H.; Poeppl, A.; Ling, V.; Beyene, J.; et al. Stem cell gene expression programs influence clinical outcome in human leukemia. *Nat. Med.* **2011**, *17*, 1086–1093. [CrossRef]
60. Moretti, S. CD123 (interleukin 3 receptor alpha chain). *J. Biol. Regul. Homeost. Agents* **2001**, *15*, 98–100.

61. Martinez-Moczygemba, M.; Huston, D.P. Biology of common beta receptor-signaling cytokines: IL-3, IL-5, and GM-CSF. *J. Allergy Clin. Immunol.* **2003**, *112*, 653–665. [PubMed]
62. Barry, S.C.; Korpelainen, E.; Sun, Q.; Stomski, F.C.; Moretti, P.A.; Wakao, H.; D'Andrea, R.J.; Vadas, M.A.; Lopez, A.F.; Goodall, G.J. Roles of the N and C terminal domains of the interleukin-3 receptor alpha chain in receptor function. *Blood* **1997**, *89*, 842–852. [PubMed]
63. Jordan, C.T.; Upchurch, D.; Szilvassy, S.J.; Guzman, M.L.; Howard, D.S.; Pettigrew, A.L.; Meyerrose, T.; Rossi, R.; Grimes, B.; Rizzieri, D.A.; et al. The interleukin-3 receptor alpha chain is a unique marker for human acute myelogenous leukemia stem cells. *Leukemia* **2000**, *14*, 1777–1784. [CrossRef] [PubMed]
64. Huang, S.; Chen, Z.; Yu, J.F.; Young, D.; Bashey, A.; Ho, A.D.; Law, P. Correlation between IL-3 receptor expression and growth potential of human CD34+ hematopoietic cells from different tissues. *Stem Cells* **1999**, *17*, 265–272. [CrossRef] [PubMed]
65. Ashmun, R.A.; Look, A.T. Metalloprotease activity of CD13/aminopeptidase N on the surface of human myeloid cells. *Blood* **1990**, *75*, 462–469. [PubMed]
66. Mina-Osorio, P. The moonlighting enzyme CD13: Old and new functions to target. *Trends Mol. Med.* **2008**, *14*, 361–371. [CrossRef] [PubMed]
67. Piedfer, M.; Dauzonne, D.; Tang, R.; N'Guyen, J.; Billard, C.; Bauvois, B. Aminopeptidase-N/CD13 is a potential proapoptotic target in human myeloid tumor cells. *FASEB J.* **2011**, *25*, 2831–2842. [CrossRef] [PubMed]
68. Bakker, A.B.; van den Oudenrijn, S.; Bakker, A.Q.; Feller, N.; van Meijer, M.; Bia, J.A.; Jongeneelen, M.A.; Visser, T.J.; Bijl, N.; Geuijen, C.A.; et al. C-type lectin-like molecule-1: A novel myeloid cell surface marker associated with acute myeloid leukemia. *Cancer Res.* **2004**, *64*, 8443–8450. [CrossRef] [PubMed]
69. Marshall, A.S.; Willment, J.A.; Lin, H.H.; Williams, D.L.; Gordon, S.; Brown, G.D. Identification and characterization of a novel human myeloid inhibitory C-type lectin-like receptor (MICL) that is predominantly expressed on granulocytes and monocytes. *J. Biol. Chem.* **2004**, *279*, 14792–14802. [CrossRef] [PubMed]
70. Ma, H.; Padmanabhan, I.S.; Parmar, S.; Gong, Y. Targeting CLL-1 for acute myeloid leukemia therapy. *J. Hematol. Oncol.* **2019**, *12*, 41. [CrossRef] [PubMed]
71. van de Donk, N.W.; Janmaat, M.L.; Mutis, T.; Lammerts van Bueren, J.J.; Ahmadi, T.; Sasser, A.K.; Lokhorst, H.M.; Parren, P.W. Monoclonal antibodies targeting CD38 in hematological malignancies and beyond. *Immunol. Rev.* **2016**, *270*, 95–112. [CrossRef] [PubMed]
72. Malavasi, F.; Deaglio, S.; Funaro, A.; Ferrero, E.; Horenstein, A.L.; Ortolan, E.; Vaisitti, T.; Aydin, S. Evolution and function of the ADP ribosyl cyclase/CD38 gene family in physiology and pathology. *Physiol. Rev.* **2008**, *88*, 841–886. [CrossRef] [PubMed]
73. Deaglio, S.; Morra, M.; Mallone, R.; Ausiello, C.M.; Prager, E.; Garbarino, G.; Dianzani, U.; Stockinger, H.; Malavasi, F. Human CD38 (ADP-ribosyl cyclase) is a counter-receptor of CD31, an Ig superfamily member. *J. Immunol.* **1998**, *160*, 395–402. [PubMed]
74. Dianzani, U.; Funaro, A.; DiFranco, D.; Garbarino, G.; Bragardo, M.; Redoglia, V.; Buonfiglio, D.; De Monte, L.B.; Pileri, A.; Malavasi, F. Interaction between endothelium and CD4+CD45RA+ lymphocytes. Role of the human CD38 molecule. *J. Immunol.* **1994**, *153*, 952–959. [PubMed]
75. Taussig, D.C.; Miraki-Moud, F.; Anjos-Afonso, F.; Pearce, D.J.; Allen, K.; Ridler, C.; Lillington, D.; Oakervee, H.; Cavenagh, J.; Agrawal, S.G.; et al. Anti-CD38 antibody-mediated clearance of human repopulating cells masks the heterogeneity of leukemia-initiating cells. *Blood* **2008**, *112*, 568–575. [CrossRef] [PubMed]
76. Lin, P.; Owens, R.; Tricot, G.; Wilson, C.S. Flow cytometric immunophenotypic analysis of 306 cases of multiple myeloma. *Am. J. Clin. Pathol.* **2004**, *121*, 482–488. [CrossRef] [PubMed]
77. Menssen, H.D.; Renkl, H.J.; Rodeck, U.; Maurer, J.; Notter, M.; Schwartz, S.; Reinhardt, R.; Thiel, E. Presence of Wilms' tumor gene (wt1) transcripts and the WT1 nuclear protein in the majority of human acute leukemias. *Leukemia* **1995**, *9*, 1060–1067. [PubMed]
78. Dao, T.; Pankov, D.; Scott, A.; Korontsvit, T.; Zakhaleva, V.; Xu, Y.; Xiang, J.; Yan, S.; de Morais Guerreiro, M.D.; Veomett, N.; et al. Therapeutic bispecific T-cell engager antibody targeting the intracellular oncoprotein WT1. *Nat. Biotechnol.* **2015**, *33*, 1079–1086. [CrossRef]
79. Ataie, N.; Xiang, J.; Cheng, N.; Brea, E.J.; Lu, W.; Scheinberg, D.A.; Liu, C.; Ng, H.L. Structure of a TCR-Mimic Antibody with Target Predicts Pharmacogenetics. *J. Mol. Biol.* **2016**, *428*, 194–205. [CrossRef]
80. Rheinlander, A.; Schraven, B.; Bommhardt, U. CD45 in human physiology and clinical medicine. *Immunol. Lett.* **2018**, *196*, 22–32. [CrossRef]

81. Hermiston, M.L.; Xu, Z.; Weiss, A. CD45: A critical regulator of signaling thresholds in immune cells. *Annu. Rev. Immunol.* **2003**, *21*, 107–137. [CrossRef] [PubMed]
82. Holmes, N. CD45: All is not yet crystal clear. *Immunology* **2006**, *117*, 145–155. [CrossRef] [PubMed]
83. Arancia, G.; Malorni, W.; Donelli, G. Cellular mechanisms of lymphocyte-mediated lysis of tumor cells. *Annali Dell'Istituto Superiore di Sanita* **1990**, *26*, 369–384. [PubMed]
84. McCann, F.E.; Vanherberghen, B.; Eleme, K.; Carlin, L.M.; Newsam, R.J.; Goulding, D.; Davis, D.M. The size of the synaptic cleft and distinct distributions of filamentous actin, ezrin, CD43, and CD45 at activating and inhibitory human NK cell immune synapses. *J. Immunol.* **2003**, *170*, 2862–2870. [CrossRef] [PubMed]
85. Podack, E.R.; Dennert, G. Assembly of two types of tubules with putative cytolytic function by cloned natural killer cells. *Nature* **1983**, *302*, 442–445. [CrossRef] [PubMed]
86. Dennert, G.; Podack, E.R. Cytolysis by H-2-specific T killer cells. Assembly of tubular complexes on target membranes. *J. Exp. Med.* **1983**, *157*, 1483–1495. [CrossRef] [PubMed]
87. Masson, D.; Zamai, M.; Tschopp, J. Identification of granzyme A isolated from cytotoxic T-lymphocyte-granules as one of the proteases encoded by CTL-specific genes. *FEBS Lett.* **1986**, *208*, 84–88. [CrossRef]
88. Masson, D.; Tschopp, J. A family of serine esterases in lytic granules of cytolytic T lymphocytes. *Cell* **1987**, *49*, 679–685. [CrossRef]
89. Sutton, V.R.; Wowk, M.E.; Cancilla, M.; Trapani, J.A. Caspase activation by granzyme B is indirect, and caspase autoprocessing requires the release of proapoptotic mitochondrial factors. *Immunity* **2003**, *18*, 319–329. [CrossRef]
90. Beresford, P.J.; Xia, Z.; Greenberg, A.H.; Lieberman, J. Granzyme A loading induces rapid cytolysis and a novel form of DNA damage independently of caspase activation. *Immunity* **1999**, *10*, 585–594. [CrossRef]
91. Saxena, R.K.; Saxena, Q.B.; Adler, W.H. Identity of effector cells participating in the reverse antibody-dependent cell-mediated cytotoxicity. *Immunology* **1982**, *46*, 459–464. [PubMed]
92. Pende, D.; Parolini, S.; Pessino, A.; Sivori, S.; Augugliaro, R.; Morelli, L.; Marcenaro, E.; Accame, L.; Malaspina, A.; Biassoni, R.; et al. Identification and molecular characterization of NKp30, a novel triggering receptor involved in natural cytotoxicity mediated by human natural killer cells. *J. Exp. Med.* **1999**, *190*, 1505–1516. [CrossRef] [PubMed]
93. Williams, B.A.; Wang, X.; Routy, B.; Cheng, R.; Maghera, S.; Keating, A. NK Cell Line Killing of Leukemia Cells Is Enhanced By Reverse Antibody Dependent Cell Mediated Cytotoxicity (R-ADCC) Via NKp30 and NKp44 and Target Fcγ Receptor II (CD32). *Blood* **2014**, *124*, 2444.
94. Ball, E.D.; McDermott, J.; Griffin, J.D.; Davey, F.R.; Davis, R.; Bloomfield, C.D. Expression of the three myeloid cell-associated immunoglobulin G Fc receptors defined by murine monoclonal antibodies on normal bone marrow and acute leukemia cells. *Blood* **1989**, *73*, 1951–1956. [PubMed]
95. Weiskopf, K.; Weissman, I.L. Macrophages are critical effectors of antibody therapies for cancer. *MAbs* **2015**, *7*, 303–310. [CrossRef] [PubMed]
96. Kurdi, A.T.; Glavey, S.V.; Bezman, N.A.; Jhatakia, A.; Guerriero, J.L.; Manier, S.; Moschetta, M.; Mishima, Y.; Roccaro, A.; Detappe, A.; et al. Antibody-Dependent Cellular Phagocytosis by Macrophages is a Novel Mechanism of Action of Elotuzumab. *Mol. Cancer* **2018**, *17*, 1454–1463. [CrossRef] [PubMed]
97. Fishelson, Z.; Kirschfink, M. Complement C5b-9 and Cancer: Mechanisms of Cell Damage, Cancer Counteractions, and Approaches for Intervention. *Front. Immunol.* **2019**, *10*, 752. [CrossRef] [PubMed]
98. He, S.Z.; Busfield, S.; Ritchie, D.S.; Hertzberg, M.S.; Durrant, S.; Lewis, I.D.; Marlton, P.; McLachlan, A.J.; Kerridge, I.; Bradstock, K.F.; et al. A Phase 1 study of the Safety, Pharmacokinetics, and Anti-leukemic Activity of the anti-CD123 monoclonal antibody, CSL360, in Relapsed, Refractory or High-Risk Acute Myeloid Leukemia (AML). *Leuk. Lymphoma* **2014**, *56*, 1406–1415. [CrossRef] [PubMed]
99. Smith, B.D.; Roboz, G.J.; Walter, R.B.; Altman, J.K.; Ferguson, A.; Curcio, T.J.; Orlowski, K.F.; Garrett, L.; Busfield, S.J.; Barnden, M.; et al. First-in Man, Phase 1 Study of CSL362 (Anti-IL3Rα/Anti-CD123 Monoclonal Antibody) in Patients with CD123+ Acute Myeloid Leukemia (AML) in CR at High Risk for Early Relapse. *Blood* **2014**, *124*, 120.
100. Schurch, C.M. Therapeutic Antibodies for Myeloid Neoplasms-Current Developments and Future Directions. *Front. Oncol.* **2018**, *8*, 152. [CrossRef] [PubMed]

101. Sekeres, M.A.; Lancet, J.E.; Wood, B.L.; Grove, L.E.; Sandalic, L.; Sievers, E.L.; Jurcic, J.G. Randomized phase IIb study of low-dose cytarabine and lintuzumab versus low-dose cytarabine and placebo in older adults with untreated acute myeloid leukemia. *Haematologica* **2013**, *98*, 119–128. [CrossRef] [PubMed]
102. Feldman, E.J.; Brandwein, J.; Stone, R.; Kalaycio, M.; Moore, J.; O'Connor, J.; Wedel, N.; Roboz, G.J.; Miller, C.; Chopra, R.; et al. Phase III randomized multicenter study of a humanized anti-CD33 monoclonal antibody, lintuzumab, in combination with chemotherapy, versus chemotherapy alone in patients with refractory or first-relapsed acute myeloid leukemia. *J. Clin. Oncol.* **2005**, *23*, 4110–4116. [CrossRef] [PubMed]
103. Vasu, S.; He, S.; Cheney, C.; Gopalakrishnan, B.; Mani, R.; Lozanski, G.; Mo, X.; Groh, V.; Whitman, S.P.; Konopitzky, R.; et al. Decitabine enhances anti-CD33 monoclonal antibody BI 836858-mediated natural killer ADCC against AML blasts. *Blood* **2016**, *127*, 2879–2889. [CrossRef] [PubMed]
104. Lonberg, N.; Taylor, L.D.; Harding, F.A.; Trounstine, M.; Higgins, K.M.; Schramm, S.R.; Kuo, C.C.; Mashayekh, R.; Wymore, K.; McCabe, J.G.; et al. Antigen-specific human antibodies from mice comprising four distinct genetic modifications. *Nature* **1994**, *368*, 856–859. [CrossRef] [PubMed]
105. Zhang, K.; Desai, A.; Zeng, D.; Gong, T.; Lu, P.; Wang, M. Magic year for multiple myeloma therapeutics: Key takeaways from the ASH 2015 annual meeting. *Oncotarget* **2017**, *8*, 10748–10759. [CrossRef] [PubMed]
106. Dos Santos, C.; Xiaochuan, S.; Chenghui, Z.; Ndikuyeze, G.H.; Glover, J.; Secreto, T.; Doshi, P.; Sasser, K.; Danet-Desnoyers, G. Anti-Leukemic Activity of Daratumumab in Acute Myeloid Leukemia Cells and Patient-Derived Xenografts. *Blood* **2014**, *124*, 2312.
107. De Weers, M.; Tai, Y.T.; Van Der Veer, M.S.; Bakker, J.M.; Vink, T.; Jacobs, D.C.; Oomen, L.A.; Peipp, M.; Valerius, T.; Slootstra, J.W.; et al. Daratumumab, a novel therapeutic human CD38 monoclonal antibody, induces killing of multiple myeloma and other hematological tumors. *J. Immunol.* **2011**, *186*, 1840–1848. [CrossRef] [PubMed]
108. Strickland, S.A.; Glenn, M.; Zheng, W.; Daskalakis, N.; Mikhael, J.R. SAR650984, a CD38 Monoclonal Antibody in Patients with Selected CD38+ Hematological Malignancies- Data From a Dose-Escalation Phase I Study. *Blood* **2013**, *122*, 284.
109. Spiess, C.; Zhai, Q.; Carter, P.J. Alternative molecular formats and therapeutic applications for bispecific antibodies. *Mol. Immunol.* **2015**, *67 Pt A*, 95–106. [CrossRef]
110. Handgretinger, R.; Zugmaier, G.; Henze, G.; Kreyenberg, H.; Lang, P.; Von Stackelberg, A. Complete remission after blinatumomab-induced donor T-cell activation in three pediatric patients with post-transplant relapsed acute lymphoblastic leukemia. *Leukemia* **2011**, *25*, 181–184. [CrossRef]
111. Topp, M.S.; Kufer, P.; Gökbuget, N.; Goebeler, M.; Klinger, M.; Neumann, S.; Horst, H.A.; Raff, T.; Viardot, A.; Schmid, M.; et al. Targeted therapy with the T-cell-engaging antibody blinatumomab of chemotherapy-refractory minimal residual disease in B-lineage acute lymphoblastic leukemia patients results in high response rate and prolonged leukemia-free survival. *J. Clin. Oncol.* **2011**, *29*, 2493–2498. [CrossRef] [PubMed]
112. Curran, E.; Stock, W. Taking a "BiTE out of ALL"—Blinatumomab approval for MRD positive ALL. *Blood* **2019**, *16*, 1715–1719. [CrossRef]
113. Krzewski, K.; Coligan, J.E. Human NK cell lytic granules and regulation of their exocytosis. *Front. Immunol.* **2012**, *3*, 335. [CrossRef] [PubMed]
114. Huehls, A.M.; Coupet, T.A.; Sentman, C.L. Bispecific T-cell engagers for cancer immunotherapy. *Immunol. Cell Biol.* **2015**, *93*, 290–296. [CrossRef] [PubMed]
115. Dreier, T.; Lorenczewski, G.; Brandl, C.; Hoffmann, P.; Syring, U.; Hanakam, F.; Kufer, P.; Riethmuller, G.; Bargou, R.; Baeuerle, P.A. Extremely potent, rapid and costimulation-independent cytotoxic T-cell response against lymphoma cells catalyzed by a single-chain bispecific antibody. *Int. J. Cancer* **2002**, *100*, 690–697. [CrossRef] [PubMed]
116. Aigner, M.; Feulner, J.; Schaffer, S.; Kischel, R.; Kufer, P.; Schneider, K.; Henn, A.; Rattel, B.; Friedrich, M.; Baeuerle, P.A.; et al. T lymphocytes can be effectively recruited for ex vivo and in vivo lysis of AML blasts by a novel CD33/CD3-bispecific BiTE antibody construct. *Leukemia* **2013**, *27*, 1107–1115. [CrossRef] [PubMed]
117. Laszlo, G.S.; Gudgeon, C.J.; Harrington, K.H.; Dell'Aringa, J.; Newhall, K.J.; Means, G.D.; Sinclair, A.M.; Kischel, R.; Frankel, S.R.; Walter, R.B. Cellular determinants for preclinical activity of a novel CD33/CD3 bispecific T-cell engager (BiTE) antibody, AMG 330, against human AML. *Blood* **2014**, *123*, 554–561. [CrossRef] [PubMed]

118. Friedrich, M.; Henn, A.; Raum, T.; Bajtus, M.; Matthes, K.; Hendrich, L.; Wahl, J.; Hoffmann, P.; Kischel, R.; Kvesic, M.; et al. Preclinical characterization of AMG 330, a CD3/CD33-bispecific T-cell-engaging antibody with potential for treatment of acute myelogenous leukemia. *Mol. Cancer* **2014**, *13*, 1549–1557. [CrossRef]
119. Harrington, K.H.; Gudgeon, C.J.; Laszlo, G.S.; Newhall, K.J.; Sinclair, A.M.; Frankel, S.R.; Kischel, R.; Chen, G.; Walter, R.B. The Broad Anti-AML Activity of the CD33/CD3 BiTE Antibody Construct, AMG 330, Is Impacted by Disease Stage and Risk. *PLoS ONE* **2015**, *10*, e0135945. [CrossRef]
120. Ravandi, F.; Stein, A.S.; Kantarjian, H.M.; Walter, R.B.; Paschka, P.; Jongen-Lavrencic, M.; Ossenkoppele, G.J.; Yang, Z.; Mehta, B.; Subklewe, M. A Phase 1 First-in-Human Study of AMG 330, an Anti-CD33 Bispecific T-Cell Engager (BiTE®) Antibody Construct, in Relapsed/Refractory Acute Myeloid Leukemia (R/R AML). *Blood* **2018**, *132* (Suppl. 1), 25.
121. Stamova, S.; Cartellieri, M.; Feldmann, A.; Arndt, C.; Koristka, S.; Bartsch, H.; Bippes, C.C.; Wehner, R.; Schmitz, M.; von Bonin, M.; et al. Unexpected recombinations in single chain bispecific anti-CD3-anti-CD33 antibodies can be avoided by a novel linker module. *Mol. Immunol.* **2011**, *49*, 474–482. [CrossRef] [PubMed]
122. Arndt, C.; Von Bonin, M.; Cartellieri, M.; Feldmann, A.; Koristka, S.; Michalk, I.; Stamova, S.; Bornhäuser, M.; Schmitz, M.; Ehninger, G.; et al. Redirection of T cells with a first fully humanized bispecific CD33-CD3 antibody efficiently eliminates AML blasts without harming hematopoietic stem cells. *Leukemia* **2013**, *27*, 964–967. [CrossRef] [PubMed]
123. Arndt, C.; Feldmann, A.; Von Bonin, M.; Cartellieri, M.; Ewen, E.M.; Koristka, S.; Michalk, I.; Stamova, S.; Berndt, N.; Gocht, A.; et al. Costimulation improves the killing capability of T cells redirected to tumor cells expressing low levels of CD33: Description of a novel modular targeting system. *Leukemia* **2014**, *28*, 59–69. [CrossRef] [PubMed]
124. Al-Hussaini, M.; Rettig, M.P.; Ritchey, J.K.; Karpova, D.; Uy, G.L.; Eissenberg, L.G.; Gao, F.; Eades, W.C.; Bonvini, E.; Chichili, G.R.; et al. Targeting CD123 in acute myeloid leukemia using a T-cell-directed dual-affinity retargeting platform. *Blood* **2016**, *127*, 122–131. [CrossRef] [PubMed]
125. Kuo, S.R.; Wong, L.; Liu, J.S. Engineering a CD123xCD3 bispecific scFv immunofusion for the treatment of leukemia and elimination of leukemia stem cells. *Protein Eng. Des. Sel.* **2012**, *25*, 561–569. [CrossRef] [PubMed]
126. Kipriyanov, S.M.; Moldenhauer, G.; Schuhmacher, J.; Cochlovius, B.; Von der Lieth, C.W.; Matys, E.R.; Little, M. Bispecific tandem diabody for tumor therapy with improved antigen binding and pharmacokinetics11Edited by J. Karn. *J. Mol. Biol.* **1999**, *293*, 41–56. [CrossRef] [PubMed]
127. Reusch, U.; Harrington, K.H.; Gudgeon, C.J.; Fucek, I.; Ellwanger, K.; Weichel, M.; Knackmuss, S.H.; Zhukovsky, E.A.; Fox, J.A.; Kunkel, L.A.; et al. Characterization of CD33/CD3 Tetravalent Bispecific Tandem Diabodies (TandAbs) for the Treatment of Acute Myeloid Leukemia. *Clin. Cancer Res.* **2016**, *22*, 5829–5838. [CrossRef]
128. Silla, L.M.; Chen, J.; Zhong, R.K.; Whiteside, T.L.; Ball, E.D. Potentiation of lysis of leukaemia cells by a bispecific antibody to CD33 and CD16 (Fc gamma RIII) expressed by human natural killer (NK) cells. *Br. J. Haematol.* **1995**, *89*, 712–718. [CrossRef]
129. Nitta, T.; Yagita, H.; Azuma, T.; Sato, K.; Okumura KBispecific, F. Bispecific F (ab')2 monomer prepared with anti-CD3 and anti-tumor monoclonal antibodies is most potent in induction of cytolysis of human T cells. *Eur. J. Immunol.* **1989**, *19*, 1437–1441. [CrossRef]
130. Oshimi, K.; Seto, T.; Oshimi, Y.; Masuda, M.; Okumura, K.O.; Mizoguchi, H. Increased lysis of patient CD10-positive leukemic cells by T cells coated with anti-CD3 Fab' antibody cross-linked to anti-CD10 Fab' antibody. *Blood* **1991**, *77*, 1044–1049.
131. Kaneko, T.; Fusauchi, Y.; Kakui, Y.; Masuda, M.; Akahoshi, M.; Teramura, M.; Motoji, T.; Okumura, K.; Mizoguchi, H.; Oshimi, K. A bispecific antibody enhances cytokine-induced killer-mediated cytolysis of autologous acute myeloid leukemia cells. *Blood* **1993**, *81*, 1333–1341. [PubMed]
132. Gaudet, F.; Nemeth, J.F.; McDaid, R.; Li, Y.; Harman, B.; Millar, H.; Teplyakov, A.; Wheeler, J.; Luo, J.; Tam, S.; et al. Development of a CD123xCD3 Bispecific Antibody (JNJ-63709178) for the Treatment of Acute Myeloid Leukemia (AML). *Blood* **2016**, *128*, 2824.
133. Van Loo, P.F.; Doornbos, R.; Dolstra, H.; Shamsili, S.; Bakker, L. Preclinical Evaluation of MCLA117, a CLEC12AxCD3 Bispecific Antibody Efficiently Targeting a Novel Leukemic Stem Cell Associated Antigen in AML. *Blood* **2015**, *126*, 325.

134. Wiernik, A.; Foley, B.; Zhang, B.; Verneris, M.R.; Warlick, E.; Gleason, M.K.; Ross, J.A.; Luo, X.; Weisdorf, D.J.; Walcheck, B.; et al. Targeting natural killer cells to acute myeloid leukemia in vitro with a CD16 × 33 bispecific killer cell engager and ADAM17 inhibition. *Clin. Cancer Res.* **2013**, *19*, 3844–3855. [CrossRef] [PubMed]
135. Gleason, M.K.; Ross, J.A.; Warlick, E.D.; Lund, T.C.; Verneris, M.R.; Wiernik, A.; Spellman, S.; Haagenson, M.D.; Lenvik, A.J.; Litzow, M.R.; et al. CD16xCD33 bispecific killer cell engager (BiKE) activates NK cells against primary MDS and MDSC CD33+ targets. *Blood* **2014**, *123*, 3016–3026. [CrossRef] [PubMed]
136. Vallera, D.A.; Felices, M.; McElmurry, R.; McCullar, V.; Zhou, X.; Schmohl, J.U.; Zhang, B.; Lenvik, A.J.; Panoskaltsis-Mortari, A.; Verneris, M.R.; et al. IL15 Trispecific Killer Engagers (TriKE) Make Natural Killer Cells Specific to CD33+ Targets While Also Inducing Persistence, In Vivo Expansion, and Enhanced Function. *Clin. Cancer Res.* **2016**, *22*, 3440–3450. [CrossRef] [PubMed]
137. Singer, H.; Kellner, C.; Lanig, H.; Aigner, M.; Stockmeyer, B.; Oduncu, F.; Schwemmlein, M.; Stein, C.; Mentz, K.; Mackensen, A.; et al. Effective elimination of acute myeloid leukemic cells by recombinant bispecific antibody derivatives directed against CD33 and CD16. *J. Immunother* **2010**, *33*, 599–608. [CrossRef] [PubMed]
138. Kügler, M.; Stein, C.; Kellner, C.; Mentz, K.; Saul, D.; Schwenkert, M.; Schubert, I.; Singer, H.; Oduncu, F.; Stockmeyer, B.; et al. A recombinant trispecific single-chain Fv derivative directed against CD123 and CD33 mediates effective elimination of acute myeloid leukaemia cells by dual targeting. *Br. J. Haematol.* **2010**, *150*, 574–586. [CrossRef] [PubMed]
139. Ghose, T.; Norvell, S.T.; Guclu, A.; MacDonald, A.S. Immunochemotherapy of human malignant melanoma with chlorambucil-carrying antibody. *Eur J. Cancer* **1975**, *11*, 321–326. [CrossRef]
140. Diamantis, N.; Banerji, U. Antibody-drug conjugates–an emerging class of cancer treatment. *Br. J. Cancer* **2016**, *114*, 362–367. [CrossRef] [PubMed]
141. Hedrich, W.D.; Fandy, T.E.; Ashour, H.M.; Wang, H.; Hassan, H.E. Antibody-Drug Conjugates: Pharmacokinetic/Pharmacodynamic Modeling, Preclinical Characterization, Clinical Studies, and Lessons Learned. *Clin. Pharm.* **2018**, *57*, 687–703. [CrossRef] [PubMed]
142. Zein, N.; Sinha, A.M.; McGahren, W.J.; Ellestad, G.A. Calicheamicin gamma 1I: An antitumor antibiotic that cleaves double-stranded DNA site specifically. *Science* **1988**, *240*, 1198–1201. [CrossRef]
143. Richardson, N.C.; Kasamon, Y.L.; Chen, H.; de Claro, R.A.; Ye, J.; Blumenthal, G.M.; Farrell, A.T.; Pazdur, R. FDA Approval Summary: Brentuximab Vedotin in First-Line Treatment of Peripheral T-Cell Lymphoma. *Oncologist* **2019**, *24*, e180–e187. [CrossRef] [PubMed]
144. Gregson, S.J.; Masterson, L.A.; Wei, B.; Pillow, T.H.; Spencer, S.D.; Kang, G.D.; Yu, S.F.; Raab, H.; Lau, J.; Li, G.; et al. Pyrrolobenzodiazepine Dimer Antibody-Drug Conjugates: Synthesis and Evaluation of Noncleavable Drug-Linkers. *J. Med. Chem* **2017**, *60*, 9490–9507. [CrossRef] [PubMed]
145. Sutherland, M.S.; Walter, R.B.; Jeffrey, S.C.; Burke, P.J.; Yu, C.; Harrington, K.H.; Stone, I.; Ryan, M.C.; Sussman, D.; Zeng, W.; et al. SGN-CD33A: A Novel CD33-Directed Antibody-Drug Conjugate, Utilizing Pyrrolobenzodiazepine Dimers, Demonstrates Preclinical Antitumor Activity Against Multi-Drug Resistant Human AML. *Blood* **2012**, *120*, 3589.
146. Smellie, M.; Bose, D.S.; Thompson, A.S.; Jenkins, T.C.; Hartley, J.A.; Thurston, D.E. Sequence-selective recognition of duplex DNA through covalent interstrand cross-linking: Kinetic and molecular modeling studies with pyrrolobenzodiazepine dimers. *Biochemistry* **2003**, *42*, 8232–8239. [CrossRef]
147. van der Velden, V.H.; te Marvelde, J.G.; Hoogeveen, P.G.; Bernstein, I.D.; Houtsmuller, A.B.; Berger, M.S.; van Dongen, J.J. Targeting of the CD33-calicheamicin immunoconjugate Mylotarg (CMA-676) in acute myeloid leukemia: In vivo and in vitro saturation and internalization by leukemic and normal myeloid cells. *Blood* **2001**, *97*, 3197–3204. [CrossRef]
148. Bross, P.F.; Beitz, J.; Chen, G.; Chen, X.H.; Duffy, E.; Kieffer, L.; Roy, S.; Sridhara, R.; Rahman, A.; Williams, G.; et al. Approval summary: Gemtuzumab ozogamicin in relapsed acute myeloid leukemia. *Clin. Cancer Res.* **2001**, *7*, 1490–1496.
149. Petersdorf, S.H.; Kopecky, K.J.; Slovak, M.; Willman, C.; Nevill, T.; Brandwein, J.; Larson, R.A.; Erba, H.P.; Stiff, P.J.; Stuart, R.K.; et al. A phase 3 study of gemtuzumab ozogamicin during induction and postconsolidation therapy in younger patients with acute myeloid leukemia. *Blood* **2013**, *121*, 4854–4860. [CrossRef]

150. Burnett, A.K.; Hills, R.K.; Milligan, D.; Kjeldsen, L.; Kell, J.; Russell, N.H.; Yin, J.A.; Hunter, A.; Goldstone, A.H.; Wheatley, K. Identification of patients with acute myeloblastic leukemia who benefit from the addition of gemtuzumab ozogamicin: Results of the MRC AML15 trial. *J. Clin. Oncol.* **2011**, *29*, 369–377. [CrossRef]
151. Burnett, A.K.; Russell, N.H.; Hills, R.K.; Kell, J.; Freeman, S.; Kjeldsen, L.; Hunter, A.E.; Yin, J.; Craddock, C.F.; Dufva, I.H.; et al. Addition of gemtuzumab ozogamicin to induction chemotherapy improves survival in older patients with acute myeloid leukemia. *J. Clin. Oncol.* **2012**, *30*, 3924–3931. [CrossRef] [PubMed]
152. Sutherland, M.S.; Walter, R.B.; Jeffrey, S.C.; Burke, P.J.; Yu, C.; Kostner, H.; Stone, I.; Ryan, M.C.; Sussman, D.; Lyon, R.P.; et al. SGN-CD33A: A novel CD33-targeting antibody-drug conjugate using a pyrrolobenzodiazepine dimer is active in models of drug-resistant AML. *Blood* **2013**, *122*, 1455–1463. [CrossRef] [PubMed]
153. Bixby, D.L.; Stein, A.S.; Fathi, A.T.; Kovacsovics, T.J.; Levy, M.Y.; Erba, H.P.; Lancet, J.E.; Jillella, A.P.; Ravandi, F.; Walter, R.B.; et al. Vadastuximab Talirine Monotherapy in Older Patients with Treatment Naive CD33-Positive Acute Myeloid Leukemia (AML). *Blood* **2016**, *128*, 590.
154. Fathi, A.T.; Erba, H.P.; Lancet, J.E.; Stein, E.M.; Ravandi, F.; Faderl, S.; Walter, R.B.; Advani, A.; DeAngelo, D.J.; Kovacsovics, T.J.; et al. Vadastuximab Talirine Plus Hypomethylating Agents: A Well-Tolerated Regimen with High Remission Rate in Frontline Older Patients with Acute Myeloid Leukemia (AML). *Blood* **2016**, *128*, 591.
155. Whiteman, K.R.; Noordhuis, P.; Walker, R.; Watkins, K.; Kovtun, Y.; Harvey, L.; Wilhelm, A.; Johnson, H.; Schuurhuis, G.J.; Ossenkoppele, G.J.; et al. The Antibody-Drug Conjugate (ADC) IMGN779 Is Highly Active in Vitro and in Vivo Against Acute Myeloid Leukemia (AML) with FLT3-ITD Mutations. *Blood* **2014**, *124*, 2321.
156. Wu, A.M.; Senter, P.D. Arming antibodies: Prospects and challenges for immunoconjugates. *Nat. Biotechnol.* **2005**, *23*, 1137–1146. [CrossRef] [PubMed]
157. Eriksson, D.; Stigbrand, T. Radiation-induced cell death mechanisms. *Tumour. Biol.* **2010**, *31*, 363–372. [CrossRef] [PubMed]
158. Dai, S.P.; Xie, C.; Ding, N.; Zhang, Y.J.; Han, L.; Han, Y.W. Targeted inhibition of genome-wide DNA methylation analysis in epigenetically modulated phenotypes in lung cancer. *Med. Oncol.* **2015**, *32*, 615. [CrossRef]
159. Aghevlian, S.; Boyle, A.J.; Reilly, R.M. Radioimmunotherapy of cancer with high linear energy transfer (LET) radiation delivered by radionuclides emitting alpha-particles or Auger electrons. *Adv. Drug Deliv. Rev.* **2017**, *109*, 102–118. [CrossRef]
160. Larson, S.M.; Carrasquillo, J.A.; Cheung, N.K.; Press, O.W. Radioimmunotherapy of human tumours. *Nat. Rev. Cancer* **2015**, *15*, 347–360. [CrossRef]
161. Rizvi, S.M.; Henniker, A.J.; Goozee, G.; Allen, B.J. In vitro testing of the leukaemia monoclonal antibody WM-53 labeled with alpha and beta emitting radioisotopes. *Leuk. Res.* **2002**, *26*, 37–43. [CrossRef]
162. Heylmann, D.; Rödel, F.; Kindler, T.; Kaina, B. Radiation sensitivity of human and murine peripheral blood lymphocytes, stem and progenitor cells. *Biochim. Biophys. Acta* **2014**, *1846*, 121–129. [CrossRef] [PubMed]
163. Kersemans, V.; Cornelissen, B.; Minden, M.D.; Brandwein, J.; Reilly, R.M. Drug-resistant AML cells and primary AML specimens are killed by 111In-anti-CD33 monoclonal antibodies modified with nuclear localizing peptide sequences. *J. Nucl. Med.* **2008**, *49*, 1546–1554. [CrossRef] [PubMed]
164. Leyton, J.V.; Gao, C.; Williams, B.; Keating, A.; Minden, M.; Reilly, R.M. A radiolabeled antibody targeting CD123(+) leukemia stem cells—initial radioimmunotherapy studies in NOD/SCID mice engrafted with primary human AML. *Leuk. Res. Rep.* **2015**, *4*, 55–59. [CrossRef] [PubMed]
165. Leyton, J.V.; Hu, M.; Gao, C.; Turner, P.V.; Dick, J.E.; Minden, M.; Reilly, R.M. Auger electron radioimmunotherapeutic agent specific for the CD123+/CD131- phenotype of the leukemia stem cell population. *J. Nucl. Med.* **2011**, *52*, 1465–1473. [CrossRef] [PubMed]
166. Leyton, J.V.; Williams, B.; Gao, C.; Keating, A.; Minden, M.; Reilly, R.M. MicroSPECT/CT imaging of primary human AML engrafted into the bone marrow and spleen of NOD/SCID mice using 111In-DTPA-NLS-CSL360 radioimmunoconjugates recognizing the CD123+/CD131- epitope expressed by leukemia stem cells. *Leuk. Res.* **2014**, *38*, 1367–1373. [CrossRef] [PubMed]
167. Gyurkocza, B.; Sandmaier, B.M. Conditioning regimens for hematopoietic cell transplantation: One size does not fit all. *Blood* **2014**, *124*, 344–353. [CrossRef] [PubMed]

168. Wallen, H.; Gooley, T.A.; Deeg, H.J.; Pagel, J.M.; Press, O.W.; Appelbaum, F.R.; Storb, R.; Gopal, A.K. Ablative allogeneic hematopoietic cell transplantation in adults 60 years of age and older. *J. Clin. Oncol.* **2005**, *23*, 3439–3446. [CrossRef] [PubMed]
169. McSweeney, P.A.; Niederwieser, D.; Shizuru, J.A.; Sandmaier, B.M.; Molina, A.J.; Maloney, D.G.; Chauncey, T.R.; Gooley, T.A.; Hegenbart, U.; Nash, R.A.; et al. Hematopoietic cell transplantation in older patients with hematologic malignancies: Replacing high-dose cytotoxic therapy with graft-versus-tumor effects. *Blood* **2001**, *97*, 3390–3400. [CrossRef]
170. Clift, R.A.; Buckner, C.D.; Appelbaum, F.R.; Bearman, S.I.; Petersen, F.B.; Fisher, L.D.; Anasetti, C.; Beatty, P.; Bensinger, W.I.; Doney, K. Allogeneic marrow transplantation in patients with acute myeloid leukemia in first remission: A randomized trial of two irradiation regimens. *Blood* **1990**, *76*, 1867–1871.
171. Clift, R.A.; Buckner, C.D.; Appelbaum, F.R.; Sullivan, K.M.; Storb, R.; Thomas, E.D. Long-term follow-Up of a randomized trial of two irradiation regimens for patients receiving allogeneic marrow transplants during first remission of acute myeloid leukemia. *Blood* **1998**, *92*, 1455–1456. [PubMed]
172. Goyal, G. Reduced-intensity conditioning allogeneic hematopoietic-cell transplantation for older patients with acute myeloid leukemia. *Adv. Hematol.* **2016**, *7*, 131–141. [CrossRef] [PubMed]
173. Storb, R.; Gyurkocza, B.; Storer, B.E.; Sorror, M.L.; Blume, K.; Niederwieser, D.; Chauncey, T.R.; Pulsipher, M.A.; Petersen, F.B.; Sahebi, F.; et al. Graft-versus-host disease and graft-versus-tumor effects after allogeneic hematopoietic cell transplantation. *J. Clin. Oncol.* **2013**, *31*, 1530–1538. [CrossRef] [PubMed]
174. Lacombe, F.; Durrieu, F.; Briais, A.; Dumain, P.; Belloc, F.; Bascans, E.; Reiffers, J.; Boisseau, M.R.; Bernard, P. Flow cytometry CD45 gating for immunophenotyping of acute myeloid leukemia. *Leukemia* **1997**, *11*, 1878–1886. [CrossRef] [PubMed]
175. Matthews, D.C.; Appelbaum, F.R.; Eary, J.F.; Fisher, D.R.; Durack, L.D.; Hui, T.E.; Martin, P.J.; Mitchell, D.; Press, O.W.; Storb, R.; et al. Phase I study of (131)I-anti-CD45 antibody plus cyclophosphamide and total body irradiation for advanced acute leukemia and myelodysplastic syndrome. *Blood* **1999**, *94*, 1237–1247. [PubMed]
176. Pagel, J.M.; Appelbaum, F.R.; Eary, J.F.; Rajendran, J.; Fisher, D.R.; Gooley, T.; Ruffner, K.; Nemecek, E.; Sickle, E.; Durack, L.; et al. 131I-anti-CD45 antibody plus busulfan and cyclophosphamide before allogeneic hematopoietic cell transplantation for treatment of acute myeloid leukemia in first remission. *Blood* **2006**, *107*, 2184–2191. [CrossRef] [PubMed]
177. Pagel, J.M.; Gooley, T.A.; Rajendran, J.; Fisher, D.R.; Wilson, W.A.; Sandmaier, B.M.; Matthews, D.C.; Deeg, H.J.; Gopal, A.K.; Martin, P.J.; et al. Allogeneic hematopoietic cell transplantation after conditioning with 131I-anti-CD45 antibody plus fludarabine and low-dose total body irradiation for elderly patients with advanced acute myeloid leukemia or high-risk myelodysplastic syndrome. *Blood* **2009**, *114*, 5444–5453. [CrossRef]
178. Mawad, R.; Gooley, T.A.; Rajendran, J.G.; Fisher, D.R.; Gopal, A.K.; Shields, A.T.; Sandmaier, B.M.; Sorror, M.L.; Deeg, H.J.; Storb, R.; et al. Radiolabeled anti-CD45 antibody with reduced-intensity conditioning and allogeneic transplantation for younger patients with advanced acute myeloid leukemia or myelodysplastic syndrome. *Biol. Blood Marrow Transpl.* **2014**, *20*, 1363–1368. [CrossRef]
179. Orozco, J.J.; Kenoyer, A.; Balkin, E.R.; Gooley, T.A.; Hamlin, D.K.; Wilbur, D.S.; Hylarides, M.D.; Frost, S.H.; Mawad, R.; O'Donnell, P.; et al. Anti-CD45 radioimmunotherapy without TBI before transplantation facilitates persistent haploidentical donor engraftment. *Blood* **2016**, *127*, 352–359. [CrossRef]
180. Orozco, J.; Zeller, J.; Pagel, J.M. Radiolabeled antibodies directed at CD45 for conditioning prior to allogeneic transplantation in acute myeloid leukemia and myelodysplastic syndrome. *Adv. Hematol.* **2011**, *3*, 5–16. [CrossRef]
181. Agura, E.D.; Gyurkocza, B.; Nath, R.; Litzow, M.R.; Tomlinson, B.K.; Abhyankar, S.; Seropian, S.; Stiff, P.J.; Choe, H.K.; Kebriaei, P.; et al. Targeted Conditioning of Iomab-B (131I-anti-CD45) Prior to Allogeneic Hematopoietic Cell Transplantation Versus Conventional Care in Relapsed or Refractory Acute Myeloid Leukemia (AML): Preliminary Feasibility and Safety Results from the Prospective, Randomized Phase 3 Sierra Trial. *Blood* **2018**, *132* (Suppl. 1), 1017.
182. Cassaday, R.D.; Press, O.W.; Pagel, J.M.; Rajendran, J.G.; Gooley, T.A.; Fisher, D.R.; Miyaoka, R.S.; Maloney, D.G.; Smith, S.D.; Till, B.G.; et al. Safety and Efficacy of Escalating Doses of 90Y-BC8-DOTA (Anti-CD45) Followed by Carmustine, Etoposide, Cytarabine, and Melphalan (BEAM) Chemotherapy and Autologous Stem Cell Transplantation (ASCT) for High- Risk Lymphoma. *Biol. Blood Marrow Transpl.* **2018**, *24*, 329. [CrossRef]

183. Glatting, G.; Müller, M.; Koop, B.; Hohl, K.; Friesen, C.; Neumaier, B.; Berrie, E.; Bird, P.; Hale, G.; Blumstein, N.M.; et al. Anti-CD45 monoclonal antibody YAML568: A promising radioimmunoconjugate for targeted therapy of acute leukemia. *J. Nucl. Med.* **2006**, *47*, 1335–1341. [PubMed]
184. Jurcic, J.G.; Larson, S.M.; Sgouros, G.; McDevitt, M.R.; Finn, R.D.; Divgi, C.R.; Ballangrud, Å.M.; Hamacher, K.A.; Ma, D.; Humm, J.L.; et al. Targeted alpha particle immunotherapy for myeloid leukemia. *Blood* **2002**, *100*, 1233–1239. [CrossRef] [PubMed]
185. Mehta, B.M.; Finn, R.D.; Larson, S.M.; Scheinberg, D.A. Pharmacokinetics and dosimetry of an alpha-particle emitter labeled antibody: 213Bi-HuM195 (anti-CD33) in patients with leukemia. *J. Nucl. Med.* **1999**, *40*, 1935–1946.
186. Jurcic, J.G.; Rosenblat, T.L.; McDevitt, M.R.; Pandit-Taskar, N.; Carrasquillo, J.A.; Chanel, S.M.; Ryan, C.; Frattini, M.G.; Cicic, D.; Larson, S.M.; et al. Phase I Trial of the Targeted Alpha-Particle Nano-Generator Actinium-225 (225Ac)-Lintuzumab (Anti-CD33; HuM195) in Acute Myeloid Leukemia (AML). *Blood* **2011**, *118*, 6516. [CrossRef]
187. Jurcic, J.G.; Ravandi, F.; Pagel, J.M.; Park, J.H.; Smith, B.D.; Douer, D.; Levy, M.Y.; Estey, E.; Kantarjian, H.M.; Earle, D.; et al. Phase I trial of a-particle therapy with actinium-225 (225Ac)-lintuzumab (anti-CD33) and low-dose cytarabine (LDAC) in older patients with untreated acute myeloid leukemia. *J. Clin. Oncol.* **2017**, *33*, 7050. [CrossRef]
188. Lagadinou, E.D.; Sach, A.; Callahan, K.; Rossi, R.M.; Neering, S.J.; Minhajuddin, M.; Ashton, J.M.; Pei, S.; Grose, V.; O'Dwyer, K.M.; et al. BCL-2 inhibition targets oxidative phosphorylation and selectively eradicates quiescent human leukemia stem cells. *Cell Stem Cell* **2013**, *12*, 329–341. [CrossRef]
189. DiNardo, C.D.; Rausch, C.R.; Benton, C.; Kadia, T.; Jain, N.; Pemmaraju, N.; Daver, N.; Covert, W.; Marx, K.R.; Mace, M.; et al. Clinical experience with the BCL2-inhibitor venetoclax in combination therapy for relapsed and refractory acute myeloid leukemia and related myeloid malignancies. *Am. J. Hematol.* **2018**, *93*, 401–407. [CrossRef]
190. Wierzbowska, A.; Robak, T.; Pluta, A.; Wawrzyniak, E.; Cebula, B.; Hołowiecki, J.; Kyrcz-Krzemień, S.; Grosicki, S.; Giebel, S.; Skotnicki, A.B.; et al. Cladribine combined with high doses of arabinoside cytosine, mitoxantrone, and G-CSF (CLAG-M) is a highly effective salvage regimen in patients with refractory and relapsed acute myeloid leukemia of the poor risk: A final report of the Polish Adult Leukemia Group. *Eur. J. Haematol.* **2008**, *80*, 115–126.
191. Muppidi, M.R.; Freyer, C.W.; Ford, L.A.; Ontiveros, E.P.; Thompson, J.E.; Griffiths, E.A.; Wang, E.S. CLAG±M (cladribine, cytarabine, granulocyte colony stimulating factor ± mitoxantrone) Results in High Response Rates in Older Patients with Secondary and Relapsed/Refractory Acute Myeloid Leukemia—A Single Institute Experience. *Blood* **2015**, *126*, 1341.
192. Li, T.; Ao, E.C.; Lambert, B.; Brans, B.; Vandenberghe, S.; Mok, G.S. Quantitative Imaging for Targeted Radionuclide Therapy Dosimetry—Technical Review. *Theranostics* **2017**, *7*, 4551–4565. [CrossRef] [PubMed]
193. Kunos, C.A.; Capala, J.; Ivy, S.P. Radiopharmaceuticals for Relapsed or Refractory Leukemias. *Front. Oncol.* **2019**, *9*, 97. [CrossRef] [PubMed]

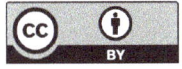

© 2019 by the authors. Licensee MDPI, Basel, Switzerland. This article is an open access article distributed under the terms and conditions of the Creative Commons Attribution (CC BY) license (http://creativecommons.org/licenses/by/4.0/).

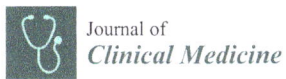

Review

Dendritic Cell-Based Immunotherapy of Acute Myeloid Leukemia

Heleen H. Van Acker [1], Maarten Versteven [1], Felix S. Lichtenegger [2], Gils Roex [1], Diana Campillo-Davo [1], Eva Lion [1], Marion Subklewe [2], Viggo F. Van Tendeloo [1], Zwi N. Berneman [1,3] and Sébastien Anguille [1,3,*]

[1] Laboratory of Experimental Hematology, Vaccine & Infectious Disease Institute, Faculty of Medicine & Health Sciences, University of Antwerp, 2610 Wilrijk, Antwerp, Belgium; heleen.vanacker@uantwerpen.be (H.H.V.A.); maarten.versteven@uantwerpen.be (M.V.); gils.roex@uantwerpen.be (G.R.); Diana.CampilloDavo@uantwerpen.be (D.C.-D.); eva.lion@uza.be (E.L.); vigske@gmail.com (V.F.V.T.); zwi.berneman@uza.be (Z.N.B.)
[2] Department of Medicine III, LMU Munich, University Hospital, 80799 Munich, Germany; F.Lichtenegger@gmx.de (F.S.L.); Marion.Subklewe@med.uni-muenchen.de (M.S.)
[3] Division of Hematology and Center for Cell Therapy & Regenerative Medicine, Antwerp University Hospital, 2650 Edegem, Antwerp, Belgium
* Correspondence: sebastien.anguille@uza.be; Tel.: +32-3-821-56-96

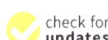

Received: 21 March 2019; Accepted: 24 April 2019; Published: 27 April 2019

Abstract: Acute myeloid leukemia (AML) is a type of blood cancer characterized by the uncontrolled clonal proliferation of myeloid hematopoietic progenitor cells in the bone marrow. The outcome of AML is poor, with five-year overall survival rates of less than 10% for the predominant group of patients older than 65 years. One of the main reasons for this poor outcome is that the majority of AML patients will relapse, even after they have attained complete remission by chemotherapy. Chemotherapy, supplemented with allogeneic hematopoietic stem cell transplantation in patients at high risk of relapse, is still the cornerstone of current AML treatment. Both therapies are, however, associated with significant morbidity and mortality. These observations illustrate the need for more effective and less toxic treatment options, especially in elderly AML and have fostered the development of novel immune-based strategies to treat AML. One of these strategies involves the use of a special type of immune cells, the dendritic cells (DCs). As central orchestrators of the immune system, DCs are key to the induction of anti-leukemia immunity. In this review, we provide an update of the clinical experience that has been obtained so far with this form of immunotherapy in patients with AML.

Keywords: dendritic cells; immunotherapy; acute myeloid leukemia

1. Introduction

Acute myeloid leukemia (AML) is a highly aggressive type of leukemia characterized by the uncontrolled clonal proliferation of abnormal myeloid cells in the bone marrow [1–3]. AML primarily affects older people; over 50% of AML patients are older than 65 [1,2]. The past decades have witnessed an increased incidence of AML, which is mainly due to the aging population [4]. Treatment of AML remains challenging, although considerable advances have been made over the last 50 years. In this context, an influential discovery in the treatment of AML was the cytarabine-based chemotherapy in association with an anthracycline or related agent during the 1970s. This combination chemotherapy regimen significantly improved the probability to induce complete remission (CR) [5] and has consequently remained the backbone of frontline AML therapy [6]. The next major development in the treatment of AML was marked by the implementation of allogeneic hematopoietic stem cell transplantation (HSCT), which transformed this disease into a potentially curable one [7].

Despite these accomplishments, the long-term outcome of adults with AML remains precarious, with a five-year overall survival (OS) rate hovering at around 25% [8]. According to data from the Surveillance, Epidemiology, and End Results (SEER) Program of the National Cancer Institute (NCI, Bethesda, MD, USA), the steady improvement in long-term survival since the mid-1970s is almost completely attributable to the decrease in mortality among patients younger than 65 years. By contrast, the prognosis of patients aged 65 years or older has not improved considerably over time, the latest reported five-year survival rate being <10% [8]. Considering the above observation that elderly patients represent a significant and rising proportion of AML patients [4], one cannot but conclude that the overall picture remains grim, and that the scientific and therapeutic progress made did not translate into an equivalent improvement in long-term survival [2].

Perhaps the most important reason for this unsatisfying outcome is the high relapse-rate in leukemia, especially in elderly AML patients. Indeed, up to 80% of the patients older than 60 years will eventually relapse, despite having initially achieved CR with conventional (poly)chemotherapy [9,10]. It is generally accepted that this relapse arises from the existence of a small reservoir of treatment-resistant leukemic (stem) cells (LSCs) that persist after chemotherapy [11], a condition known as minimal residual disease (MRD), which may evolve to a full clinical relapse [12,13]. Allogeneic HSCT can be used effectively to clear MRD and has a positive impact on relapse rate and survival. Unfortunately, HSCT is still associated with significant morbidity and mortality, generally limiting its use to younger patients with fewer co-morbidities [2]. For patients with no transplant donor available or for older patients who are usually deemed unfit for HSCT, there is currently no standard post-remission therapy to control MRD and avoid relapse [1,4,6,14].

The above observations emphasize the need for more effective and less aggressive treatment alternatives to improve the long-term outcome of AML, especially in elderly patients. It is within this context that immunotherapy has come to the fore in recent years [12,15–17]. From the experience with allogeneic HSCT, we have learned that immune cells are indeed capable of recognizing and eliminating AML cells—the so-called "graft-versus-leukemia" (GvL) effect [12,16]. Leukemia antigen-specific CD8+ cytotoxic T-lymphocytes (CTLs) and natural killer (NK) cells are the main immune effector cells responsible for attacking and killing AML cells (Figure 1) [12]. As conductors of the immunological orchestra, dendritic cells (DCs) are endowed with the potent and unique ability to harness the anti-leukemia activity of both immune effector cell types. It is therefore not surprising that DCs have attracted much interest in recent years as tools for immunotherapy of AML [12,18,19]. In this review, we summarize the clinical experience that has been obtained with this form of immunotherapy in AML.

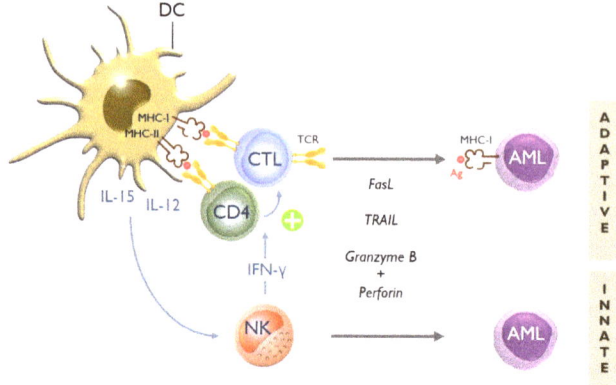

Figure 1. Dendritic cells are key to the induction of adaptive and innate anti-leukemia immunity. Dendritic

cells (DCs) can stimulate both adaptive and innate immune responses against acute myeloid leukemia (AML) cells [12]. There exist two types of adaptive immune responses: humoral or B-cell-mediated (not shown in this figure), and cellular or T-cell-mediated immune responses. The initiation of the latter type of immune response involves the presentation of AML-related antigens (Ag) by DCs via major histocompatibility complex (MHC) class I and II molecules to $CD8^+$ cytotoxic T-lymphocytes (CTLs) and $CD4^+$ helper T cells, respectively. If appropriately stimulated, naive $CD4^+$ T cells (T_H0) can be polarized into T helper type 1 (T_H1) cells, which in turn support the generation of antigen-specific CTLs (+). These CTLs—via their specific T-cell receptor (TCR)—are capable of recognizing AML cells that display the particular antigen(s) to which the CTLs are directed [12]. CTLs possess different tools in their armamentarium to kill AML cells, such as death receptor ligands (e.g., Fas ligand (FasL) and tumor necrosis factor-related apoptosis-inducing ligand (TRAIL)) and cytolytic proteins released from intracytoplasmic granules (e.g., granzyme B and perforin) [16]. The innate arm of the immune system is unequivocally important for mounting effective anti-leukemia immunity [20]. Innate effector cells, predominantly natural killer (NK) cells, are able to eradicate AML cells in a non-antigen-specific, non-MHC-restricted manner. NK cells can utilize the same cytolytic tools as CTLs [16]. In addition to their direct cytotoxic activity, NK cells also play an immunoregulatory role by secreting cytokines such as interferon (IFN)-γ. Through this so-called "helper" function, NK cells can support the generation of T_H1 and CTL responses [21,22]. Several DC-derived cytokines are known to be involved in DC-mediated NK-cell activation, including interleukin (IL)-12 and IL-15 [23]. The latter is usually not secreted by the DCs, but "trans-presented" on the DC surface via IL-15 receptor-α [24,25].

2. Clinical Use of DCs for Immunotherapy of AML

The feasibility, safety/toxicity and immunogenicity of DC vaccination in AML has been reviewed elsewhere (see Ref. [26]) and are outside the scope of this review. In addition, our group has previously done a cost–benefit analysis and found that DC therapy following chemotherapy is a cost-effective treatment [27]. Tables 1–3 provide an overview of all DC-based clinical studies performed so far in AML. As of 31 December 2018, nearly 200 patients with AML have been treated with this form of immunotherapy.

As shown in Tables 1–3 most studies have relied on DCs derived from autologous peripheral blood monocytes (moDCs), although allogeneic DCs have also been used [26]. In some studies, autologous leukemic blast cells were used as precursor cells for DC generation (AML-DCs) [26]. In one clinical trial, AML-DCs were generated from a leukemic cell line [28]. One drawback of the use of AML-DCs is their limited yield compared to moDCs, making clinical implementations more cumbersome [29]. In addition, in a head-to-head comparison between AML-DCs and moDCs, Draube and colleagues [29] found that moDCs were more effective in activating autologous leukemia-specific T cells than AML-DCs. Several arguments exist that could explain these findings. It has been postulated that AML-DCs lack the expression of 4-1BBL, an important ligand for co-stimulation [30]. Alternatively, indoleamine 2,3-dioxygenase 1 (IDO-1) expression by leukemic blasts can result in DCs with a more tolerogenic functionality [31]. Combined, these findings provide a preference of the use of moDCs over AML-DCs. On the other hand, AML-DCs have the advantage over moDCs in the sense that they present the full antigen repertoire of the leukemic blasts from which they are derived, thereby obviating the need for an antigen-loading step [26]. MoDCs, by contrast, require to be loaded with one or more AML antigens. This can be done by exogenous pulsing with a peptide (e.g., Wilms' tumor 1 [WT1] peptide) [32–36], by pulsing with apoptotic AML cells or lysates [37–40], by fusing the DCs with leukemic blasts (so-called fusion hybrids) [41,42], or by messenger RNA (mRNA) electroporation [8,43–45]. Messenger RNA electroporation involves the application of a brief electrical pulse to make the DC plasma membrane transiently permeable allowing the antigen-encoding mRNA to enter the cytosol. The mRNA will then be translated by the DCs into full-length antigenic protein. The translated antigen is further degraded into small peptide fragments, which are presented on the DC surface via major histocompatibility complex (MHC) molecules to the T cells. This technique has been used to load moDCs with one of the following leukemia-associated antigens: WT1, human telomerase reverse transcriptase (hTERT) and preferentially expressed antigen in melanoma (PRAME) [8,43–45]. mRNA electroporation is a non-viral gene transfer method; only one study implemented an (adeno)viral transduction approach for gene transfer of the leukemia-associated antigens survivin and MUC1 [46].

Table 1. Overview of DC (dendric cell) vaccine studies for AML (acute myeloid leukemia) in the post-HSCT setting.

	DC Type (Auto/Allo)	Antigen (Loading)	Immunological Effects	Clinical Effects
$n = 1$ [37]	CD34$^+$ DCs (allogeneic)	Apo-AML cells (pulsing)	Positive DTH ↑ T-cell reactivity to DCs	↓ AML cell load (morphological)
$n = 1$ [32]	moDCs (allogeneic)	WT1$_{235}$ (pulsing)	Positive DTH ↔ WT1-specific T cells	Absent
$n = 1$ [47]	MoDCs * (allogeneic)	Unloaded	Allo-MLR response to DCs	Absent
$n = 1$ [34]	moDCs (allogeneic)	WT1$_{37;126;187}$ (pulsing)	Absence of WT1 response	Absent
$n = 2$ [38]	moDCs (autologous)	AML cell lysate (pulsing)	Positive DTH ↑ T-cell reactivity to DCs	Absent
$n = 19/23$ [46]	MoDCs ** (autologous)	survivin/MUC1 (adenovirus)	ND	Induction of CR (13) Favorable OS (48.9% at 3 years)
$n = 12$ [46]	MoDCs ** (autologous)	survivin/MUC1 (adenovirus)	ND	Induction of CR (10)

Abbreviations: HSCT, hematopoietic stem cell transplantation; n, number of DC-treated patients; DC type, type of DC used; auto, DCs from autologous origin; allo, DCs from allogeneic origin; CD34$^+$ DCs, DCs derived from CD34$^+$ hematopoietic progenitor cells; moDCs, monocyte-derived DCs; *, in combination with donor lymphocyte infusions (DLI); **, in combination with cytokine-induced killer cells; Antigen, antigenic material used to load DCs; loading, antigen-loading method used; Apo-AML cells, apoptotic AML cells; WT1$_{37;126;187;235}$, designated epitope derived from Wilms' tumor 1 (WT1) antigen; MUC1, mucin 1; DTH, delayed-type hypersensitivity test; ↑, increase; ↔, steady state; allo-MLR, allogeneic mixed lymphocyte reaction; ND, no data; ↓, decrease; CR, complete remission; (number), number of patients in whom the designated clinical effect was observed; OS, overall survival.

Table 2. Overview of DC vaccine studies for AML in an advanced disease setting.

	DC Type (Auto/Allo)	Antigen (Loading)	Immunological Effects	Clinical Effects
$n = 1$ [41]	moDCs (allogeneic)	AML cells (fusion hybrids)	ND	Disease stabilization
$n = 4$ [39]	moDCs‖ (autologous)	Apo-AML cells (pulsing)	↑ AML-reactive T cells (2/4) ↑ WT1/hTERT-specific T cells (1/1)	Disease stabilization (2/4)
$n = 5$ [48]	AML-DCs (autologous)	NA	↑ PRAME-specific T cells (1/3) ↑ IFN-γ by CD4$^+$ T cells (2/3) T$_H$1/T$_H$2 cytokine profile	Disease stabilization (1) ↓ AML cell load (2) (morphological)
$n = 8$ † [35,36]	moDCs ‖ (autologous)	WT1 peptide (pulsing)	↑ WT1-specific T cells (in clinical responders) ↓ T$_{reg}$ cells and MDSCs (in clinical responders)	Disease stabilization (3) ↓ AML cell load (2) (molecular)
$n = 21$ [49]	AML-DCs ** (autologous)	NA	↑ CD4$^+$ and CD8$^+$ T cells ↑ T$_H$1 cytokines	Induction of CR (6) Induction of PR (9)

Abbreviations: n, number of DC-treated patients; †, including two patients with acute lymphoblastic leukemia (ALL); DC type, type of DC used; auto, DCs from autologous origin; allo, DCs from allogeneic origin; moDCs, monocyte-derived DCs; ‖, in combination with systemic administration of the Toll-like receptor agonist OK432; AML-DCs, AML cell-derived DCs; **, in combination with cytokine-induced killer cells and low-dose chemotherapy (for further details, see [49]); Antigen, antigenic material used to load DCs; loading, antigen-loading method used; Apo-AML cells, apoptotic AML cells; NA, not applicable; WT1, Wilms' tumor 1 antigen; ND, no data; ↑, increase; hTERT, human telomerase reverse transcriptase; PRAME, preferentially expressed antigen in melanoma; IFN-, interferon; T$_H$1/T$_H$2, T helper type 1 or 2; ↓, decrease; T$_{reg}$, regulatory T cells; MDSCs, myeloid-derived suppressor cells; CR, complete remission; PR, partial remission; (number), number of patients in whom the designated immunological or clinical effect was observed.

Table 3. Overview of DC vaccine studies for AML in a post-remission setting.

	DC Type (Auto/Allo)	Antigen (Loading)	Immunological Effects	Clinical Effects
n = 3 [ ]	moDCs ◊ (autologous)	WT1$_{235}$ (pulsing)	Positive DTH (2/3) ↑ WT1-specific T cells (2/2) No ↑ γδ T cells	Disease stabilization (1/3) ↓ AML cell load (1/3) (morphological)
n = 5 [,]	moDCs (autologous)	WT1/PRAME (mRNA EP)	Positive DTH (4) ↑ Ag-specific T cells (2)	Continued CR (21, 25, 33 m) (3)
n = 5 [ ]	AML-DCs (autologous)	NA	Minimal or absent DTH ↑ AML-reactive T cells (4/4) ↑ WT1-specific T cells (1/1) No ↑ T$_{reg}$ cells	Continued CR (13–16 m) (2)
n = 5 [ ]	moDCs (autologous)	Apo-AML cells (pulsing)	ND	Continued CR (+13 m) (1)
n = 12 [ ]	AML-DCs (allogeneic)	NA	Positive DTH ↑ WT1/PRAME-specific T cells	Disease stabilization (1) Disease stabilization (1) Favorable OS in patients without circulating blasts
n = 10/13 [ ]	moDCs (autologous)	WT1/PRAME/ CMVpp65 (mRNA EP)	Local immune response (10) ↑ Ag-specific T cells WT1 (2/10) PRAME (4/10) CMV (9/10)	Favorable RFS (1084 days vs. 396 days in matched cohort) Prolonged RFS and OS in immune responders
n = 17 [ ]	moDCs (autologous)	AML cells (fusion hybrids)	↑ AML-reactive T cells (6) ↑ AML Ag-specific T cells (2) (i.e., MUC1, WT1 or PRAME)	Favorable RFS (71% at 57 m)
n = 21 [ ]	moDCs (autologous)	hTERT (mRNA EP)	Positive DTH ↑ hTERT-specfic T cells (11/19)	Favorable RFS (58% at 52 m)
n = 30 [,]	moDCs (autologous)	WT1 (mRNA EP)	Positive DTH ↑ WT1-specific T cells (in clinical responders) NK activation (4/10)	Induction of CMR (9) Disease stabilization (4) Favorable RFS in responders Favorable OS

Abbreviations: n, number of DC-treated patients; DC type, type of DC used; auto, DCs from autologous origin; allo, DCs from allogeneic origin; moDCs, monocyte-derived DCs; ◊, pulsed with zoledronic acid in an attempt to induce γδ T-cell anti-leukemia immunity; AML-DCs, AML cell-derived DCs; Antigen, antigenic material used to load DCs; loading, antigen-loading method used; WT1$_{235}$, designated epitope derived from Wilms' tumor 1 (WT1) antigen; PRAME, preferentially expressed antigen in melanoma; mRNA EP, messenger RNA electroporation; NA, not applicable; Apo-AML cells, apoptotic AML cells; CMVpp65, Cytomegalovirus pp65 peptide; hTERT, human telomerase reverse transcriptase; DTH, delayed-type hypersensitivity test; ↑, increase; Ag, antigen; T$_{reg}$, regulatory T cells; ND, no data; MUC1, mucin 1; NK, natural killer cell; ↓, decrease; CR, complete remission; CMR, complete molecular remission; RFS, relapse-free survival; OS, overall survival; (number), number of patients in whom the designated immunological or clinical effect was observed; (number m), follow-up time in months.

Non-specific and antigen-specific immunological effects have been obtained in a considerable number of DC-treated AML patients. These effects include delayed-type hypersensitivity (DTH) skin test reactions, which essentially confirms the ability of the DCs to elicit T-cell-mediated immunity in vivo [ ]. Other (non-specific) signs of the immunogenicity of DC therapy that have been observed include: increases in CD4$^+$ and/or CD8$^+$ T-cell frequencies during or after DC administration [,], enhanced activation of CD4$^+$ T cells, as evidenced by their increased IFN-γ production following DC therapy [ ], and elevations in plasma levels of immunostimulatory or T$_H$1-polarizing cytokines (such as interleukin (IL)-2) [, ,]. Regarding the increased IFN-γ expression, it should be mentioned that IFN-γ can in turn have an effect on DCs. It is known that IFN-γ can induce IDO expression in subsets of DCs [ ] and that this can induce tolerance in the DCs under specific circumstances. This might serve as an explanation why IDO-1 expression correlates with poor clinical outcome in patients with AML [–]. To date, studies have focused on the effects of IDO-expression in AML-blasts. Therefore, during the generation of AML-DCs derived from AML-blasts, their IDO-1 expression status might need to be taken into consideration. In contrast, the effect of IDO-expression on the phenotype and function of moDCs has not been studied yet. Several studies listed in Tables 1– have provided proof-of-principle that antigen-loaded DCs can induce leukemia antigen-specific T-cell immunity in patients with AML.

Specific T-cell responses have been demonstrated by direct ex vivo tetramer analysis and/or following in vitro antigenic restimulation experiments towards the following AML-related tumor antigens: WT1 [33,35,36,39,44,51–53,58,59], PRAME [44,48,53,59], hTERT [39,60,61], and MUC1 [59]. It was also shown that DC-induced T-cell immune responses within a single patient can be directed against multiple antigens (e.g., WT1 and PRAME [44,53], or WT1 and hTERT [39]) and/or multiple epitopes a particular antigen (e.g., $WT1_{37-45}$, $WT1_{126-134}$, $WT1_{187-195}$, and $WT1_{235-243}$) [52]. This ability to induce multi-antigen- or multi-epitope-specific T-cell immunity is important, as this reduces the likelihood of tumor escape from T-cell recognition due to antigen loss (i.e., loss of expression of a single antigen/epitope) [62] or antigenic drift (i.e., mutations leading to epitope changes resulting in failure of the CTLs to recognize the original epitope) [63]. Theoretically, the use of DCs loaded with multiple antigens or AML lysates could also involve a higher risk of autoimmunity, for example, towards non-malignant cells that also express low levels of leukemia-associated antigens [64]. In clinical trials, treatment with multiple antigen-loaded DCs are well tolerated, and no or minor autoimmune reactions are normally observed [38]. Several studies have shown that DC therapy can also elicit leukemia antigen-specific T cells in the bone marrow compartment [39,59], which is of special importance in view of the observation that the bone marrow is the primary site where high-avidity AML-reactive CTLs reside [65].

In AML, DC vaccines have been applied in three different clinical settings: (a) in the context of HSCT, usually for treatment of relapsed AML after allogeneic HSCT (Table 1); (b) in an advanced disease setting, for example, for patients with refractory disease or relapsed AML for whom conventional treatment options have been exhausted (Table 2); and (c) after chemotherapy-induced remission of AML to prevent or delay relapse (Table 3). In the post-transplant relapse setting (Setting a), one study merits further discussion. Here, multi-genetically modified moDCs (Ad-siSSF DCs) were manufactured based on an adenovirus delivering: (i) secretory flagellin, a Toll-like receptor (TLR)-5 agonist inducing DC maturation; (ii) a survivin-MUC1 fusion protein, two leukemia-associated antigens; and (iii) SOCS1 shRNA, an RNA interference moiety overriding the intracellular immune checkpoint molecule SOCS1 [46]. Forty-eight patients with a post-transplant acute leukemia relapse (all AML, except for seven patients with acute lymphoblastic leukemia) were treated with either Ad-siSSF DCs or donor lymphocyte infusions (DLI). The vaccine was not only found to be safe but also induced a three-year OS of 48.9% compared with 27.5% in the DLI group. Thirteen out of 23 (57%) patients treated with the Ad-siSSF DCs achieved CR versus 12 out of 25 (48%) treated with DLI. In a second phase, 12 AML patients with early molecular relapse after HSCT were treated with Ad-siSSF DCs. Here, DC vaccination induced a CR rate of 83% (10 out of 12 patients). It should, however, be pointed out that the patients also received two subsequent infusions of cytokine-induced killer cells (CIKs), potentially contributing to the clinical effects of the DC vaccine. Moreover, all 12 patients were in early (molecular) relapse and efficacy would likely be lower in full-blown relapse [66,67]. This is supported by a mouse model of DC-based immunotherapy of AML [68], indicating that the therapeutic utility of DC vaccines is limited in the case of a high leukemic cell load.

In patients with relapsed/refractory AML (Setting b), clinical responses were usually limited to temporary disease stabilizations before further progression [39,41,48] and/or transient reductions in leukemic cell load [35,36,48]. The latter was evidenced either morphologically by demonstration of decreases in blast counts [48], or molecularly by demonstration of decreases in WT1 tumor marker transcript levels (as measured by quantitative reverse-transcriptase polymerase chain reaction (qRT-PCR) [35,36]. WT1 is a transcription factor used as a molecular marker for the monitoring of minimal residual disease in leukemia, especially in myeloid leukemias and myelodysplastic syndrome [69]. It is also a predictive factor of imminent relapse in AML patients, including those that received allo-SCT, even when other markers are not available [70–73]. Only one study [49] reported CR and partial remissions (PR) in the relapsed/refractory setting. It is important to note, however, that these patients also received chemotherapy and CIKs, making it difficult to draw conclusions about the effectiveness of DCs as a stand-alone treatment for advanced AML. In patients with advanced AML, immunosuppressive cells (T$_{reg}$ cells and myeloid-derived suppressor cells (MDSCs)) may prevail over anti-tumor immune effector cells (CTLs and NK cells), explaining the higher likelihood of treatment failure when applying immunotherapy in the context of a high tumor burden [67,74].

The most obvious proof of clinical activity of DC vaccination in monotherapy has indeed been gathered in patients with low disease burden or MRD (Setting c). The concept is to administer DC vaccines as consolidation therapy to prevent or postpone relapse. Sustained and longer than usual CRs were reported in all post-remission DC vaccine studies, but the single-arm design of these studies precludes drawing firm conclusions on the true efficacy with respect to relapse prevention [28,40,43,44,50,51]. Nevertheless, several clinical trials have reported exceptionally long progression-free survival (PFS) times [42,44,45], indicating that DC vaccination can be an effective strategy to prevent/delay relapse. In the study by Rosenblatt et al. [42], 17 AML patients who achieved remission after chemotherapy, were vaccinated with moDCs fused to AML cells. This resulted in a 71% relapse-free survival at a median follow-up of 57 months. Moreover, the treatment was well tolerated and adverse events were transient and minor (grade 1–2 intensity). It should, however, be noted that the selection bias for long-term survivors requires careful interpretation of the data [42]. The achieved prevention of relapse is nonetheless remarkable when comparing to the treatment of patients aged 60–70 years with reduced intensity conditioning HSCT or chemotherapy alone resulting in three-year relapse-free survival of 68% and 19%, respectively [75]. In a study by Khoury et al. [45], 22 intermediate- or high-risk AML patients (median age of 58 years) were treated with human telomerase reverse transcriptase (hTERT)-expressing DCs. Given the central role of telomerase activity in maintaining self-renewal of leukemic stem cells, hTERT-DC vaccination may be ideally suited to target the small reservoir of residual leukemic stem cells that persist after chemotherapy. hTERT-DC vaccines administered in the post-remission setting were well tolerated and, after 52 months, 58% of the patients were free of disease recurrence. This compares favorably to the reported three-year relapse rates of 60% and 90% for patients with intermediate- and high-risk AML, respectively [76].

The group of Dr Felix Lichtenegger and Prof Marion Subklewe from Munich, Germany, used TLR-7/8-matured DCs loaded with *WT1*, *PRAME* and *CMVpp65* mRNA in 10 AML patients who were in remission after intensive chemotherapy, but at high risk of relapse. The vaccination proved to be safe and resulted in local inflammatory responses with dense T-cell infiltration. Increased antigen-specific CD8$^+$ T cells were seen in peripheral blood for all three antigens. PFS was 1084 days, comparing favorably to a closely matched cohort from a patient registry of the same study group (Table 3). Median overall survival was not reached at the end of observation. In particular, excellent survival was seen in the immune responders (Ref. [44] and personal communication).

Our group has also shown that DC vaccination can confer an OS benefit in remission patients with AML. In a recently completed phase II clinical trial [8], we treated 30 AML patients with autologous, *WT1* mRNA-electroporated moDCs following standard induction chemotherapy; 27 of them were in CR and three were in PR. Two out of these three patients in PR were brought into CR by DC therapy. Most patients did not have morphologically demonstrable disease prior to the start of DC therapy but had evidence of residual disease at the molecular level (i.e., elevated *WT1* transcript levels in blood and/or marrow, as determined by qRT-PCR). In nine patients who had an increased level of the WT1 tumor marker at the start of DC therapy, *WT1* transcript levels returned to normal during DC vaccination, compatible with the induction of complete molecular remission (CMR). Five of these nine patients are still in CMR now more than five years after diagnosis and can be probably considered as cured. Apart from induction of morphological and/or molecular remission, four patients experienced disease stabilization for a period of time, a situation that is highly uncommon in AML given the aggressive behavior of this disease. The objective clinical response rate was 43%. PFS was significantly different in responders vs. non-responders. OS compared favorable to controls from the SEER and Swedish Acute Leukemia Registry, in patients ≤65 as well as >65 years, and was linked to the induction of WT1-specific CD8$^+$ T-cell immunity [8]. Eleven out of 30 patients were alive in CR with a median OS from diagnosis of eight years (range 72.6–125.5 months), at the time of publication.

These encouraging results have led us to embark on a follow-up randomized clinical trial comparing *WT1* mRNA-electroporated DC vaccination with standard-of-care in the post-remission setting of AML. The study is open for inclusion (Clinicaltrials.gov identifier NCT01686334).

3. Conclusions and Future Perspectives

Taken together, it can be concluded that DC-based immunotherapy has the potential to bring about demonstrable clinical responses in patients with AML. This holds particularly true in the post-remission setting of AML where treatment with DCs can produce durable remissions and prevent or delay relapse in some high-risk patients. Unfortunately, not all patients experience overt clinical benefit from this form of immunotherapy, underscoring the need to delve further into the possible reasons for therapeutic success or failure. In all studies listed in Tables 1–3 patients who failed to mount an immune response to DC vaccination had an inferior clinical outcome as compared to immune responders, indicating that the elicitation of (anti-leukemia) immunity by DCs is required to obtain a clinical response. For example, in our phase II clinical trial of WT1-targeted DC vaccination as a post-remission treatment for AML, only patients in whom DC vaccination elicited a poly-epitope WT1-specific CD8$^+$ T-cell immune response experienced sustained CR [52,58]. There was also evidence in our study for a correlation between DC-induced NK cell activation and clinical activity [52]. As becomes evident from the data summarized in Tables 1–3 there is also a considerable number of patients who do not mount a clinical response despite the presence of DC-induced immune changes. One possible explanation for this observation is that the DCs currently used for immunotherapy are too weakly immunogenic to evoke clinically beneficial immune responses and/or that they do not induce the "right" type of immunity, i.e.:

- The immunostimulatory activity of the DCs may be too weak to induce high-avidity, long-lived leukemia-specific CTLs capable of mediating cytotoxicity of AML cells [33,39].
- The immunostimulatory activity of the DCs may be too weak to activate NK cells or γδ T-cells and harness innate immunity against AML cells [77–82].
- The immunostimulatory activity of the DCs may be too weak to overcome the immunosuppressive action of T_{reg} cells and MDSCs [35,36,51,83].
- The DCs used for therapy may favor the induction of a T_H2 response over a T_H1 response [84,85], which is otherwise the type of immunity that would be preferred in the setting of cancer immunotherapy [48].
- The DCs used for therapy may favor immune tolerance and produce undesired immune effects such as induction of T_{reg} cells and MDSCs [35,36,86].

These observations explain the impetus behind the many research efforts that are currently being undertaken to optimize the immunostimulatory properties of DCs in order to increase the likelihood of inducing protective anti-leukemia immunity in AML patients and, consequently, also the likelihood of therapeutic success [87]. One of the promising next-generation DC product candidates are IL-15-differentiated DCs [88]. In contrast to conventional IL-4 moDC vaccines, IL-15 DCs proved to be superior antigen-presenting cells, capable of direct tumoricidal activity [89], and, via expression of IL-15, capable of harnessing both NK cells and γδ T cells in the anti-tumor immune response [82,90].

Combining DC therapy with immune checkpoint targeting strategies, currently evoking a renaissance in the cancer immunotherapy field [91,92], is another avenue to unlock the full therapeutic potential of DC vaccines for AML. Moving beyond the combination of DC vaccines with systemic monoclonal antibodies, interceding programmed death (PD)-1/PD-L signaling in the DCs themselves reinforces the DC-mediated T cell and NK cell activation and prevents T_{reg} cell stimulation [91,92].

Another potential approach to enhance efficacy of DC therapy is combination with AML-specific monoclonal antibodies. Leukemia-specific mAb targets include CD33, CD123 and CD56, as reviewed in [93,94]. Especially ADCC-eliciting antibodies are interesting in the context of combination with DC vaccination, as ADCC-mediated killing results in the release of tumor neoantigens that can be taken up and cross-presented by tumor-residing DCs [95]. However, as of now, there are no studies combining such mAbs with DC therapy in AML.

Finally, there is an increasing interest to combine DC vaccination with conventional therapies, given the potential synergism between both. In our phase II clinical trial of *WT1* mRNA-electroporated DC vaccination, we observed unexpectedly high second remission rates and OS times to subsequent salvage treatment (i.e., chemotherapy and/or allogeneic HSCT) in vaccinated patients that experienced the first relapse. This may indicate that DC vaccination can potentiate the response to subsequent treatment, an observation that has also been made in the solid tumor vaccine field [67,96]. Hypomethylating agents (HMAs), which are being increasingly applied in the frontline treatment of elderly AML patients, have also shown synergistic activity with DC vaccination; one of the mechanisms underlying this synergism involves reduction of PD-1 expression on T cells and inhibition of MDSCs [97]. A phase II randomized clinical trial (Clinicaltrials.gov identifier NCT01686334) is currently ongoing to evaluate the effectiveness of combined HMA treatment and *WT1* mRNA-targeted DC vaccination.

Author Contributions: Conceptualization, H.H.V.A. and S.A.; Methodology, H.H.V.A., M.V., F.S.L., G.R., D.C.-D. and S.A.; Writing—Original Draft Preparation, H.H.V.A., M.V., F.S.L. and S.A.; Writing—Review and Editing, E.L., M.V., D.C.-D., M.S., V.F.V.T., Z.N.B. and S.A.; Visualization, S.A.; Supervision, E.L., M.S., V.F.V.T., Z.N.B. and S.A.; Project Administration, E.L.; and Funding Acquisition, E.L., V.F.V.T., Z.N.B. and S.A.

Funding: This work was supported by grants from the Fund for Scientific Research Flanders (FWO Vlaanderen, grants G.0535.18N and 1524919N), the Baillet-Latour Fund, Kom op Tegen Kanker (KoTK) and the Belgian Foundation against Cancer (Stichting tegen Kanker, grant 2016-138 FAF-C/2016/764). We also received support from a Methusalem Fund from the University of Antwerp, from the Kaushik Bhansali Fund, and from the Belgian public utility foundations VOCATIO and Horlait-Dapsens. H.H.V.A. held a Ph.D. fellowship of the FWO (grant 11ZL518N). MV holds a Doctoral Grant Strategic Basic Research of the FWO (grant 1S24517N). G.R. receives a doctoral scholarship from the University of Antwerp. D.C.D. is supported by a DOC-PRO Ph.D. grant of the Special Research Fund (BOF) of the University of Antwerp.

Conflicts of Interest: V.F.V.T. and Z.N.B. are co-inventors of a patent covering the messenger RNA electroporation technique (WO/2003/000907; improved transfection of eukaryotic cells with linear polynucleotides by electroporation). The remaining authors declare no competing financial interests.

References

1. Estey, E.; Doehner, H. Acute myeloid leukaemia. *Lancet* **2006**, *368*, 1894–1907. [CrossRef]
2. Ferrara, F.; Schiffer, C.A. Acute myeloid leukaemia in adults. *Lancet* **2013**, *381*, 484–495. [CrossRef]
3. De Veirman, K.; Van Valckenborgh, E.; Lahmar, Q.; Geeraerts, X.; De Bruyne, E.; Menu, E.; Van Riet, I.; Vanderkerken, K.; Van Ginderachter, J.A. Myeloid-derived suppressor cells as therapeutic target in hematological malignancies. *Front. Oncol.* **2014**, *4*, 349. [CrossRef] [PubMed]
4. Sekeres, M.A. Treatment of older adults with acute myeloid leukemia: state of the art and current perspectives. *Haematologica* **2008**, *93*, 1769–1772. [CrossRef] [PubMed]
5. Tallman, M.S.; Gilliland, D.G.; Rowe, J.M. Drug therapy for acute myeloid leukemia. *Blood* **2005**, *106*, 1154–1163. [CrossRef]
6. Rowe, J.M.; Tallman, M.S. How I treat acute myeloid leukemia. *Blood* **2010**, *116*, 3147–3156. [CrossRef]
7. Peccatori, J.; Ciceri, F. Allogeneic stem cell transplantation for acute myeloid leukemia. *Haematologica* **2010**, *95*, 857–859. [CrossRef]
8. Anguille, S.; Van de Velde, A.L.; Smits, E.L.; Van Tendeloo, V.F.; Juliusson, G.; Cools, N.; Nijs, G.; Stein, B.; Lion, E.; Van Driessche, A.; et al. Dendritic cell vaccination as postremission treatment to prevent or delay relapse in acute myeloid leukemia. *Blood* **2017**, *130*, 1713–1721. [CrossRef] [PubMed]
9. Buchner, T.; Berdel, W.E.; Haferlach, C.; Schnittger, S.; Haferlach, T.; Serve, H.; Mueller-Tidow, C.; Braess, J.; Spiekermann, K.; Kienast, J.; et al. Long-term results in patients with acute myeloid leukemia (AML): The influence of high-dose AraC, G-CSF priming, autologous transplantation, prolonged maintenance, age, history, cytogenetics, and mutation status. Data of the AMLCG 1999 trial. *Blood* **2009**, *114*, 200–201.
10. Stone, R.M.; Berg, D.T.; George, S.L.; Dodge, R.K.; Paciucci, P.A.; Schulman, P.P.; Lee, E.J.; Moore, J.O.; Powell, B.L.; Baer, M.R.; et al. Postremission therapy in older patients with de novo acute myeloid leukemia: a randomized trial comparing mitoxantrone and intermediate-dose cytarabine with standard-dose cytarabine. *Blood* **2001**, *98*, 548–553. [CrossRef]

11. Snauwaert, S.; Vandekerckhove, B.; Kerre, T. Can immunotherapy specifically target acute myeloid leukemic stem cells? *Oncoimmunology* **2013**, *2*, e22943. [CrossRef]
12. Schurch, C.M.; Riether, C.; Ochsenbein, A.F. Dendritic cell-based immunotherapy for myeloid leukemias. *Front. Immunol.* **2013**, *4*, 496. [CrossRef]
13. Hourigan, C.S.; Karp, J.E. Minimal residual disease in acute myeloid leukaemia. *Nat. Rev. Clin. Oncol.* **2013**, *10*, 460–471. [CrossRef] [PubMed]
14. Vasu, S.; Kohlschmidt, J.; Mrozek, K.; Eisfeld, A.K.; Nicolet, D.; Sterling, L.J.; Becker, H.; Metzeler, K.H.; Papaioannou, D.; Powell, B.L.; et al. Ten-year outcome of patients with acute myeloid leukemia not treated with allogeneic transplantation in first complete remission. *Blood Adv.* **2018**, *2*, 1645–1650. [CrossRef]
15. Smits, E.L.J.M.; Berneman, Z.N.; Van Tendeloo, V.F.I. Immunotherapy of acute myeloid leukemia: current approaches. *Oncologist* **2009**, *14*, 240–252. [CrossRef]
16. Barrett, A.J.; Le Blanc, K. Immunotherapy prospects for acute myeloid leukaemia. *Clin. Exp. Immunol.* **2010**, *161*, 223–232. [CrossRef]
17. Martner, A.; Thoren, F.B.; Aurelius, J.; Hellstrand, K. Immunotherapeutic strategies for relapse control in acute myeloid leukemia. *Blood Rev.* **2013**, *27*, 209–216. [CrossRef] [PubMed]
18. Tesfatsion, D.A. Dendritic cell vaccine against leukemia: advances and perspectives. *Immunotherapy* **2014**, *6*, 485–496. [CrossRef] [PubMed]
19. Pyzer, A.R.; Avigan, D.E.; Rosenblatt, J. Clinical trials of dendritic cell-based cancer vaccines in hematologic malignancies. *Hum. Vaccin. Immunother.* **2014**, *10*, 3125–3131. [CrossRef]
20. Rey, J.; Veuillen, C.; Vey, N.; Bouabdallah, R.; Olive, D. Natural killer and gamma delta T cells in haematological malignancies: enhancing the immune effectors. *Trends Mol. Med.* **2009**, *15*, 275–284. [CrossRef]
21. Hardy, M.Y.; Kassianos, A.J.; Vulink, A.; Wilkinson, R.; Jongbloed, S.L.; Hart, D.N.; Radford, K.J. NK cells enhance the induction of CTL responses by IL-15 monocyte-derived dendritic cells. *Immunol. Cell Biol.* **2009**, *87*, 606–614. [CrossRef]
22. Pampena, M.B.; Levy, E.M. Natural killer cells as helper cells in dendritic cell cancer vaccines. *Front. Immunol.* **2015**, *6*, 13. [CrossRef]
23. Chijioke, O.; Munz, C. Dendritic cell derived cytokines in human natural killer cell differentiation and activation. *Front. Immunol.* **2013**, *4*, 365. [CrossRef] [PubMed]
24. Lucas, M.; Schachterle, W.; Oberle, K.; Aichele, P.; Diefenbach, A. Dendritic cells prime natural killer cells by trans-presenting interleukin 15. *Immunity* **2007**, *26*, 503–517. [CrossRef] [PubMed]
25. Mortier, E.; Woo, T.; Advincula, R.; Gozalo, S.; Ma, A. IL-15Ralpha chaperones IL-15 to stable dendritic cell membrane complexes that activate NK cells via trans presentation. *J. Exp. Med.* **2008**, *205*, 1213–1225. [CrossRef] [PubMed]
26. Anguille, S.; Willemen, Y.; Lion, E.; Smits, E.L.; Berneman, Z.N. Dendritic cell vaccination in acute myeloid leukemia. *Cytotherapy* **2012**, *14*, 647–656. [CrossRef]
27. Van de Velde, A.L.; Beutels, P.; Smits, E.L.; Van Tendeloo, V.F.; Nijs, G.; Anguille, S.; Verlinden, A.; Gadisseur, A.P.; Schroyens, W.A.; Dom, S.; et al. Medical costs of treatment and survival of patients with acute myeloid leukemia in Belgium. *Leuk. Res.* **2016**, *46*, 26–29. [CrossRef] [PubMed]
28. van de Loosdrecht, A.A.; van Wetering, S.; Santegoets, S.; Singh, S.K.; Eeltink, C.M.; den Hartog, Y.; Koppes, M.; Kaspers, J.; Ossenkoppele, G.J.; Kruisbeek, A.M.; et al. A novel allogeneic off-the-shelf dendritic cell vaccine for post-remission treatment of elderly patients with acute myeloid leukemia. *Cancer Immunol. Immunother.* **2018**, *67*, 1505–1518. [CrossRef] [PubMed]
29. Draube, A.; Beyer, M.; Wolf, J. Activation of autologous leukemia-specific T cells in acute myeloid leukemia: monocyte-derived dendritic cells cocultured with leukemic blasts compared with leukemia-derived dendritic cells. *Eur. J. Haematol.* **2008**, *81*, 281–288. [CrossRef]
30. Houtenbos, I.; Westers, T.M.; Dijkhuis, A.; de Gruijl, T.D.; Ossenkoppele, G.J.; van de Loosdrecht, A.A. Leukemia-specific T-cell reactivity induced by leukemic dendritic cells is augmented by 4-1BB targeting. *Clin. Cancer Res.: Off. J. Am. Assoc. Cancer Res.* **2007**, *13*, 307–315. [CrossRef] [PubMed]
31. Curti, A.; Pandolfi, S.; Valzasina, B.; Aluigi, M.; Isidori, A.; Ferri, E.; Salvestrini, V.; Bonanno, G.; Rutella, S.; Durelli, I.; et al. Modulation of tryptophan catabolism by human leukemic cells results in the conversion of CD25- into CD25+ T regulatory cells. *Blood* **2007**, *109*, 2871–2877. [CrossRef]
32. Kitawaki, T.; Kadowaki, N.; Kondo, T.; Ishikawa, T.; Ichinohe, T.; Teramukai, S.; Fukushima, M.; Kasai, Y.; Maekawa, T.; Uchiyama, T. Potential of dendritic-cell immunotherapy for relapse after allogeneic

hematopoietic stem cell transplantation, shown by WT1 peptide- and keyhole-limpet-hemocyanin-pulsed, donor-derived dendritic-cell vaccine for acute myeloid leukemia. *Am. J. Hematol.* **2008**, *83*, 315–317. [CrossRef]
33. Kitawaki, T.; Kadowaki, N.; Fukunaga, K.; Kasai, Y.; Maekawa, T.; Ohmori, K.; Kondo, T.; Maekawa, R.; Takahara, M.; Nieda, M.; et al. A phase I/IIa clinical trial of immunotherapy for elderly patients with acute myeloid leukaemia using dendritic cells co-pulsed with WT1 peptide and zoledronate. *Br. J. Haematol.* **2011**, *153*, 796–799. [CrossRef]
34. Shah, N.N.; Loeb, D.M.; Khuu, H.; Stroncek, D.; Ariyo, T.; Raffeld, M.; Delbrook, C.; Mackall, C.L.; Wayne, A.S.; Fry, T.J. Induction of Immune Response after Allogeneic Wilms' Tumor 1 Dendritic Cell Vaccination and Donor Lymphocyte Infusion in Patients with Hematologic Malignancies and Post-Transplantation Relapse. *Biol. Blood Marrow Transpl.* **2016**, *22*, 2149–2154. [CrossRef] [PubMed]
35. Ota, S.; Ogasawara, M. Vaccination of acute leukemia patients with WT1 peptide-pulsed dendritic cells induces immunological and clinical responses: a pilot study. *Blood* **2014**, *124*, 2319.
36. Ogasawara, M.; Ota, S. Dendritic cell vaccination in acute leukemia patients induces reduction of myeloid-derived suppressor cells: immunological analysis of a pilot study. *Blood* **2014**, *124*, 1113.
37. Fujii, S.; Shimizu, K.; Fujimoto, K.; Kiyokawa, T.; Tsukamoto, A.; Sanada, I.; Kawano, F. Treatment of post-transplanted, relapsed patients with hematological malignancies by infusion of HLA-matched, allogeneic-dendritic cells (DCs) pulsed with irradiated tumor cells and primed T cells. *Leuk. Lymphoma* **2001**, *42*, 357–369. [CrossRef]
38. Lee, J.J.; Kook, H.; Park, M.S.; Nam, J.H.; Choi, B.H.; Song, W.H.; Park, K.S.; Lee, I.K.; Chung, I.J.; Hwang, T.J.; et al. Immunotherapy using autologous monocyte-derived dendritic cells pulsed with leukemic cell lysates for acute myeloid leukemia relapse after autologous peripheral blood stem cell transplantation. *J. Clin. Apher.* **2004**, *19*, 66–70. [CrossRef] [PubMed]
39. Kitawaki, T.; Kadowaki, N.; Fukunaga, K.; Kasai, Y.; Maekawa, T.; Ohmori, K.; Itoh, T.; Shimizu, A.; Kuzushima, K.; Kondo, T.; et al. Cross-priming of CD8(+) T cells in vivo by dendritic cells pulsed with autologous apoptotic leukemic cells in immunotherapy for elderly patients with acute myeloid leukemia. *Exp. Hematol.* **2011**, *39*, 424–433. [CrossRef]
40. Chevallier, P.; Saiagh, S.; Dehame, V.; Guillaume, T.; Peterlin, P.; Garnier, A.; Le Bris, Y.; Bercegeay, S.; Coulais, D.; Rambaud, M.A.; et al. A Phase I/II Study of Vaccination By Autologous Leukemic Apoptotic Corpse Pulsed Dendritic Cells for Elderly Acute Myeloid Leukemia Patients in First or Second Complete Remission (LAM DC trial). *Blood* **2016**, *128*, 2821.
41. Massumoto, C.; Sousa-Canavez, J.M.; Leite, K.R.; Camara-Lopes, L.H. Stabilization of acute myeloid leukemia with a dendritic cell vaccine. *Hematol. Oncol. Stem Cell* **2008**, *1*, 239–240. [CrossRef]
42. Rosenblatt, J.; Stone, R.M.; Uhl, L.; Neuberg, D.; Joyce, R.; Levine, J.D.; Arnason, J.; McMasters, M.; Luptakova, K.; Jain, S.; et al. Individualized vaccination of AML patients in remission is associated with induction of antileukemia immunity and prolonged remissions. *Sci. Transl. Med.* **2016**, *8*, 368ra171. [CrossRef] [PubMed]
43. Bigalke, I.; Fløisand, Y.; Solum, G.; Hønnåshagen, K.; Lundby, M.; Anderson, K.; Sæbøe-Larssen, S.; Inderberg, E.-M.; Eckl, J.; Schendel, D.J.; et al. AML Patients in Minimal Residual Disease Vaccinated with a Novel Generation of Fast Dendritic Cells Expressing WT-1 and PRAME Mount Specific Immune Responses That Relate to Clinical Outcome. *Blood* **2015**, *126*, 3798.
44. Lichtenegger, F.S.; Deiser, K.; Rothe, M.; Schnorfeil, F.M.; Krupka, C.; Augsberger, C.; Kohnke, T.; Bucklein, V.L.; Altmann, T.; Moosmann, A.; et al. Induction of Antigen-Specific T-Cell Responses through Dendritic Cell Vaccination in AML: Results of a Phase I/II Trial and Ex Vivo Enhancement By Checkpoint Blockade. *Blood* **2016**, *128*, 5.
45. Khoury, H.J.; Collins, R.H., Jr.; Blum, W.; Stiff, P.S.; Elias, L.; Lebkowski, J.S.; Reddy, A.; Nishimoto, K.P.; Sen, D.; Wirth, E.D., 3rd; et al. Immune responses and long-term disease recurrence status after telomerase-based dendritic cell immunotherapy in patients with acute myeloid leukemia. *Cancer* **2017**, *123*, 3061–3072. [CrossRef]
46. Wang, D.H.; Huang, X.F.; Hong, B.X.; Song, X.T.; Hu, L.D.; Jiang, M.; Zhang, B.; Ning, H.M.; Li, Y.H.; Xu, C.; et al. Efficacy of intracellular immune checkpoint-silenced DC vaccine. *JCI Insight* **2018**, *3*. [CrossRef]
47. Ho, V.T.; Kim, H.T.; Kao, G.; Cutler, C.; Levine, J.; Rosenblatt, J.; Joyce, R.; Antin, J.H.; Soiffer, R.J.; Ritz, J.; et al. Sequential infusion of donor-derived dendritic cells with donor lymphocyte infusion for relapsed

hematologic cancers after allogeneic hematopoietic stem cell transplantation. *Am. J. Hematol.* **2014**, *89*, 1092–1096. [CrossRef]
48. Li, L.; Giannopoulos, K.; Reinhardt, P.; Tabarkiewicz, J.; Schmitt, A.; Greiner, J.; Rolinski, J.; Hus, I.; Dmoszynska, A.; Wiesneth, M.; et al. Immunotherapy for patients with acute myeloid leukemia using autologous dendritic cells generated from leukemic blasts. *Int. J. Oncol.* **2006**, *28*, 855–861. [CrossRef] [PubMed]
49. Dong, M.; Liang, D.; Li, Y.; Kong, D.; Kang, P.; Li, K.; Ping, C.; Zhang, Y.; Zhou, X.; Zhang, Y.; et al. Autologous dendritic cells combined with cytokine-induced killer cells synergize low-dose chemotherapy in elderly patients with acute myeloid leukaemia. *J. Int. Med Res.* **2012**, *40*, 1265–1274. [CrossRef] [PubMed]
50. Przespolewski, A.; Szeles, A.; Wang, E.S. Advances in immunotherapy for acute myeloid leukemia. *Future Oncol. (Lond. Engl.)* **2018**, *14*, 963–978. [CrossRef]
51. Roddie, H.; Klammer, M.; Thomas, C.; Thomson, R.; Atkinson, A.; Sproul, A.; Waterfall, M.; Samuel, K.; Yin, J.; Johnson, P.; et al. Phase I/II study of vaccination with dendritic-like leukaemia cells for the immunotherapy of acute myeloid leukaemia. *Br. J. Haematol.* **2006**, *133*, 152–157. [CrossRef]
52. Van Tendeloo, V.F.; Van de Velde, A.; Van Driessche, A.; Cools, N.; Anguille, S.; Ladell, K.; Gostick, E.; Vermeulen, K.; Pieters, K.; Nijs, G.; et al. Induction of complete and molecular remissions in acute myeloid leukemia by Wilms' tumor 1 antigen-targeted dendritic cell vaccination. *Proc. Natl. Acad. Sci. USA* **2010**, *107*, 13824–13829. [CrossRef]
53. de Gruijl, T.D.; Santegoets, S.; van Wetering, S.; Singh, S.K.; Hall, A.; van den Loosdrecht, A.A.; Kruisbeek, A.M. Allogeneic dendritic cell (DC) vaccination as an "off the shelf" treatment to prevent or delay relapse in elderly acute myeloid leukemia patients: Results of phase I/IIa safety and feasibility study. *J. Immunother. Cancer* **2013**, *1*, P205. [CrossRef]
54. Mellor, A.L.; Lemos, H.; Huang, L. Indoleamine 2,3-Dioxygenase and Tolerance: Where Are We Now? *Front. Immunol.* **2017**, *8*, 1360. [CrossRef]
55. Chamuleau, M.E.; van de Loosdrecht, A.A.; Hess, C.J.; Janssen, J.J.; Zevenbergen, A.; Delwel, R.; Valk, P.J.; Lowenberg, B.; Ossenkoppele, G.J. High INDO (indoleamine 2,3-dioxygenase) mRNA level in blasts of acute myeloid leukemic patients predicts poor clinical outcome. *Haematologica* **2008**, *93*, 1894–1898. [CrossRef] [PubMed]
56. Folgiero, V.; Goffredo, B.M.; Filippini, P.; Masetti, R.; Bonanno, G.; Caruso, R.; Bertaina, V.; Mastronuzzi, A.; Gaspari, S.; Zecca, M.; et al. Indoleamine 2,3-dioxygenase 1 (IDO1) activity in leukemia blasts correlates with poor outcome in childhood acute myeloid leukemia. *Oncotarget* **2014**, *5*, 2052–2064. [CrossRef] [PubMed]
57. Mangaonkar, A.; Mondal, A.K.; Fulzule, S.; Pundkar, C.; Park, E.J.; Jillella, A.; Kota, V.; Xu, H.; Savage, N.M.; Shi, H.; et al. A novel immunohistochemical score to predict early mortality in acute myeloid leukemia patients based on indoleamine 2,3 dioxygenase expression. *Sci. Rep.* **2017**, *7*, 12892. [CrossRef]
58. Berneman, Z.N.; Van de Velde, A.L.; Willemen, Y.; Anguille, S.; Saevels, K.; Germonpré, P.; Huizing, M.T.; Peeters, M.; Snoeckx, A.; Parizel, P.; et al. Vaccination with WT1 mRNA-electroporated dendritic cells: report of clinical outcome in 66 cancer patients. *Blood* **2014**, *124*, 310.
59. Rosenblatt, J.; Stone, R.M.; Uhl, L.; Neuberg, D.; Vasir, B.; Somaiya, P.; Joyce, R.; Levine, J.D.; Boussiotis, V.A.; Zwicker, J.; et al. Clinical trial evaluating DC/AML fusion cell vaccination in AML patients who achieve a chemotherapy-induced remission. *Biol. Blood Marrow Transpl.* **2014**, *20*, S50. [CrossRef]
60. DiPersio, J.F.; Collins, R.H., Jr.; Blum, W.; Devetten, M.P.; Stiff, P.; Elias, L.; Reddy, A.; Smith, J.A.; Khoury, H.J. Immune Responses in AML Patients Following Vaccination with GRNVAC1, Autologous RNA Transfected Dendritic Cells Expressing Telomerase Catalytic Subunit hTERT. *Blood* **2009**, *114*, 262.
61. Khoury, H.J.; Collins, R.H., Jr.; Blum, W.; Maness, L.; Stiff, P.; Kelsey, S.M.; Reddy, A.; Smith, J.A.; DiPersio, J.F. Prolonged administration of the telomerase vaccine GRNVAC1 is well tolerated and appears to be associated with favorable outcomes in high-risk acute myeloid leukemia (AML). *Blood* **2010**, *116*, 904.
62. Teague, R.M.; Kline, J. Immune evasion in acute myeloid leukemia: current concepts and future directions. *J. Immunother. Cancer* **2013**, *1*, 13. [CrossRef]
63. Bai, X.F.; Liu, J.; Li, O.; Zheng, P.; Liu, Y. Antigenic drift as a mechanism for tumor evasion of destruction by cytolytic T lymphocytes. *J. Clin. Invest.* **2003**, *111*, 1487–1496. [CrossRef] [PubMed]
64. Anguille, S.; Van Tendeloo, V.F.; Berneman, Z.N. Leukemia-associated antigens and their relevance to the immunotherapy of acute myeloid leukemia. *Leukemia* **2012**, *26*, 2186–2196. [CrossRef]

65. Melenhorst, J.J.; Scheinberg, P.; Chattopadhyay, P.K.; Gostick, E.; Ladell, K.; Roederer, M.; Hensel, N.F.; Douek, D.C.; Barrett, A.J.; Price, D.A. High avidity myeloid leukemia-associated antigen-specific CD8(+) T cells preferentially reside in the bone marrow. *Blood* **2009**, *113*, 2238–2244. [CrossRef]
66. Gulley, J.L.; Madan, R.A.; Schlom, J. Impact of tumour volume on the potential efficacy of therapeutic vaccines. *Curr. Oncol. (Tor. Ont.)* **2011**, *18*, e150–e157. [CrossRef]
67. Anguille, S.; Smits, E.L.; Lion, E.; van Tendeloo, V.F.; Berneman, Z.N. Clinical use of dendritic cells for cancer therapy. *Lancet Oncol* **2014**, *15*, e257–e267. [CrossRef]
68. Pawlowska, A.B.; Hashino, S.; McKenna, H.; Weigel, B.J.; Taylor, P.A.; Blazar, B.R. In vitro tumor-pulsed or in vivo Flt3 ligand-generated dendritic cells provide protection against acute myelogenous leukemia in nontransplanted or syngeneic bone marrow-transplanted mice. *Blood* **2001**, *97*, 1474–1482. [CrossRef]
69. Menssen, H.D.; Siehl, J.M.; Thiel, E. Wilms tumor gene (WT1) expression as a panleukemic marker. *Int. J. Hematol.* **2002**, *76*, 103–109. [CrossRef] [PubMed]
70. Trka, J.; Kalinova, M.; Hrusak, O.; Zuna, J.; Krejci, O.; Madzo, J.; Sedlacek, P.; Vavra, V.; Michalova, K.; Jarosova, M.; et al. Real-time quantitative PCR detection of WT1 gene expression in children with AML: prognostic significance, correlation with disease status and residual disease detection by flow cytometry. *Leukemia* **2002**, *16*, 1381–1389. [CrossRef] [PubMed]
71. Ogawa, H.; Tamaki, H.; Ikegame, K.; Soma, T.; Kawakami, M.; Tsuboi, A.; Kim, E.H.; Hosen, N.; Murakami, M.; Fujioka, T.; et al. The usefulness of monitoring WT1 gene transcripts for the prediction and management of relapse following allogeneic stem cell transplantation in acute type leukemia. *Blood* **2003**, *101*, 1698–1704. [CrossRef] [PubMed]
72. Garg, M.; Moore, H.; Tobal, K.; Liu Yin, J.A. Prognostic significance of quantitative analysis of WT1 gene transcripts by competitive reverse transcription polymerase chain reaction in acute leukaemia. *Br. J. Haematol.* **2003**, *123*, 49–59. [CrossRef] [PubMed]
73. Cilloni, D.; Renneville, A.; Hermitte, F.; Hills, R.K.; Daly, S.; Jovanovic, J.V.; Gottardi, E.; Fava, M.; Schnittger, S.; Weiss, T.; et al. Real-time quantitative polymerase chain reaction detection of minimal residual disease by standardized WT1 assay to enhance risk stratification in acute myeloid leukemia: a European LeukemiaNet study. *J. Clin. Oncol. Off. J. Am. Soc. Clin. Oncol.* **2009**, *27*, 5195–5201. [CrossRef] [PubMed]
74. Widen, K.; Mozaffari, F.; Choudhury, A.; Mellstedt, H. Overcoming immunosuppressive mechanisms. *Ann. Oncol. Off. J. Eur. Soc. Med Oncol. / Esmo* **2008**, *19*, vii241–vii247. [CrossRef]
75. Farag, S.S.; Maharry, K.; Zhang, M.J.; Perez, W.S.; George, S.L.; Mrozek, K.; DiPersio, J.; Bunjes, D.W.; Marcucci, G.; Baer, M.R.; et al. Comparison of reduced-intensity hematopoietic cell transplantation with chemotherapy in patients age 60-70 years with acute myelogenous leukemia in first remission. *Biol. Blood Marrow Transpl.* **2011**, *17*, 1796–1803. [CrossRef] [PubMed]
76. Byrd, J.C.; Mrozek, K.; Dodge, R.K.; Carroll, A.J.; Edwards, C.G.; Arthur, D.C.; Pettenati, M.J.; Patil, S.R.; Rao, K.W.; Watson, M.S.; et al. Pretreatment cytogenetic abnormalities are predictive of induction success, cumulative incidence of relapse, and overall survival in adult patients with de novo acute myeloid leukemia: results from Cancer and Leukemia Group B (CALGB 8461). *Blood* **2002**, *100*, 4325–4336. [CrossRef] [PubMed]
77. Lion, E.; Willemen, Y.; Berneman, Z.N.; Van Tendeloo, V.F.I.; Smits, E.L.J. Natural killer cell immune escape in acute myeloid leukemia. *Leukemia* **2012**, *26*, 2019–2026. [CrossRef] [PubMed]
78. Lion, E.; Smits, E.L.; Berneman, Z.N.; Van Tendeloo, V.F. NK cells: key to success of DC-based cancer vaccines? *Oncologist* **2012**, *17*, 1256–1270. [CrossRef] [PubMed]
79. Van Acker, H.H.; Anguille, S.; Van Tendeloo, V.F.; Lion, E. Empowering gamma delta T cells with antitumor immunity by dendritic cell-based immunotherapy. *Oncoimmunology* **2015**, *4*, e1021538. [CrossRef]
80. van Beek, J.J.; Gorris, M.A.; Skold, A.E.; Hatipoglu, I.; Van Acker, H.H.; Smits, E.L.; de Vries, I.J.; Bakdash, G. Human blood myeloid and plasmacytoid dendritic cells cross activate each other and synergize in inducing NK cell cytotoxicity. *Oncoimmunology* **2016**, *5*, e1227902. [CrossRef] [PubMed]
81. Van Acker, H.H.; Beretta, O.; Anguille, S.; De Caluwe, L.; Papagna, A.; Van den Bergh, J.M.; Willemen, Y.; Goossens, H.; Berneman, Z.N.; Van Tendeloo, V.F.; et al. Desirable cytolytic immune effector cell recruitment by interleukin-15 dendritic cells. *Oncotarget* **2017**, *8*, 13652–13665. [CrossRef]
82. Van Acker, H.H.; Anguille, S.; De Reu, H.; Berneman, Z.N.; Smits, E.L.; Van Tendeloo, V.F. Interleukin-15-Cultured Dendritic Cells Enhance Anti-Tumor Gamma Delta T Cell Functions through IL-15 Secretion. *Front. Immunol.* **2018**, *9*, 658. [CrossRef]

83. van Ee, T.J.; Van Acker, H.H.; van Oorschot, T.G.; Van Tendeloo, V.F.; Smits, E.L.; Bakdash, G.; Schreibelt, G.; de Vries, I.J.M. BDCA1+CD14+ Immunosuppressive Cells in Cancer, a Potential Target? *Vaccines (Basel)* **2018**, *6*, 65. [CrossRef] [PubMed]
84. Ueno, H.; Schmitt, N.; Klechevsky, E.; Pedroza-Gonzalez, A.; Matsui, T.; Zurawski, G.; Oh, S.; Fay, J.; Pascual, V.; Banchereau, J.; et al. Harnessing human dendritic cell subsets for medicine. *Immunol. Rev.* **2010**, *234*, 199–212. [CrossRef] [PubMed]
85. Palucka, K.; Banchereau, J. Cancer immunotherapy via dendritic cells. *Nat. Rev. Cancer* **2012**, *12*, 265–277. [CrossRef]
86. Curti, A.; Trabanelli, S.; Onofri, C.; Aluigi, M.; Salvestrini, V.; Ocadlikova, D.; Evangelisti, C.; Rutella, S.; De Cristofaro, R.; Ottaviani, E.; et al. Indoleamine 2,3-dioxygenase-expressing leukemic dendritic cells impair a leukemia-specific immune response by inducing potent T regulatory cells. *Haematologica* **2010**, *95*, 2022–2030. [CrossRef]
87. Anguille, S.; Lion, E.; Smits, E.; Berneman, Z.N.; van Tendeloo, V.F.I. Dendritic cell vaccine therapy for acute myeloid leukemia: questions and answers. *Hum. Vaccines* **2011**, *7*, 579–584. [CrossRef]
88. Anguille, S.; Smits, E.L.; Cools, N.; Goossens, H.; Berneman, Z.N.; Van Tendeloo, V.F. Short-term cultured, interleukin-15 differentiated dendritic cells have potent immunostimulatory properties. *J. Transl. Med.* **2009**, *7*, 109. [CrossRef] [PubMed]
89. Anguille, S.; Lion, E.; Tel, J.; de Vries, I.J.; Coudere, K.; Fromm, P.D.; Van Tendeloo, V.F.; Smits, E.L.; Berneman, Z.N. Interleukin-15-induced CD56(+) myeloid dendritic cells combine potent tumor antigen presentation with direct tumoricidal potential. *Plos ONE* **2012**, *7*, e51851. [CrossRef]
90. Anguille, S.; Van Acker, H.H.; Van den Bergh, J.; Willemen, Y.; Goossens, H.; Van Tendeloo, V.F.; Smits, E.L.; Berneman, Z.N.; Lion, E. Interleukin-15 Dendritic Cells Harness NK Cell Cytotoxic Effector Function in a Contact- and IL-15-Dependent Manner. *PLoS ONE* **2015**, *10*, e0123340. [CrossRef]
91. Versteven, M.; Van den Bergh, J.M.J.; Marcq, E.; Smits, E.L.J.; Van Tendeloo, V.F.I.; Hobo, W.; Lion, E. Dendritic Cells and Programmed Death-1 Blockade: A Joint Venture to Combat Cancer. *Front. Immunol.* **2018**, *9*, 394. [CrossRef]
92. Giannopoulos, K. Targeting Immune Signaling Checkpoints in Acute Myeloid Leukemia. *J. Clin. Med.* **2019**, *8*, 236. [CrossRef]
93. Masarova, L.; Kantarjian, H.; Garcia-Mannero, G.; Ravandi, F.; Sharma, P.; Daver, N. Harnessing the Immune System Against Leukemia: Monoclonal Antibodies and Checkpoint Strategies for AML. *Adv. Exp. Med. Biol.* **2017**, *995*, 73–95.
94. Liu, Y.; Bewersdorf, J.P.; Stahl, M.; Zeidan, A.M. Immunotherapy in acute myeloid leukemia and myelodysplastic syndromes: The dawn of a new era? *Blood Rev.* **2019**, *34*, 67–83. [CrossRef]
95. Lee, S.C.; Srivastava, R.M.; Lopez-Albaitero, A.; Ferrone, S.; Ferris, R.L. Natural killer (NK): dendritic cell (DC) cross talk induced by therapeutic monoclonal antibody triggers tumor antigen-specific T cell immunity. *Immunol. Res.* **2011**, *50*, 248–254. [CrossRef] [PubMed]
96. Gribben, J.G.; Ryan, D.P.; Boyajian, R.; Urban, R.G.; Hedley, M.L.; Beach, K.; Nealon, P.; Matulonis, U.; Campos, S.; Gilligan, T.D.; et al. Unexpected association between induction of immunity to the universal tumor antigen CYP1B1 and response to next therapy. *Clin. Cancer Res. Off. J. Am. Assoc. Cancer Res.* **2005**, *11*, 4430–4436. [CrossRef]
97. Nahas, M.R.; Stroopinsky, D.; Rosenblatt, J.; Cole, L.; Pyzer, A.R.; Anastasiadou, E.; Sergeeva, A.; Ephraim, A.; Washington, A.; Orr, S.; et al. Hypomethylating agent alters the immune microenvironment in acute myeloid leukaemia (AML) and enhances the immunogenicity of a dendritic cell/AML vaccine. *Br. J. Haematol.* **2019**. [CrossRef]

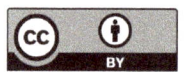

© 2019 by the authors. Licensee MDPI, Basel, Switzerland. This article is an open access article distributed under the terms and conditions of the Creative Commons Attribution (CC BY) license (http://creativecommons.org/licenses/by/4.0/).

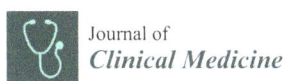

Review

Targeting Immune Signaling Checkpoints in Acute Myeloid Leukemia

Krzysztof Giannopoulos [1,2]

1. Department of Experimental Hematooncology, Medical University of Lublin, 20-093 Lublin, Poland; krzysztof.giannopoulos@gmail.com or krzysztof.giannopoulos@umlub.pl; Tel.: +48-81-448-66-32; Fax: +48-81-448-66-34
2. Department of Hematology, St John's Cancer Centre, 20-093 Lublin, Poland

Received: 15 January 2019; Accepted: 5 February 2019; Published: 12 February 2019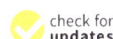

Abstract: The modest successes of targeted therapies along with the curative effects of allogeneic hematopoietic stem cell transplantation (alloHSCT) in acute myeloid leukemia (AML) stimulate the development of new immunotherapies. One of the promising methods of immunotherapy is the activation of immune response by the targeting of negative control checkpoints. The two best-known inhibitory immune checkpoints are cytotoxic T-lymphocyte antigen-4 (CTLA-4) and the programmed cell death protein 1 receptor (PD-1). In AML, PD-1 expression is observed in T-cell subpopulations, including T regulatory lymphocytes. Increased PD-1 expression on CD8+ T lymphocytes may be one of the factors leading to dysfunction of cytotoxic T cells and inhibition of the immune response during the progressive course of AML. Upregulation of checkpoint molecules was observed after alloHSCT and therapy with hypomethylating agents, pointing to a potential clinical application in these settings. Encouraging results from recent clinical trials (a response rate above 50% in a relapsed setting) justify further clinical use. The most common clinical trials employ two PD-1 inhibitors (nivolumab and pembrolizumab) and two anti-PD-L1 (programmed death-ligand 1) monoclonal antibodies (atezolizumab and durvalumab). Several other inhibitors are under development or in early phases of clinical trials. The results of these clinical trials are awaited with great interest in, as they may allow for the established use of checkpoint inhibitors in the treatment of AML.

Keywords: acute myeloid leukemia; immunotherapy; programmed cell death protein 1 receptor/programmed death-ligand 1 (PD-1/PD-L1) signaling

1. Introduction

The modest successes of targeted therapies in acute myeloid leukemia (AML) and the proven power of the immune system to fight effectively against leukemic blasts in the context of the graft-versus-leukemia effect, stimulate the development of new immunotherapies. One of the promising methods of immunotherapy is the activation of immune response by the targeting of negative control checkpoints on the surface of immune cells or by eliminating the regulatory proteins present in the tumor microenvironment [1]. The homeostasis of the stimulating and inhibiting signals of the immune response is regulated by immunological control checkpoints, which allow the activation of cytotoxic response against pathogens, while maintaining a tolerance to the organism's own cells.

To avoid autoimmunity, the process of T-cell activation must be strictly regulated. For stimulation, T cells require at least two different signals from antigen presenting cells (APC). The first signal is the recognition of the antigen, and more specifically its immunogenic part—an epitope presented by the major histocompatibility complex (MHC), located on the APC and recognized by the T-cell receptor (TCR) (Figure 1a). The second signal is the result of costimulation, mainly by the interaction of the CD28 molecule of the T-lymphocyte with CD80 (B7.1) or CD86 (B7.2) molecules, on the APC.

The stimulation of T cells is also closely related to other stimulatory signals sent to the cell as a result of the combination of specific receptor pairs and their ligands, including the glucocorticoid-induced TNF (tumor necrosis factor) receptor and its specific ligand, and also the interaction between the transmembrane 4-1BB receptor (CD137) and its ligand, 4-1BBL (CD137L) [2–4].

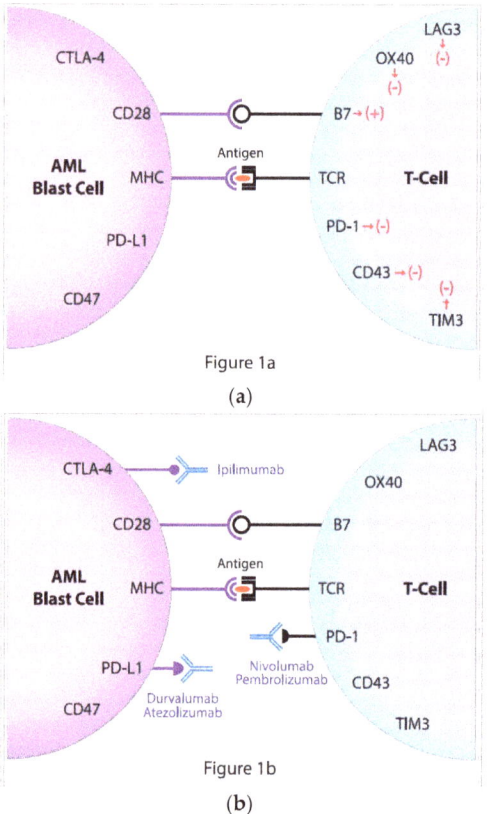

Figure 1. (**a**) The regulation of antileukemic immune response; the activation of an immune response requires two signals. The first is responsible for the specific recognition of antigen (peptide) located in the great groove of the major histocompatibility complex (MHC) by the T-cell receptor (TCR). The second is the costimulatory signal that is transmitted by the interaction of CD28 and B7 molecules. These signals are regulated by many negative receptors including the lymphocyte-activation gene 3 (LAG3), OX40, programmed cell death protein 1 receptor (PD-1), CD43 as well as T-cell immunoglobulin domain and mucin domain 3 (TIM3) on the T cell that interacts with ligands on acute myeloid leukemia (AML) blasts, i.e., CD47, programmed death-ligand 1 (PD-L1) and Cytotoxic T-lymphocyte Antigen-4 (CTLA-4). (**b**) The restoration of antileukemic immune response by the targeting of the negative control checkpoints. In order to restore the antileukemic immune response, two inhibitory immune checkpoint molecules might be targeted by treatment with specific monoclonal antibodies directed against the cytotoxic T-lymphocyte antigen-4 (CTLA-4), ipilimumab, and the programmed cell death protein 1, nivolumab and pembrolizumab as well as PD-L1, atezolizumab and durvalumab.

The two best-known inhibitory immune checkpoints are cytotoxic T-lymphocyte antigen-4 (CTLA-4) and the programmed cell death protein 1 receptor(PD-1) (Figure 1a) [1]. On T cells, the CTLA-4 receptor inhibits T cell maturation and differentiation by competing with the costimulatory receptor CD28, for CD80 (B7.1) and CD86 (B7.2) [5]. Although the increased CD80 and CD86 expressions that are associated with poor outcome were reported in AML, treatment with the anti-CTLA-4 monoclonal antibody ipilimumab, proved limited clinical activity [6-8]. Encouraging results from trials on solid tumors have turned the attention of researchers to the potential that blocking the PD-1 signaling pathway may have potential applications in the field of hematology–oncology. Those new therapies might target the immune synapse of patients irrespective of the PD-1 expression and thereby could be proposed for a majority of AML patients (Figure 1b).

2. The Role of PD-1/PD-L1 Signaling Pathway

PD-1 is a surface glycoprotein cell receptor that belongs to the CD28 family. PD-1 is composed of 288 amino acids, and its molecular weight ranges from 50 to 55 kDa2. PD-1 exhibits approximately 31–33% homology with CTLA-4, CD28, and Inducible T-cell COStimulator (ICOS) molecules. PD-1 interactions with ligands prevent autoimmunity on the one hand, by inducing apoptosis of autoantigen-specific T cells and on the other hand, by inhibiting regulatory T cell (Treg) apoptosis. The expressions of PD-1 on T and B cells is a consequence of the activation of the signaling pathway TCR or the B-cell receptor (BCR), respectively [9].

The PD-1 protein is encoded by the *PDCD-1* gene, located on chromosome 2 (2q.37.3) [10]. *PDCD-1* consists of five exons. Exon 1 encodes a leader peptide that is extracellular. Exon 2 encodes the immunoglobulin (Ig) variable (V-like domain. Amino acid fragments (ca. 20) are located at the IgV-like domain, that separates it from the cell membrane. A transmembrane domain encapsulated by exon 3 is anchored within the cell membrane. Exons 4 and 5 encode an intracellular domain, in which we distinguish two tyrosines, located in two amino acid motifs—proximal (tyrosine-based motif inhibitors—ITIM) and distal (a tyrosine immunoreceptor-based switch motif—ITSM) [11]. The tyrosines mentioned above play a fundamental role in the function of PD-1 as an inhibitor [12]. Under physiological conditions, PD-1 is expressed on the cells of the immune system, including mature CD4+ and CD8+ T cells, as well as on B cells and T cells during their thymus development [13,14]. In addition, PD-1 expression is found on natural killer (NK) cells, some dendritic cell (DC) subpopulations, and monocytes [15,16]. In a form unrelated to the cell membrane, PD-1 may be present in the cytoplasm of Treg and naïve CD4+ cells. PD-1 can be regulated by various factors, including hormones, cytokines or suppressor genes, such as Phosphatase and tensin homolog (*PTEN*) and liver kinase B1 (*LKB1*) [17]. The cytokines that stimulate the expression of PD-1 are interleukin 2 (IL-2), IL-7, IL-15 and IL-21. It has been shown that in the induction of PD-1 expression in T cells, there is a significant role played by the nuclear factor of stimulated Tc1 cells (NF-ATc1). It has also been proven that the specific inhibition of this factor, consisting in the abolition of its translocation to the nucleus, results in the reduction of PD-1 expression, and the mutation of the gene encoding NF-ATc1 results in the complete lack of receptor expression [18]. The transmission of the signal through TCR after its stimulation leads to the binding of NFAT to the promoter region of the *PDCD1* gene [18]. PD-1 expression in B-lymphocytes is induced by the molecules that stimulate the activation and the proliferation of these lymphocytes, including anti-IgM, anti-CD40 and lipopolysaccharide (LPS) [9]. The interaction with toll-like receptors (TLRs) such as TLR2, TLR3, TLR4 and the nucleotide-binding oligomerization domain (NOD) has a stimulating effect on the expression of PD-1 in DC. In turn, IL-4 and TLR9 act to inhibit the expression of PD-1 in DC [19]. In macrophages, PD-1 expression is stimulated by an interferon-stimulated response element (ISRE), signal transducers and activators of transcription (STAT), including STAT1 and STAT2, and interferon α (IFNα), through ISRE [20].

The programmed death-ligand 1 (PD-L1), also referred to as B7-H1 or CD274, is a transmembrane type I glycoprotein, made up of 290 amino acids, belonging to the B7 family. This protein has two extracellular IgV- and Ig constant (C)-like domains, wherein the IgV-like domain allows for interaction with the analogous domain of the PD-1 receptor. The cytoplasmic domain of the PD-L1 ligand is short, and its exact role in the transmission of intracellular signals has not yet been determined [21]. The expression of PD-L1 at the mRNA level is detected in almost all cells. The expression of the PD-L1 protein on hematopoietic cells is limited primarily to antigen-presenting cells, such as dendritic cells, macrophages, and B28 lymphocytes. PD-L1 is also expressed in activated T cells [12]. PD-L1 is also found in tissues not belonging to the immune system, including pancreatic islet cells, hepatic stellate cells, vascular endothelial cells and placental trophoblast cells [18,22]. The expression of PD-L1 on B cells is stimulated by anti-IgM antibodies, LPS, type I and II IFNs, TNF and IL-21. In the case of T cells, the inducers of PD-L1 expression are anti-CD3 antibodies or cytokines, such as IL-2, IL-7, IL-15, IFN and TNF. The expression of PD-L1 on macrophages is stimulated by a granulocyte-macrophage-colony-stimulating factor (GM-CSF), monocytes by IL-10, and on DC by IFN-γ, IL-4, IL-12 and GM-CSF [23].

Programmed death-ligand 2 (PD-L2), also referred to as B7-DC and CD273, is the second ligand able to attach to the PD-1 receptor [24]. PD-L2 has extracellular Ig-V- and IgC-like domains, and a short intracellular domain. The expression of PD-L2, as compared with PD-L1, is not as common and is limited to macrophages, DC, and some B-cell subpopulations [25–27]. The partial presence of PD-L2 was also demonstrated on mast cells of myeloid origin, T-lymphocytes and vascular endothelial cells [28,29]. The PD-1 receptor interacts with its specific ligands—PD-L1 and PD-L2. Ligands compete with each other for binding to PD-1, but PD-L1 plays a major role in regulating the PD-1/PD-L1/PD-L2 pathway. Although PD-L2 has a stronger affinity for PD-1 compared to PD-L1, the extent of expression of this molecule is limited [30]. The expression of PD-1 on lymphocytes may be induced by the contact of the lymphocyte receptor with an antigen [1,31]. The interaction of PD-1 with ligands results in the activation of phosphotyrosine phosphatase, containing the SH2 domain (SHP2) and the decrease in Bcl-xL expression, leading to the inhibition of phosphatidylinositol 3-kinase/serine-threonine protein kinase—(PI3K/AKT). Functionally, elevated levels of PD-1 expression are observed on tumor-infiltrating lymphocytes (TILs) that interact with tumor cells by linking to the PD-L1 and PD-L2 ligands present on them, which in turn could lead to a lymphocyte depletion. This phenomenon leads to the inhibition of the effector functions of T cells, which lose the cytotoxic ability to kill tumor cells. PD-1 also plays a significant role in T-cell adhesion, which is activated upon contact with APC. The interaction of these cells may be impaired by PD-1-derived inhibitory signals that are necessary for its interaction with PD-L1. This hypothesis is reinforced by experimental in vitro studies showing lower T-cell mobility and improved T-cell interactions with APC after blocking with PD-1 or PD-L1 antibodies [32]. Furthermore, PD-1 could inhibit T-cell adhesion and the formation of the immunological synapse [33,34].

3. PD-1/PD-L1 Expression in Leukemias

The expression of PD-1 in hematological malignancies has been the subject of many studies in recent years. In patients with chronic lymphocytic leukemia (CLL), PD-1 expression is observed on T lymphocytes, but also on leukemic cells [35–37]. In addition, we proved earlier that PD-1 expression on leukemic cells in CLL patients was higher compared to the healthy group, both at the level of the transcript and in the form of membrane protein. However, the significance of PD-1 and PD-L1 expression in the prognostic context has not been confirmed [35]. In addition, in CLL patients with an advanced disease (stage III and IV, according to the Rai classification), a higher percentage of CD4+PD-1+ T lymphocytes was observed than in patients with a less advanced disease [38].

In AML, PD-1 expression was observed in T-cell subpopulations, including CD4+ T-effector cells, Tregs and CD8+ T cells, both in untreated patients and in patients with a recurrent disease [39]. An increased PD-1 expression on CD8+ T cells may be one of the factors leading to the dysfunction of cytotoxic T cells and the inhibition of the immune response during the progressive course of AML [40]. Knaus et al. [41] characterized the T-cell exhaustion in AML at diagnosis, that diverged between responders and non-responders upon treatment. Response to therapy correlated with the upregulation of costimulatory T-cell signaling pathways, and the downregulation of inhibitory T-cell signaling pathways, indicative of the restoration of T-cell function. Notably, CD8+ T-cell dysfunction was, in part, reversible upon PD-1 blockade in vitro. By contrast, a similar expression of inhibitory molecules on T cells from patients at AML diagnosis and from age-matched healthy controls were observed [42]. However, when observed at relapse after allogeneic hematopoietic stem-cell transplantation (alloHSCT), the PD-1 expression was significantly increased, compared with its expression at diagnosis, in both CD4+ and CD8+ T cells. Notably, bone marrow CD8 T cells consisted of a higher frequency of PD-1+ cells compared with those from peripheral blood [43]. These cells were also functionally deficient, as was the case in the functional model of WT-1-specific leukemia-reactive CD8+ cells from bone marrow that released lower levels of IFN-γ, granzyme B and TNF, when compared with those from peripheral blood.

Most studies suggest that in newly diagnosed AML patients, PD-L1 expression on blasts is usually not observed [44]. However, it might depend on the detection method, since in one study the PD-L1 was expressed in 24 out of 75 AML patients [45]. The appearance of PD-L1 on AML blasts was associated with the negative course of the disease [44]. The PD-L1 overexpression in AML usually occurred during therapy, after alloHSCT and at the relapse of the disease. The PD-L1 positive rate in the relapsed/refractory group was higher than that in the de novo patient group (56.3% vs. 25.4%, $p = 0.019$). In 59 de novo patients, the complete remission (CR) rate of the PD-L1 positive group after one course of chemotherapy, was lower than that of the PD-L1 negative group (66.7% vs. 71.4%); the CR rate of PD-L1 positive group after 2 two courses of chemotherapy, was also lower than that of PD-L1 negative group (70% vs. 88.6%). The relapse rate and the proportion of refractory patients in PD-L1 positive group were higher than those in the PD-L1 negative group [45].

The factors that stimulate the expression of PD-L1 in AML were cytokines, particularly IFN-γ [46,47]. In addition, we reported that TP53 might specifically modulate the immune response to tumor antigens by regulating PD-L1 via *miR-34* and blocking its expression [48]. The *PD-L1* expression was elevated in the AML group with *TP53* mut, compared with the *TP53* wt group, with a median expression of 9.1 vs. 8.3, $p < 0.001$. In line with this finding, Goltz et al. [49], analyzing gene methylation status in AML patients, found that low PD-L1 methylation was found in the *TP53* mut group. Wang et al. [50] have shown that *PD-L1* was overexpressed in the AML samples and that the expression level was reversely correlated with *miR-34a* expression, that directly targets the 3' untranslated region of PD-L1, thereby modulating PD-L1 expression. We also found that the highest expression of PD-L1 was in a group with a poor prognosis, compared with favorable and intermediate groups, as defined by The Cancer Genome Atlas research network's risk stratification. The expression of PD-L1 was also associated with the number of recurrent mutations. Possibly, an increased number of driver mutations created more neoantigens, which in turn, modified the immune microenvironment and caused an increase in PD-L1 expression [51]. The expression of PD-L1 in AML is therefore associated with adverse gene mutations that affect the microenvironment of the tumor and may lead to an unfavorable clinical course of the disease [45].

4. Inhibition of PD-1/PD-L1 in AML

The PD-1/PD-L1/PD-L2 pathway may be inhibited by blocking the PD-1 receptor or its ligands. Blocking the PD-1 molecule itself prevents its interaction with PD-L1 and PD-L2, which is considered the most effective activation of the immune response (Figure 1b). By contrast, PD-L1 blockade affects only the PD-1/PD-L1 axis, and considering its widespread expression, the activation of the immune response might be significant. Due to the limited expression of the PD-L2 ligand, it is not suitable target for therapies that use monoclonal antibodies [52]. Thus, in actions directed toward the PD-1/PD-L1 pathway, anti-PD-1 antibodies, as well as anti-PD-L1, are used [30]. The most common clinical trials employ two PD-1 inhibitors (nivolumab and pembrolizumab) and two anti-PD-L1 monoclonal antibodies (atezolizumab and durvalumab) (Table 1). Several others are under development or are in early phases of clinical trials. The key mechanism of action in anti-PD-1 and anti-PD-L1 monoclonal antibodies, relies on blocking PD-1 interaction with PD-L1 and/or PD-L2 ligands. To minimize the side effects mediated by the recognition of fragment crystallizable (Fc) region, atezolizumab and durvalumab have a point mutation in the Fc domain; thus, they did not induce the cytotoxicity of the antibody-dependent cellular cytotoxicity, nor the complement-dependent cytotoxicity. The upregulation of checkpoint molecules was observed after alloHSCT and therapy with hypomethylating agents, pointing to a potential clinical application in these settings [53,54]. Moreover, a higher PD-1 expression on T cells was strongly associated with leukemia relapse, post-alloHSCT [55]. This was especially the case in the subpopulation of CD8+ T cells that, characterized by the expression of two exhaustion markers, PD-1 and the T-cell immunoglobulin domain and mucin domain 3 (TIM-3), presented the strongest predictive value for leukemia relapse, post-alloHSCT. The median frequencies of CD8+ PD-1+TIM-3+ in relapsed AML were 8.6%, compared with 0.5% in patients maintaining remission. Notably, the increase of PD-1+ TIM-3+ CD8+ T cells occurred before a clinical diagnosis of leukemia relapse, suggesting their predictive value. This study might provide an early diagnostic approach and a therapeutic target for leukemia relapse, post-transplantation.

The expression of PD-1 is regulated by DNA methylation. The demethylation of the PD-1 promoter correlated with an increase in PD-1 expression. The demethylation of the PD-1 promoter correlated with a significantly worse overall response rate (8% vs. 60%, $p = 0.014$), and a trend towards a shorter overall survival (OS) ($p = 0.11$) was observed [56]. In a cohort of patients treated with hypomethylating therapy, PD-L1, PD-L2, PD-1 and CTLA4 expressions were upregulated [54]. The treatment of leukemia cells with a hypomethylating agent, decitabine, resulted in the dose-dependent upregulation of PD-L1, PD-L2, PD-1 and CTLA4. Decitabine could also increase the expression of genes involved in antigen processing and presentation by the respective promoter, demethylation. In a mouse model of colorectal cancer, a significantly larger inhibition of tumor growth and a prolongation of survival were observed after treatment with a combination of PD-1 blockade and decitabine, than in mice treated with decitabine or PD-1 blockade alone [57]. These results suggest that PD-1 signaling may be involved in resistance mechanisms to hypomethylating agents, and provide evidence that checkpoint inhibition could be a potential therapy for treating AML.

In recently published results from a phase II study, relapsed/refractory AML patients were treated with nivolumab and azacytidine [58]. The overall response rate (ORR) was 33%, including 15 (22%) patients with complete remission/complete remission with insufficient count recovery (CRi), one patient with a partial response, and seven patients with hematologic improvements (HI) that were maintained for >6 months. Six patients (9%) exhibited a stable disease for >6 months. The highest ORR (58%) was observed in hypomethylating agent-naive patients. Grades 2–4 immune-related adverse events (irAE) occurred in 16 (23%) patients. Fourteen of the 16 (88%) patients with toxicities responded to steroids, and these 14 patients were safely rechallenged with nivolumab. In this study, a total of 13% of the patients had to discontinue nivolumab (all discontinuations were due to grades 3/4 irAE; no discontinuations were due to grade 2 irAE) and were subsequently kept only on azacitidine.

The preliminary results of a phase-II study (NCT02532231) of nivolumab maintenance in high-risk AML patients, who have achieved CR following induction and consolidation chemotherapy, also showed promising results, with the rates for a 6- and a 12-month CR duration being 79% and 71%, respectively [59]. In a series of case reports, Albring et al. [60] reported three AML patients who, at relapse after alloHSCT, were treated with nivolumab. In one patient, the therapy led to CR; in another, it led to disease stabilization; a third patient failed to respond to nivolumab. The only side effects were the irAE of pancytopenia and a graft-versus-host disease of the skin in one patient, as well as muscle and joint pain in another patient.

Table 1. The first agents for PD-1/PD-L1 inhibition in AML.

Monoclonal Antibody	Target/Type	First Registration
Nivolumab	PD-1, IgG4	Melanoma—06.2015
Pembrolizumab	PD-1, IgG4	Melanoma—08.2014
Atezolizumab	PD-L1, IgG1 modified Fc region	Urothelial carcinoma—05.2016
Durvalumab	PD-L1, IgG1 modified Fc region	Urothelial carcinoma—05.2017

PD-1: programmed cell death protein 1 receptor; PD-L1: programmed death-ligand 1; AML: acute myeloid leukemia; IgG: Intravenous Gamma Globulin.

5. Future Treatment Modalities with Checkpoint Inhibitors in AML

The era of immunotherapy in AML started several years ago when the curative potential of alloHSCT, due to the graft-versus-leukemia effect, was discovered. Nowadays, chimeric antigen receptor (CAR)T-cell therapy replaces the defective immune system and the checkpoint inhibitors restore function to the antileukemia immune response (Figure 1b). Several phases I/II clinical trials for checkpoint inhibitors in monotherapy or combined treatment for AML have started in the last few years (Figure 2) [61,62]. The results of larger clinical trials are needed to determine the role that checkpoint inhibition plays in AML. It seems that the clinical setting can be complex, starting from combined therapy with hypomethylating drugs for patients who are ineligible for transplantation, followed by combined therapy with other modifiers of the immune system and finally, to the augmentation of the graft-versus-leukemia effect, post-alloHSCT, in either monotherapy or polytherapy. In this regard, the double blockade of CTLA-4 and PD-1/PD-L1 presents an interesting treatment option, in boosting antileukemic immunity. Recent results in solid tumors proved that in advanced melanoma, combined therapy was effective in 57% of patients, compared with 43% for patients treated with nivolumab monotherapy and 19% for patients in the ipilimumab monotherapy arm [63]. The first clinical trials on the ipilimumab and nivolumab combined treatment in patients with relapsed AML, post-alloHSCT, have been initiated. Another approach is a double blockade of TIM-3 and PD-1 that is being evaluated in an ongoing clinical trial. Furthermore, checkpoint inhibitors might be effective in combination with cellular therapies, including chimeric antigen receptor T cells (CART) or vaccination strategies [64,65]. This is an evolving field since anti-PD1/PD-L1 therapy along with vaccination could expand the pre-existing specific T cells and induce functionally active antileukemic cytotoxic T cells. The results from clinical trials in melanoma have not provided clear support for this approach, since similar clinical activity was observed irrespective of vaccination [66]. Similarly, PD-1 inhibition in combination with CART did not further enhance the expansion or persistence of CART [64]. Further results from these clinical trials and others are awaited with great interest, as they may allow for the established use of checkpoint inhibitors in the treatment of AML.

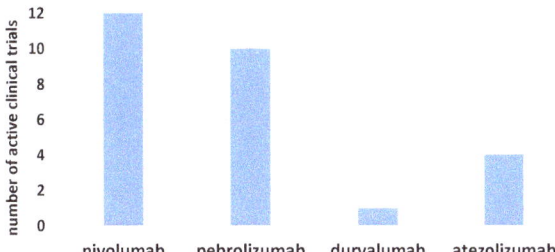

Figure 2. The numbers of active clinical trials for checkpoints inhibitors in acute myeloid leukemia.

Figure 2 displays the number of active clinical trials for checkpoint inhibitors in AML both in monotherapy and in combination with chemotherapy. The histogram presents trials registered on clinicaltrial.gov [62].

Funding: The studies on PD-1/PD-L1 function in AML were supported by the Polish National Science Centre, grant no 2013/10/M/NZ5/00313. The APC was funded by Medical University of Lublin grant No. 462.

Acknowledgments: Author would like to thank Dominika Iwanek and Jacek Przesmycki for technical support in the preparation of figures.

Conflicts of Interest: The author declares no conflict of interest.

References

1. Pianko, M.J.; Liu, Y.; Bagchi, S.; Lesokhin, A.M. Immune checkpoint blockade for hematologic malignancies: A review. *Stem Cell Investig.* **2017**, *4*, 32. [CrossRef] [PubMed]
2. Chen, J.; Jiang, C.C.; Jin, L.; Zhang, X.D. Regulation of PD-L1: A novel role of pro-survival signalling in cancer. *Ann. Oncol.* **2016**, *27*, 409–416. [CrossRef] [PubMed]
3. Lee, H.W.; Park, S.J.; Choi, B.K.; Kim, H.H.; Nam, K.O.; Kwon, B.S. 4-1BB promotes the survival of CD8+ T lymphocytes by increasing expression of Bcl-xL and Bfl-1. *J. Immunol.* **2002**, *169*, 4882–4888. [CrossRef] [PubMed]
4. Ronchetti, S.; Zollo, O.; Bruscoli, S.; Agostini, M.; Bianchini, R.; Nocentini, G.; Ayroldi, E.; Riccardi, C. GITR, a member of the TNF receptor superfamily, is costimulatory to mouse T lymphocyte subpopulations. *Eur. J. Immunol.* **2004**, *34*, 613–622. [CrossRef]
5. Sehgal, A.; Whiteside, T.L.; Boyiadzis, M. Programmed death-1 checkpoint blockade in acute myeloid leukemia. *Expert Opin. Biol. Ther.* **2015**, *15*, 1191–1203. [CrossRef] [PubMed]
6. Costello, R.T.; Mallet, F.; Sainty, D.; Maraninchi, D.; Gastaut, J.A.; Olive, D. Regulation of CD80/B7-1 and CD86/B7-2 molecule expression in human primary acute myeloid leukemia and their role in allogenic immune recognition. *Eur. J. Immunol.* **1998**, *28*, 90–103. [CrossRef]
7. Graf, M.; Reif, S.; Hecht, K.; Pelka-Fleischer, R.; Kroell, T.; Pfister, K.; Schmetzer, H. High expression of costimulatory molecules correlates with low relapse-free survival probability in acute myeloid leukemia (AML). *Ann. Hematol.* **2005**, *84*, 287–297. [CrossRef]
8. Alatrash, G.; Daver, N.; Mittendorf, E.A. Targeting immune checkpoints in hematologic malignancies. *Pharmacol. Rev.* **2016**, *68*, 1014–1025. [CrossRef]
9. Yamazaki, T.; Akiba, H.; Iwai, H.; Matsuda, H.; Aoki, M.; Tanno, Y.; Shin, T.; Tsuchiya, H.; Pardoll, D.M.; Okumura, K.; et al. Expression of programmed death 1 ligands by murine T cells and APC. *J. Immunol.* **2002**, *169*, 5538–5545. [CrossRef]
10. Shinohara, T.; Taniwaki, M.; Ishida, Y.; Kawaichi, M.; Honjo, T. Structure and chromosomal localization of the human PD-1 gene (PDCD1). *Genomics* **1994**, *23*, 704–706. [CrossRef]
11. Ishida, Y.; Agata, Y.; Shibahara, K.; Honjo, T. Induced expression of PD-1, a novel member of the immunoglobulin gene superfamily, upon programmed cell death. *EMBO J.* **1992**, *11*, 3887–3895. [CrossRef] [PubMed]
12. Dougall, W.C.; Kurtulus, S.; Smyth, M.J.; Anderson, A.C. TIGIT and CD96: New checkpoint receptor targets for cancer immunotherapy. *Immunol. Rev.* **2017**, *276*, 112–120. [CrossRef] [PubMed]
13. Liang, S.C.; Latchman, Y.E.; Buhlmann, J.E.; Tomczak, M.F.; Horwitz, B.H.; Freeman, G.J.; Sharpe, A.H. Regulation of PD-1, PD-L1, and PD-L2 expression during normal and autoimmune responses. *Eur. J. Immunol.* **2003**, *33*, 2706–2716. [CrossRef]
14. Nishimura, H.; Agata, Y.; Kawasaki, A.; Sato, M.; Imamura, S.; Minato, N.; Yagita, H.; Nakano, T.; Honjo, T. Developmentally regulated expression of the PD-1 protein on the surface of double-negative (CD4-CD8-) thymocytes. *Int. Immunol.* **1996**, *8*, 773–780. [CrossRef] [PubMed]
15. Kobayashi, M.; Kawano, S.; Hatachi, S.; Kurimoto, C.; Okazaki, T.; Iwai, Y.; Honjo, T.; Tanaka, Y.; Minato, N.; Komori, T.; et al. Enhanced expression of programmed death-1 (PD-1)/PD-L1 in salivary glands of patients with Sjögren's syndrome. *J. Rheumatol.* **2005**, *32*, 2156–2163. [PubMed]
16. Agata, Y.; Kawasaki, A.; Nishimura, H.; Ishida, Y.; Tsubata, T.; Yagita, H.; Honjo, T. Expression of the PD-1 antigen on the surface of stimulated mouse T and B lymphocytes. *Int. Immunol.* **1996**, *8*, 765–772. [CrossRef] [PubMed]
17. Francisco, L.M.; Salinas, V.H.; Brown, K.E.; Vanguri, V.K.; Freeman, G.J.; Kuchroo, V.K.; Sharpe, A.H. PD-L1 regulates the development, maintenance, and function of induced regulatory T cells. *J. Exp. Med.* **2009**, *206*, 3015–3029. [CrossRef]
18. Oestreich, K.J.; Yoon, H.; Ahmed, R.; Boss, J.M. NFATc1 regulates PD-1 expression upon T cell activation. *J. Immunol.* **2008**, *181*, 4832–4839. [CrossRef]
19. Yao, S.; Wang, S.; Zhu, Y.; Luo, L.; Zhu, G.; Flies, S.; Xu, H.; Ruff, W.; Broadwater, M.; Choi, I.H.; et al. PD-1 on dendritic cells impedes innate immunity against bacterial infection. *Blood* **2009**, *113*, 5811–5818. [CrossRef]

20. Cho, H.Y.; Lee, S.W.; Seo, S.K.; Choi, I.W.; Choi, I.; Lee, S.W. Interferon-sensitive response element (ISRE) is mainly responsible for IFN-alpha-induced upregulation of programmed death-1 (PD-1) in macrophages. *Biochim. Biophys. Acta* **2008**, *1779*, 811–819. [CrossRef]
21. Iwai, Y.; Hamanishi, J.; Chamoto, K.; Honjo, T. Cancer immunotherapies targeting the PD-1 signaling pathway. *J. Biomed. Sci.* **2017**, *24*, 26. [CrossRef] [PubMed]
22. Stewart, R.; Morrow, M.; Hammond, S.A.; Mulgrew, K.; Marcus, D.; Poon, E.; Watkins, A.; Mullins, S.; Chodorge, M.; Andrews, J.; et al. Identification and Characterization of MEDI4736, an Antagonistic Anti-PD-L1 Monoclonal Antibody. *Cancer Immunol. Res.* **2015**, *3*, 1052–1062. [CrossRef] [PubMed]
23. Kinter, A.L.; Godbout, E.J.; McNally, J.P.; Sereti, I.; Roby, G.A.; O'Shea, M.A.; Fauci, A.S. The common gamma-chain cytokines IL-2, IL-7, IL-15, and IL-21 induce the expression of programmed death-1 and its ligands. *J. Immunol.* **2008**, *181*, 6738–6746. [CrossRef] [PubMed]
24. Messal, N.; Serriari, N.E.; Pastor, S.; Nunès, J.A.; Olive, D. PD-L2 is expressed on activated human T cells and regulates their function. *Mol. Immunol.* **2011**, *48*, 2214–2219. [CrossRef] [PubMed]
25. Hawkes, E.A.; Grigg, A.; Chong, G. Programmed cell death-1 inhibition in lymphoma. *Lancet Oncol.* **2015**, *16*, e234–e245. [CrossRef]
26. Latchman, Y.; Wood, C.R.; Chernova, T.; Chaudhary, D.; Borde, M.; Chernova, I.; Iwai, Y.; Long, A.J.; Brown, J.A.; Nunes, R.; et al. PD-L2 is a second ligand for PD-1 and inhibits T cell activation. *Nat. Immunol.* **2001**, *2*, 261–268. [CrossRef] [PubMed]
27. Zhong, X.; Tumang, J.R.; Gao, W.; Bai, C.; Rothstein, T.L. PD-L2 expression extends beyond dendritic cells/macrophages to B1 cells enriched for V(H)11/V(H)12 and phosphatidylcholine binding. *Eur. J. Immunol.* **2007**, *37*, 2405–2410. [CrossRef]
28. Keir, M.E.; Butte, M.J.; Freeman, G.J.; Sharpe, A.H. PD-1 and its ligands in tolerance and immunity. *Annu. Rev. Immunol.* **2008**, *26*, 677–704. [CrossRef]
29. Salmaninejad, A.; Khoramshahi, V.; Azani, A.; Soltaninejad, E.; Aslani, S.; Zamani, M.R.; Zal, M.; Nesaei, A.; Hosseini, S.M. PD-1 and cancer: Molecular mechanisms and polymorphisms. *Immunogenetics* **2018**, *70*, 73–86. [CrossRef]
30. Ohaegbulam, K.C.; Assal, A.; Lazar-Molnar, E.; Yao, Y.; Zang, X. Human cancer immunotherapy with antibodies to the PD-1 and PD-L1 pathway. *Trends Mol. Med.* **2015**, *21*, 24–33. [CrossRef]
31. Chemnitz, J.M.; Parry, R.V.; Nichols, K.E.; June, C.H.; Riley, J.L. SHP-1 and SHP-2 associate with immunoreceptor tyrosine-based switch motif of programmed death 1 upon primary human T cell stimulation, but only receptor ligation prevents T cell activation. *J. Immunol.* **2004**, *173*, 945–954. [CrossRef] [PubMed]
32. Fife, B.T.; Pauken, K.E.; Eagar, T.N.; Obu, T.; Wu, J.; Tang, Q.; Azuma, M.; Krummel, M.F.; Bluestone, J.A. Interactions between PD-1 and PD-L1 promote tolerance by blocking the TCR-induced stop signal. *Nat. Immunol.* **2009**, *10*, 1185–1192. [CrossRef] [PubMed]
33. Patsoukis, N.; Sari, D.; Boussiotis, V.A. PD-1 inhibits T cell proliferation by upregulating p27 and p15 and suppressing Cdc25A. *Cell Cycle* **2012**, *11*, 4305–4309. [CrossRef]
34. Zinselmeyer, B.H.; Heydari, S.; Sacristán, C.; Nayak, D.; Cammer, M.; Herz, J.; Cheng, X.; Davis, S.J.; Dustin, M.L.; McGavern, D.B. PD-1 promotes immune exhaustion by inducing antiviral T cell motility paralysis. *J. Exp. Med.* **2013**, *210*, 757–774. [CrossRef] [PubMed]
35. Grzywnowicz, M.; Zaleska, J.; Mertens, D.; Tomczak, W.; Wlasiuk, P.; Kosior, K.; Piechnik, A.; Bojarska-Junak, A.; Dmoszynska, A.; Giannopoulos, K. Programmed death-1 and its ligand are novel immunotolerant molecules expressed on leukemic B cells in chronic lymphocytic leukemia. *PLoS ONE* **2012**, *7*, e35178. [CrossRef] [PubMed]
36. Xerri, L.; Chetaille, B.; Serriari, N.; Attias, C.; Guillaume, Y.; Arnoulet, C.; Olive, D. Programmed death 1 is a marker of angioimmunoblastic T-cell lymphoma and B-cell small lymphocytic lymphoma/chronic lymphocytic leukemia. *Hum. Pathol.* **2008**, *39*, 1050–1058, Erratum in **2010**, *41*, 1655. [CrossRef] [PubMed]
37. Grzywnowicz, M.; Karabon, L.; Karczmarczyk, A.; Zajac, M.; Skorka, K.; Zaleska, J.; Wlasiuk, P.; Chocholska, S.; Tomczak, W.; Bojarska-Junak, A.; et al. The function of a novel immunophenotype candidate molecule PD-1 in chronic lymphocytic leukemia. *Leuk. Lymphoma* **2015**, *56*, 2908–2913. [CrossRef] [PubMed]
38. Rusak, M.; Eljaszewicz, A.; Bołkun, Ł.; Łuksza, E.; Łapuć, I.; Piszcz, J.; Singh, P.; Dąbrowska, M.; Bodzenta-Łukaszyk, A.; Kłoczko, J.; et al. Prognostic significance of PD-1 expression on peripheral blood CD4+ T cells in patients with newly diagnosed chronic lymphocytic leukemia. *Pol. Arch. Med. Wewn.* **2015**, *125*, 553–559. [CrossRef]

39. Williams, P.; Basu, S.; Garcia-Manero, G.; Hourigan, C.S.; Oetjen, K.A.; Cortes, J.E.; Ravandi, F.; Jabbour, E.J.; Al-Hamal, Z.; Konopleva, M.; et al. The distribution of T-cell subsets and the expression of immune checkpoint receptors and ligands in patients with newly diagnosed and relapsed acute myeloid leukemia. *Cancer* **2018**. [CrossRef]
40. Tan, J.; Chen, S.; Lu, Y.; Yao, D.; Xu, L.; Zhang, Y.; Yang, L.; Chen, J.; Lai, J.; Yu, Z.; et al. Higher PD-1 expression concurrent with exhausted CD8+ T cells in patients with de novo acute myeloid leukemia. *Chin. J. Cancer Res.* **2017**, *29*, 463–470. [CrossRef]
41. Knaus, H.A.; Berglund, S.; Hackl, H.; Blackford, A.L.; Zeidner, J.F.; Montiel-Esparza, R.; Mukhopadhyay, R.; Vanura, K.; Blazar, B.R.; Karp, J.E.; et al. Signatures of CD8+ T cell dysfunction in AML patients and their reversibility with response to chemotherapy. *JCI Insight.* **2018**, *3*. [CrossRef] [PubMed]
42. Schnorfeil, F.M.; Lichtenegger, F.S.; Emmerig, K.; Schlueter, M.; Neitz, J.S.; Draenert, R.; Hiddemann, W.; Subklewe, M. T cells are functionally not impaired in AML: Increased PD-1 expression is only seen at time of relapse and correlates with a shift towards the memory T cell compartment. *J. Hematol. Oncol.* **2015**, *8*, 93. [CrossRef] [PubMed]
43. Jia, B.; Wang, L.; Claxton, D.F.; Ehmann, W.C.; Rybka, W.B.; Mineishi, S.; Rizvi, S.; Shike, H.; Bayerl, M.; Schell, T.D.; et al. Bone marrow CD8 T cells express high frequency of PD-1 and exhibit reduced anti-leukemia response in newly diagnosed AML patients. *Blood Cancer J.* **2018**, *8*, 34. [CrossRef] [PubMed]
44. Annibali, O.; Crescenzi, A.; Tomarchio, V.; Pagano, A.; Bianchi, A.; Grifoni, A.; Avvisati, G. PD-1 /PD-L1 checkpoint in hematological malignancies. *Leuk. Res.* **2018**, *67*, 45–55. [CrossRef] [PubMed]
45. Zhang, Z.F.; Zhang, Q.T.; Xin, H.Z.; Gan, S.L.; Ma, J.; Liu, Y.F.; Xie, X.S.; Sun, H. Expression of Programmed Death Ligand-1 (PD-L1) in Human Acute Leukemia and Its Clinical Significance. *Zhongguo Shi Yan Xue Ye Xue Za Zhi* **2015**, *23*, 930–934. [CrossRef] [PubMed]
46. Krönig, H.; Kremmler, L.; Haller, B.; Englert, C.; Peschel, C.; Andreesen, R.; Blank, C.U. Interferon-induced programmed death-ligand 1 (PD-L1/B7-H1) expression increases on human acute myeloid leukemia blast cells during treatment. *Eur. J. Haematol.* **2014**, *92*, 195–203. [CrossRef]
47. Jelinek, T.; Mihalyova, J.; Kascak, M.; Duras, J.; Hajek, R. PD-1/PD-L1 inhibitors in haematological malignancies: Update 2017. *Immunology* **2017**, *152*, 357–371. [CrossRef]
48. Zajac, M.; Zaleska, J.; Dolnik, A.; Bullinger, L.; Giannopoulos, K. Expression of CD274 (PD-L1) is associated with unfavourable recurrent mutations in AML. *Br. J. Haematol.* **2018**, *183*, 822–825. [CrossRef]
49. Goltz, D.; Gevensleben, H.; Grünen, S.; Dietrich, J.; Kristiansen, G.; Landsberg, J.; Dietrich, D. PD-L1 (CD274) promoter methylation predicts survival in patients with acute myeloid leukemia. *Leukemia* **2017**, *31*, 738–743. [CrossRef]
50. Wang, X.; Li, J.; Dong, K.; Lin, F.; Long, M.; Ouyang, Y.; Wei, J.; Chen, X.; Weng, Y.; He, T.; et al. Tumor suppressor miR-34a targets PD-L1 and functions as a potential immunotherapeutic target in acute myeloid leukemia. *Cell Signal* **2015**, *27*, 443–452. [CrossRef]
51. Le, D.T.; Uram, J.N.; Wang, H.; Bartlett, B.R.; Kemberling, H.; Eyring, A.D.; Skora, A.D.; Luber, B.S.; Azad, N.S.; Laheru, D.; et al. D-1 Blockade in Tumors with Mismatch-Repair Deficiency. *N. Engl. J. Med.* **2015**, *372*, 2509–2520. [CrossRef] [PubMed]
52. Rotte, A.; Jin, J.Y.; Lemaire, V. Mechanistic overview of immune checkpoints to support the rational design of their combinations in cancer immunotherapy. *Ann. Oncol.* **2018**, *29*, 71–83. [CrossRef] [PubMed]
53. Liu, L.; Chang, Y.J.; Xu, L.P.; Zhang, X.H.; Wang, Y.; Liu, K.Y.; Huang, X.J. Reversal of T Cell Exhaustion by the First Donor Lymphocyte Infusion Is Associated with the Persistently Effective Antileukemic Responses in Patients with Relapsed AML after Allo-HSCT. *Biol. Blood Marrow Transplant.* **2018**, *24*, 1350–1359. [CrossRef] [PubMed]
54. Yang, H.; Bueso-Ramos, C.; DiNardo, C.; Estecio, M.R.; Davanlou, M.; Geng, Q.R.; Fang, Z.; Nguyen, M.; Pierce, S.; Wei, Y.; et al. Expression of PD-L1, PD-L2, PD-1 and CTLA4 in myelodysplastic syndromes is enhanced by treatment with hypomethylating agents. *Leukemia* **2014**, *28*, 1280–1288. [CrossRef] [PubMed]
55. Kong, Y.; Zhang, J.; Claxton, D.F.; Ehmann, W.C.; Rybka, W.B.; Zhu, L.; Zeng, H.; Schell, T.D.; Zheng, H. PD-1(hi)TIM-3(+) T cells associate with and predict leukemia relapse in AML patients post allogeneic stem cell transplantation. *Blood Cancer J.* **2015**, *5*, e330. [CrossRef] [PubMed]
56. Ørskov, A.D.; Treppendahl, M.B.; Skovbo, A.; Holm, M.S.; Friis, L.S.; Hokland, M.; Grønbæk, K. Hypomethylation and up-regulation of PD-1 in T cells by azacitidine in MDS/AML patients: A rationale for combined targeting of PD-1 and DNA methylation. *Oncotarget.* **2015**, *6*, 9612–9626. [CrossRef] [PubMed]

57. Yu, G.; Wu, Y.; Wang, W.; Xu, J.; Lv, X.; Cao, X.; Wan, T. Low-dose decitabine enhances the effect of PD-1 blockade in colorectal cancer with microsatellite stability by re-modulating the tumor microenvironment. *Cell Mol. Immunol.* **2018**. [CrossRef]
58. Daver, N.; Garcia-Manero, G.; Basu, S.; Boddu, P.C.; Alfayez, M.; Cortes, J.E.; Konopleva, M.; Ravandi-Kashani, F.; Jabbour, E.; Kadia, T.M.; et al. Efficacy, Safety, and Biomarkers of Response to Azacitidine and Nivolumab in Relapsed/Refractory Acute Myeloid Leukemia: A Non-randomized, Open-label, Phase 2 Study. *Cancer Discov.* **2018**. [CrossRef]
59. Kadia, T.M.; Cortes, J.E.; Ghorab, A.; Ravandi, F.; Jabbour, E.; Daver, N.G.; Alvarado, Y.; Ohanian, M.; Konopleva, M.; Kantarjian, H.M. Nivolumab (Nivo) maintenance (maint) in high-risk (HR) acute myeloid leukemia (AML) patients. *J. Clin. Oncol.* **2018**, *36* (Suppl. 15), 7014. [CrossRef]
60. Albring, J.C.; Inselmann, S.; Sauer, T.; Schliemann, C.; Altvater, B.; Kailayangiri, S.; Rössig, C.; Hartmann, W.; Knorrenschild, J.R.; Sohlbach, K.; et al. PD-1 checkpoint blockade in patients with relapsed AML after allogeneic stem cell transplantation. *Bone Marrow Transplant.* **2017**, *52*, 317–320. [CrossRef]
61. Liu, Y.; Bewersdorf, J.P.; Stahl, M.; Zeidan, A.M. Immunotherapy in acute myeloid leukemia and myelodysplastic syndromes: The dawn of a new era? *Blood Rev.* **2018**. [CrossRef] [PubMed]
62. ClinicalTrials.gov. Available online: https://clinicaltrials.gov/ (accessed on 11 January 2019).
63. Larkin, J.; Hodi, F.S.; Wolchok, J.D. Combined Nivolumab and Ipilimumab or Monotherapy in Untreated Melanoma. *N. Engl. J. Med.* **2015**, *373*, 1270–1271. [CrossRef] [PubMed]
64. Heczey, A.; Louis, C.U.; Savoldo, B.; Dakhova, O.; Durett, A.; Grilley, B.; Liu, H.; Wu, M.F.; Mei, Z.; Gee, A.; et al. CAR T Cells Administered in Combination with Lymphodepletion and PD-1 Inhibition to Patients with Neuroblastoma. *Mol. Ther.* **2017**, *25*, 2214–2224. [CrossRef] [PubMed]
65. Gibney, G.T.; Kudchadkar, R.R.; DeConti, R.C.; Thebeau, M.S.; Czupryn, M.P.; Tetteh, L.; Eysmans, C.; Richards, A.; Schell, M.J.; Fisher, K.J.; et al. Safety, correlative markers, and clinical results of adjuvant nivolumab in combination with vaccine in resected high-risk metastatic melanoma. *Clin. Cancer Res.* **2015**, *21*, 712–720. [CrossRef] [PubMed]
66. Weber, J.S.; Kudchadkar, R.R.; Yu, B.; Gallenstein, D.; Horak, C.E.; Inzunza, H.D.; Zhao, X.; Martinez, A.J.; Wang, W.; Gibney, G.; et al. Safety, efficacy, and biomarkers of nivolumab with vaccine in ipilimumab-refractory or -naive melanoma. *J. Clin. Oncol.* **2013**, *31*, 4311–4318. [CrossRef] [PubMed]

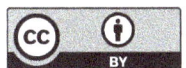

© 2019 by the author. Licensee MDPI, Basel, Switzerland. This article is an open access article distributed under the terms and conditions of the Creative Commons Attribution (CC BY) license (http://creativecommons.org/licenses/by/4.0/).

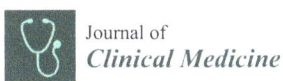

Review

Chimeric Antigen Receptor (CAR) T Cell Therapy in Acute Myeloid Leukemia (AML)

Susanne Hofmann [1,*], Maria-Luisa Schubert [1], Lei Wang [1], Bailin He [1], Brigitte Neuber [1], Peter Dreger [1,2], Carsten Müller-Tidow [1,2] and Michael Schmitt [1,2]

[1] Department of Internal Medicine V (Hematology/Oncology/Rheumatology), University Hospital Heidelberg, 69120 Heidelberg, Germany; Maria-Luisa.Schubert@med.uni-heidelberg.de (M.-L.S.); Lei.Wang@med.uni-heidelberg.de (L.W.); hebailin1990@gmail.com (B.H.); Brigitte.Neuber@med.uni-heidelberg.de (B.N.); Peter.Dreger@med.uni-heidelberg.de (P.D.); Carsten.Mueller-Tidow@med.uni-heidelberg.de (C.M.-T.) Michael.Schmitt@med.uni-heidelberg.de (M.S.)
[2] National Center for Tumor Diseases (NCT), 69120 Heidelberg, Germany
* Correspondence: susanne.hofmann@med.uni-heidelberg.de; Tel.: +49-6221-56-6614

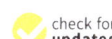

Received: 9 January 2019; Accepted: 3 February 2019; Published: 6 February 2019

Abstract: Despite high response rates after initial chemotherapy in patients with acute myeloid leukemia (AML), relapses occur frequently, resulting in a five-year-survival by <30% of the patients. Hitherto, allogeneic hemotopoietic stem cell transplantation (allo-HSCT) is the best curative treatment option in intermediate and high risk AML. It is the proof-of-concept for T cell-based immunotherapies in AML based on the graft-versus-leukemia (GvL)-effect, but it also bears the risk of graft-versus-host disease. CD19-targeting therapies employing chimeric antigen receptor (CAR) T cells are a breakthrough in cancer therapy. A similar approach for myeloid malignancies is highly desirable. This article gives an overview on the state-of-the art of preclinical and clinical studies on suitable target antigens for CAR T cell therapy in AML patients.

Keywords: AML; CAR T cell; immunotherapy

1. Introduction

With conventional chemotherapy employing anthracycline and cytarabine, high complete remission (CR) rates of 60% to 80% in younger adults and 40% to 60% in older adults (>60 years) can be achieved [1,2]. Despite these successful response rates, relapse after conventional therapy is common, mainly due to the chemorefractoriness of leukemic stem cells [3,4]. The estimated five-year survival of acute myeloid leukemia (AML) patients in the years 2008–2014 was 27.4% [5]. Until now, allogeneic hemotopoietic stem cell transplantation (allo-HSCT) was the best curative treatment option in intermediate and high risk AML. However, allo-HSCT is not suitable for every patient and bears the risk of non-relapse mortality as well as relapse. Allo-HSCT and donor lymphocyte infusion (DLI) also suggest that cellular immunotherapy is effective in AML. Both allo-HSCT and DLI bear curative potential based on the graft-versus-leukemia (GvL) effect but endow the danger of life-threatening graft-versus-host disease (GvHD). The remaining challenge is to separate GvL from GvHD and to find ways to enhance GvL without inducing GvHD. This underlines the urgent need for novel effective treatment options that mediate enduring eradication of the leukemic tumor burden including leukemic stem cells (LSCs).

Fueled by the success of immunotherapeutic strategies in other malignant hematologic entities, e.g., the anti-CD20 antibody rituximab in Non-Hodgkin's-lymphoma (NHL) or the CD19-specific chimeric antigen receptor (CAR)-T-cell therapies in acute lymphoblastic leukemia (ALL) and NHL, several efforts have been made to develop antibody-based or cellular immunotherapies for AML.

The key for successful targeted immunotherapies, either in form of an antibody or a targeted cellular approach, is the identification of a suitable target antigen. Cheever et al. summarized the features of an ideal target antigen, namely having a potential to induce clinical effects, being immunogenic, and playing a critical role in cell differentiation and proliferation of the malignant cells. Its expression should be restricted to malignant cells; it should be expressed in all malignant cells including malignant stem cells. A high number of patients should test positive for the antigen. The antigen should comprise multiple antigenic epitopes and be on the surface of malignant cells [6].

While for ALL, several other approaches, like bispecific antibodies and CAR-T-cells targeting CD19, are already in clinical practice, for AML identification of a good target antigen is more difficult. It is known from patients treated with rituximab that it is possible to live for some time with few B-cells, given the option that immunoglobulins can be substituted. Expression of antigens by AML blasts and leukemic stem cells is not exclusively restricted to those cells but overlaps with normal hematopoiesis, which can cause severe hematotoxicity of antigen-targeting therapies.

The following paragraphs focus on CAR-T cell approaches in AML.

2. Adoptive Cellular Therapies

Based on the finding that cytotoxic T cells are key players in mediating GvL in allo-HSCT, concepts of adoptive T cell therapy were initially developed, such as tumor-infiltrating lymphocytes or donor lymphocyte infusion (DLI) [7–9]. Later, genetically engineered T cells were tested in clinical trials. Two main technologies of genetically engineered T cells exist—T cell receptor (TCR) engineered T cells and chimeric antigen receptor (CAR) transduced T cells.

Both approaches directly place the T cell in the vicinity to the antigen-bearing target cell. One main difference is that a T cell receptor (TCR) recognizes intracellularly and extracelluary expressed antigens in the context of human leukocyte antigen (HLA)- receptors, whereas CAR T cells are HLA-independent and only recognize surface antigens in an antibody-specific manner (Figure 1).

CAR T-cells combine the strong feature of an antibody in target recognition and the effector, and long-term function of the T-cell and the effector cell is directly brought to the cancer cell. CARs (Figure 1) are artificial receptors composed of three domains, (1) an extracellular antigen-specific binding domain that is derived from an antibody's single chain variable fragment (scFv), (2) a hinge and transmembrane segment usually derived from CD8alpha [10] or IgG domain [11], and (3) an intracellular T-cell signaling domain.

CAR T cells are genetically engineered to express CARs via viral (retroviral, lentiviral, adenoviral) or non-viral technologies such as electroporation, transposon-based, or gene-editing systems.

Addition of co-stimulation signals to the intracellular domain in second and third generation CARs aim to improve the survival of engineered T cells (Figure 1A). First-generation CARs contain only the tyrosine-based zeta-signal-transducing subunit from the TCR/CD3 receptor complex [12–14]. Adjacent to this zeta-domain, second-generation CARs harbor one and third-generation CARs two additional costimulatory molecules [15] such as CD28 [16], CD27, DAP-12 [17], 10 4-1BB (CD137), OX40 (CD134) [18], or inducible T cell costimulator (ICOS) [19]. Indeed, depending on the introduced costimulatory signal, second and third generation CARs mediate superior activation, proliferation, and in vivo persistence of T cells [20,21]. Third generation CARs show increased tumor-lytic activity as well as reduced activation-induced cell death compared to first-generation CARs [22,23].

When relapse occurs after antibody or CAR therapy, tumor cells often lose the targeted antigen. This problem is addressed by CAR T cells targeting multiple antigens, either by simultaneous co-administration of several monospecific CARs [24] or by one distinct CAR T cell targeting several antigens (Figure 1B). These CAR T cells are called dual-targeting T cells (when one CAR T cell expresses two different antigen-specific CARs [25]) or bispecific CAR T cells (when one CAR is specific for two different targets [26]). This combinatorial CAR therapy approach was recently put forward by Perna et al. With the help of high-throughput surfaceome expression data, they identified pairs of target antigens and defined ideal features of CAR targets to reduce the risks of antigen escape and off-tumor toxicity. The features for an ideal pair are: no overlapping expression in normal tissues to minimize systemic off-tumor toxicity, very low level expression in CD34+CD38- hematopoietic stem cells (HSCs) to minimize cytotoxicity, very low expression in normal resting and activated T cells to minimize T cell reactivity, expression (for the combination) in all tumor cells to overcome clonal heterogeneity, expression in LSCs, and co-expression in tumor-cells to prevent antigen escape [27]. Besides antigen escape, loss of CAR T cells and autoantibody development are important mechanisms of CAR T cell therapy failure [28].

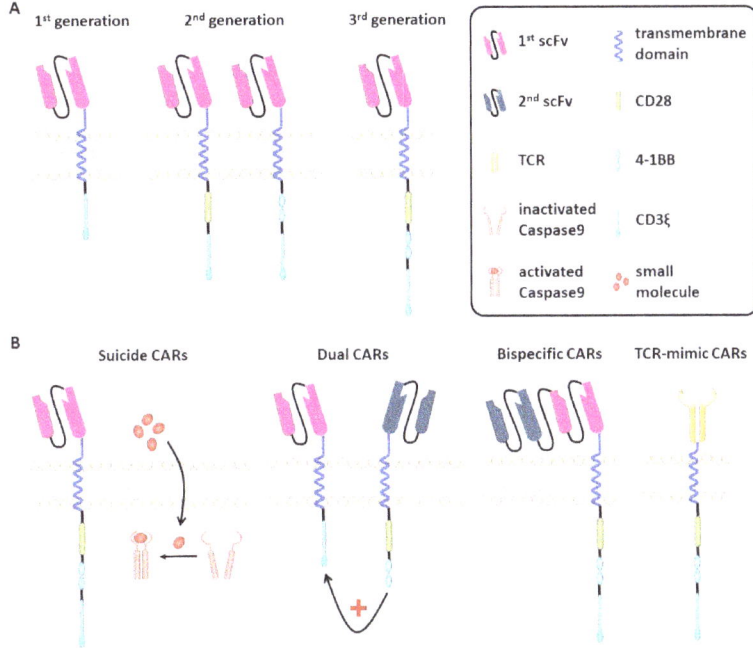

Figure 1. (**A**) Chimeric antigen receptor (CAR). CARs consist of an extracellular domain generated by joining the heavy and light chain variable regions of a monoclonal antibody with a linker to form a single-chain Fv (scFv) molecule. The antigen-specific domain binds its antigen on the surface of target cells. The scFv is attached via a hinge region to the transmembrane and intracellular receptor portion. In first-generation CARs, the signaling domain is composed of the zeta- domain of a T cell receptor (TCR)/CD3 receptor complex. In second- and third-generation CARs, one or two costimulatory signaling domains are added (e.g., CD28, 4-1BB (CD137), OX-40 (CD137), or inducible T cell costimulatory (ICOS)) within their intracellular domain, respectively. (**B**) Innovative CAR design. Suicide gene strategies are investigated as control mechanisms for better toxicity management of CAR T cells. One example is the inducible caspase 9 (iCasp9). When the small molecule AP1903 is administered, iCasp9 domains dimerize and activate apoptosis independently of CAR activation. Dual-targeting CARs express two different antigen-specific CARs, whereas bispecific CARs bear two linked scFV within one CAR construct. To address human leukocyte antigen (HLA)-presented antigens, TCR-mimic (TCRm) CARs directing the scFv domain against a peptide-HLA complex have been developed.

To date, in the context of AML, only few CARs have been investigated in clinical trials, and in contrast to B-cell malignancies, no licensing authority approved CAR therapy for AML exists. In the following sections, we give an overview of antigen candidates that are already investigated in clinical trials (Table 1), as well as those that are potentially suitable for CAR therapy in AML (Figure 2).

Table 1. Chimeric antigen receptor (CAR) trials in acute myeloid leukemia (AML) [29].

Trial ID	Status	Phase	Target	Indication	Institution
NCT03585517	R	I	CD123	CD123+ AML	Xian Lu, Beijing, China
NCT03114670	R	I	CD123	recurred AML after allo	Fengtai District, Beijing Shi, China
NCT03556982	R	I/II	CD123	R/R AML	307 Hospital of PLA, Beijing, Beijing, China
NCT02623582	terminated	I	CD123	R/R AML	Abramson Cancer Center of the University of Pennsylvania, Philadelphia, Pennsylvania, United States
NCT02159495	R	I	CD123	R/R AML, Persistent/Recurrent Blastic Plasmacytoid Dendritic Cell Neoplasm	City of Hope Medical Center, Duarte, California, United States
NCT03672851	R	I	CD123	R/R AML	Second Affiliated Hospital of Xi'an Jiaotong University, Xi'an, Shaanxi, China
NCT03766126	R	I	CD123	R/R AML	University of Pennsylvania, Philadelphia, Pennsylvania, United States
NCT01864902	R	I	UCART 123	R/R AML, newly diagnosed high-risk AML	Weill Cornell Medical College, New York, New York, United States MD Anderson Cancer Center, Houston, Texas, United States
NCT03631576	R	II/III	CD123/CLL1	R/R AML	Fujian Medical University Union Hospital, Fuzhou, Fujian, China
NCT03126864	R	I	CD33	R/R CD33+ AML	University of Texas MD Anderson Cancer Center, Houston, Texas, United States
NCT02799680	unknown	I	CD33	R/R AML	Affiliated Hospital of Academy of Military Medical Sciences, Beijing, Beijing, China l Chinese PLA General Hospital, Beijing, Beijing, China
NCT01864902	unknown	I/II	CD33	R/R AML	Biotherapeutic Department and Pediatrics Department of Chinese PLA General Hospital, Hematological Department, Affiliated Hospital of Changzhi Medical College, Beijing, Beijing, China
NCT02944162	unknown	I/II	anti-CD33 NK CAR	R/R CD33+ AML	PersonGen BioTherapeutics (Suzhou) Co., Ltd., Suzhou, Jiangsu, China

Table 1. Cont.

Trial ID	Status	Phase	Target	Indication	Institution
NCT03291444	R	I	CD33, CD38 CD56, CD117, CD123, CD34, and Muc1 for AML and MDS	R/R AML, MDS; ALL	Zhujiang Hospital, Southern Medical University, Guangzhou, Guangdong, China
NCT03473457	R	n.a.	single CAR-T or double CAR-T cells with CD33, CD38, CD56, CD123, CD117, CD133, CD34, or Muc1	R/R AML	Southern Medical University Zhujiang Hospital, Guangdong, Guangdong, China
NCT03222674	R	I/II	Muc1/CLL1/CD33/CD38/CD56/CD123	AML	Zhujiang Hospital of Southern Medical University, Guangzhou, Guangdong, China | Shenzhen Geno-immune Medical Institute, Shenzhen, Guangdong, China | Yunnan Cancer Hospital & The Third Affiliated Hospital of Kunming Medical University & Yunnan Cancer Center, KunMing, Yunnan, China
NCT02203825	completed	I	NKG2D	AML, MDS-RAEB, and Multiple Myeloma.	Dana-Farber Cancer Institute, Boston, Massachusetts, United States
NCT03018405	R	I/II	NKR2 (NKG2D)	R/R AML, AML, Myeloma	Tampa, Florida, United States | Buffalo, New York, United States | Brussels, Belgium | Brussels, Belgium | Ghent, Belgium
NCT03018405	unknown	I/II	CD7/NK92 cell	CD7+ R/R Leukemia and Lymphoma	PersonGen BioTherapeutics (Suzhou) Co., Ltd., Suzhou, Jiangsu, China
NCT01716364	unknown	I	Lewis Y	Myeloma, AML, MDS	Peter MacCallum Cancer Centre, Melbourne, Victoria, Australia

Abbreviations: R, recruiting; r/r relapsed/refractory; AML, acute myeloid leukemia; ALL, acute lymphoblastic leukemia; MDS, myelodysplastic syndrome. Note: Search term: CAR, AML (as by 12 December 2018). Source: [24].

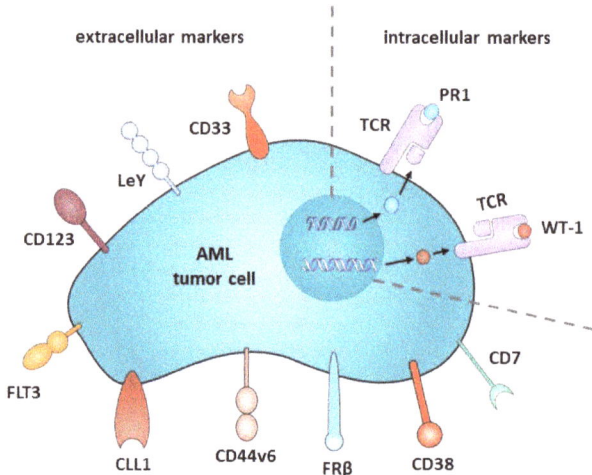

Figure 2. Potential target antigens for CAR therapy in AML.

3. CD33

CD33 is expressed in up to 90% of leukemic blast cells but also on healthy myeloid and myeloid progenitor cells [30,31]. It is not expressed on early pluripotent CD34-positive hematopoietic stem cells [32], but it is also expressed by hepatocytes, which can explain extrahematological toxicity in the form of veno-occlusive liver disease (VOD) [33,34]. A restriction is that CD34+CD33- negative leukemic stem cells have been reported [35]. CD33 is an attractive target for immunotherapy against AML. This was shown by the development of Gemtuzumab (Mylotarg®, Pfizer, Berlin, Germany), a humanized drug-conjugated anti-CD33-antibody. Although first approved in 2000 by the US Food and Drug Administration (FDA), it was withdrawn from the European and US markets in 2010 due to bone-marrow toxicity and VOD. It was reintroduced in 2018 after a meta-analysis by Hills et al. demonstrated that a low, fractionated dose of Mylotarg® in combination with chemotherapy led to an improved overall-survival of 280 treated AML patients [36].

Due to this experiment and the high expression of CD33 in myeloid leukemia, there are currently many activities considering anti-CD33 CAR therapy (Table 1). To date, one report of a patient with r/r AML who was treated with anti-CD33 CARs has been published [37]. In this phase I trial, the patient received a total of 1.12×10^9 autologous T-cells (38% CAR transduced) and suffered from cytokine release syndrome (CRS) as well as pancytopenia and disease progression nine weeks after cell infusion.

Due to the CD33 expression in healthy myelopoiesis, it is necessary to develop new safety concepts with anti-CD33 CAR transfusion.

One approach is the transient expression of anti-CD33 CAR, which was tested in an in vivo model of AML-xenotransplanted NOD scid gamma (NSG) mice [38]. Only transient cytotoxicity was observed. Another interesting method recently published is the generation of leukemia specificity by genetic knock-out of CD33 in normal hematopoietic stem and progenitor cells. Thereby, an artificial resistance against anti-CD33 CAR T cell therapy is created. In xenograft immunodeficient mice, CD33-deficient human HSPCs engrafted and differentiated normally. In rhesus macaques, anti-CD33 CAR T cell therapy transfused after autologous CD33 knock-out HSPC transplantation was effective in eliminating leukemia cells without any signs of myelotoxicity [39].

4. Lewis Y (LeY)

Lewis Y (LeY) is a carbohydrate antigen that is overexpressed by a wide variety of epithelial cancers [40] and hematological malignancies including AML [41,42] but with only limited expression on normal tissue [43].

In 2010, Peinert and colleagues published the results of the first phase I CAR- T cell trial for relapsed LeY-expressing AML [44]. They investigated an autologous second-generation anti-LeY CAR in four patients who received up to 1.3×10^9 total T cells (14–38% with anti-LeY CAR expression). No grade three or four toxicity was observed. The best response was transient cytogenetic remission in one patient; another patient showed a transient reduction of blasts, and two patients showed stable disease. All patients relapsed after 28 days to 23 months after adoptive cell therapy. CAR T cell persistence was demonstrated for up to 10 months.

5. CD123

CD123 is the transmembrane alpha chain of the interleukin 3 receptor. Due to its surface expression and its overexpression on AML blasts and LSCs, as well as its low expression on normal hematopoeietic stem cells, CD123 qualifies as a suitable target [45,46]. However, similar to CD33 targeted therapy, the problem of myelotoxicity in CD123 targeted therapy remains.

At the time of writing this manuscript, CD123 is being studied in 11 clinical trials for AML (Table 1).

CARs normally encode in its scFvs a VH and VL chain from one monoclonal antibody in the extracellular antigen binding domain. In an experimental AML model, hematopoietic toxicity was shown after treatment with anti-CD123 CAR T cells. When using VH and VL chains derived from different CD123-specific mAbs for CAR engineering, one specific combination showed less lysis of the normal hematopoietic stem cells while preserving the toxicity [47].

6. FLT3 (CD135)

FLT3-ITD mutations are found in about 20% (and FLT3-TKD in about 7%) of all AML patients [48]. In a preclinical model, second-generation anti-FLT3-41BB CARs were tested [49]. Specific cytotoxicity against FLT3+ leukemia cell lines and primary cell lines in vitro, as well as little off-tumor cytotoxicity on normal hematopoietic stem cells, was observed. In a xenograft mouse model, prolonged survival was seen in FLT3+ mice that were treated with the anti-FLT3 CARs. Compared to anti-CD33 CAR T cells, less toxicity to hematopoietic stem cells and multipotent myeloid progenitor cells and equivalent toxicity to common myeloid progenitor and granulocyte-macrophage progenitor cells was described, suggesting a lower hematologic toxicity with anti-FLT3 CAR T cells. In a second preclinical study, second-generation 4-1BB CARs that target the FLT3-ligand (FLT3L) were tested [50]. For anti-FLT3L, little off-tumor cytotoxicity on normal hematopoietic stem and progenitor cells was observed. A xenograft mouse model also showed a significantly prolonged survival in FLT3+ leukemia bearing mice after anti-FLT3L CAR T cells [50].

7. CLL1

The myeloid surface antigen C-type lectin-like molecule 1 (CLL1 or CLEC12A) is a glycoprotein highly expressed by the majority of AML patients. It is expressed on AML blasts and on normally differentiated myeloid cells. Relatively low amounts are expressed on CD34+ progenitor cells. It is not expressed on normal hematopoietic stem cells [51]. CLL 1 therefore qualifies as a promising CAR T cell target suggesting low "off-tumor" toxicity.

Four research groups generated anti-CLL1 CAR T cells, three second generation [52–54] and one third generation CAR [55]. All four showed potent activity against CLL1+ AML cell lines, as well as primary CLL1+ AML blasts in vitro and in xenograft mouse models, while sparing normal myeloid precursor cells. Tashiro et al. went a step further and introduced the inducible caspase-9 suicide gene system into the CARs and could successfully control anti-CLL1 CAR T cell activity in vitro and in vivo.

8. CD44v6

CD44v6 is the isoform variant 6 of the hyaluronic acid receptor CD44, a class I membrane glycoprotein overexpressed in hematologic malignancies including AML [56] and epithelial tumors [57]. It is absent in hematopoietic stem cells [58] and shows low expression levels on normal cells. Casucci and colleagues designed a second generation anti-CD44v6 CAR with cytotoxicity against AML cells while sparing normal hematopoietic stem cells [59]. Monocytopenia was the dose limiting toxicity in this preclinical study. To control this adverse event, the clinical-grade suicide genes, thymidine kinase [60] and the nonimmunogenic inducible Caspase 9 (iC9) [61], were coexpressed in the anti-CD44v6 CARs with iC9 successfully eradicating the CAR T cells within hours.

9. Folate Receptor ß (FRß)

Folate receptor ß (FRß) is primarily expressed on myeloid-lineage hematopoietic cells [62] and is expressed on about 70% of primary AML cells [63]. The expression of FRß on AML blasts can be increased by all-trans retinoic acid (ATRA) and enhanced the efficacy of folate-conjugated drug therapy in a preclinical study [64,65]. Preclinical models showed the efficacy of anti-FRß CAR T cells and an even better efficacy of high-affinity anti-FRß CAR T cells against AML cells in vitro and in vivo without toxicity against healthy hematopoietic progenitor/stem cells (HPSCs) [66,67].

10. CD38

CD38 is expressed on the majority of AML blasts but not healthy human hematopoietic stem cells [68,69]. Due to the modest expression level of CD38 in AML, the combination of ATRA and second generation anti-CD38 CAR T cells to enhance the CD38 expression was tested [70]. In this study, ATRA enhanced the cytotoxicity of anti-CD38 CAR T cells on AML cells with the augmented CD38 expression in vitro.

11. CD7

CD7 is expressed by T cells and natural killer cells [71]; it is also expressed in over 90% of lymphoblastic T cell leukemia and lymphoma [72,73] and in about 30% of AML cases [74,75], but is absent in normal myeloid and erythroid cells. An anti-CD7 CAR in CD7 knock-out T cells to prevent fratricide can effectively eliminate CD7 + AML cell lines as well as primary AML cells while sparing normal myeloid and erythroid progenitor cells [76–78].

12. Intracellular Targets: PR1/HLA-A2; WT1/HLA-A2

The majority of leukemia-associated-antigens and neoantigens are intracellularly processed and presented by HLA class II molecules. To address HLA-presented antigens, TCR-mimic (TCRm) CARs directing the scFv domain against a peptide-HLA complex were developed. Proteinase 1 (PR1) is a HLA A2-restricted nonamer derived from the leukemia associated antigen proteinase 3 and neutrophil elastase. Both proteases are expressed in the primary azurophilic granules of neutrophils and are overexpressed in myeloid leukemic blasts [79,80]. A second-generation CAR construct targeting HLA-A2/PR1 was preferentially cytotoxic against human AML cell lines and primary AML blasts in vitro [81]. The second TCRm CAR published targets the leukemia associated antigen Wilms tumor 1 (WT1) in the context of HLA-A2 and has demonstrated efficacy in vivo in an AML mouse model [82]. WT1 is overexpressed in AML, chronic myeloid leukemia (CML), and several solid tumors [83–85]. Another antigen candidate is PRAME (preferentially expressed antigen in melanoma). It is a so-called cancer-testis antigen and is therefore exclusively expressed in the testes and ovaries in healthy tissue. However, in several malignant tissues—and in about 20–40% of AML cases—it is intracellularly expressed and presented on the cell surface via human leukocyte antigen (HLA)-I. Chang et al. developed a TCRm human IgG1 antibody that recognizes a decamer peptide derived from PRAME in the context with HLA-A. It showed therapeutical effectiveness against mouse xenograft models of human leukemia [86]. In addition, a multicenter phase I/II clinical trial is currently testing autologous T cells that are transduced with a PRAME-specific HLA-A*02:01-restricted TCR (NCT03503968).

Whether autoimmune reactions as off-tumor toxicity occur with TCRm CAR application has to be investigated in further studies.

13. Safety Affairs

Relevant side effects of CARs are tumor-lysis syndrome and cytokine release syndrome, as well as "on-target but off-tumor" toxicity. "On-target but off-tumor" toxicity occurs when the target antigen is not only expressed on the target cells but also on normal tissues. This is the case for HER2, which is expressed in epithelial cells in the gastrointestinal, respiratory, reproductive, urinary tract, skin, breast, placenta, and normal hematopoietic cells [87]. A clinical trial investigating a third generation CAR targeting HER2 reported of one patient who developed respiratory distress within 15 min after receiving a single dose of 10^10 CAR T cells, followed by cardiac arrest [88]. This study underlines how important the target antigen selection is. Other aspects of reducing toxicity, mainly cytokine storm, are the number of infused CARs as well as the use of immunosuppressive agents and an introduced control mechanism into the CARs (Figure 1B). As control mechanisms, several suicide gene strategies were investigated, including thymidine kinase gene of the herpes simplex virus thymidine kinase (HSV-TK) [89] and the inducible caspase 9 (iCasp9) [90]. An elegant approach to limit "off-tumor" toxicity is to modify the CAR scFvs affinity of the antibody [91]. For high affinity HER2 CAR T cells, it was demonstrated that in dependence of the antigen density on the surface of the target cell, a high-affinity CAR is reactive against a malignant (high density) but not a normal (low density) cell [91].

14. Conclusions

Although in B-cell malignancies, CAR T cells now begin to build one therapeutic column in clinical practice, the value of CAR T cell therapy for AML still has to be determined.

There are major hurdles to take, e.g., finding the right antigen with low "off-tumor" toxicity and supplementing strategies to minimize "off-tumor" toxicity. Several attempts have already been made, such as suicidal control of CAR T cells, temporary expression of the CAR, and improvement of the affinity of the CAR. The CAR race has started and will hopefully improve and enrich the therapeutic armentarium against AML.

Acknowledgments: We thank M. Hinkelbein for support with editing text and references.

Conflicts of Interest: The authors declare no conflicts of interest.

References

1. Döhner, H.; Weisdorf, D.J.; Bloomfield, C.D. Acute myeloid leukemia. *N. Engl. J. Med.* **2015**, *373*, 1136–1152. [CrossRef] [PubMed]
2. Döhner, H.; Estey, E.H.; Amadori, S.; Appelbaum, F.R.; Büchner, T.; Burnett, A.K.; Dombret, H.; Fenaux, P.; Grimwade, D.; Larson, R.A.; et al. Diagnosis and management of acute myeloid leukemia in adults: Recommendations from an international expert panel, on behalf of the european leukemianet. *Blood* **2010**, *115*, 453–474. [CrossRef] [PubMed]
3. Eppert, K.; Takenaka, K.; Lechman, E.R.; Waldron, L.; Nilsson, B.; van Galen, P.; Metzeler, K.H.; Poeppl, A.; Ling, V.; Beyene, J.; et al. Stem cell gene expression programs influence clinical outcome in human leukemia. *Nat. Med.* **2011**, *17*, 1086–1093. [CrossRef] [PubMed]
4. Bonnet, D.; Dick, J.E. Human acute myeloid leukemia is organized as a hierarchy that originates from a primitive hematopoietic cell. *Nat. Med.* **1997**, *3*, 730–737. [CrossRef]
5. Available online: https://seer.cancer.gov/statfacts/html/amyl.html (accessed on 5 February 2019).

6. Cheever, M.A.; Allison, J.P.; Ferris, A.S.; Finn, O.J.; Hastings, B.M.; Hecht, T.T.; Mellman, I.; Prindiville, S.A.; Viner, J.L.; Weiner, L.M.; et al. The prioritization of cancer antigens: A national cancer institute pilot project for the acceleration of translational research. *Clin. Cancer Res.* **2009**, *15*, 5323–8337. [CrossRef] [PubMed]
7. Kolb, H.J.; Mittermuller, J.; Clemm, C.; Holler, E.; Ledderose, G.; Brehm, G.; Heim, M.; Wilmanns, W. Donor leukocyte transfusions for treatment of recurrent chronic myelogenous leukemia in marrow transplant patients. *Blood* **1990**, *76*, 2462–2465. [PubMed]
8. Kolb, H.J.; Schattenberg, A.; Goldman, J.M.; Hertenstein, B.; Jacobsen, N.; Arcese, W.; Ljungman, P.; Ferrant, A.; Verdonck, L.; Niederwieser, D.; et al. Graft-versus-leukemia effect of donor lymphocyte transfusions in marrow grafted patients. *Blood* **1995**, *86*, 2041–2050.
9. Kolb, H.J.; Schmid, C.; Barrett, A.J.; Schendel, D.J. Graft-versus-leukemia reactions in allogeneic chimeras. *Blood* **2004**, *103*, 767–776. [CrossRef]
10. Maude, S.L.; Frey, N.; Shaw, P.A.; Aplenc, R.; Barrett, D.M.; Bunin, N.J.; Chew, A.; Gonzalez, V.E.; Zheng, Z.; Lacey, S.F.; et al. Chimeric antigen receptor t cells for sustained remissions in leukemia. *N. Engl. J. Med.* **2014**, *371*, 1507–1517. [CrossRef]
11. Turtle, C.J.; Hanafi, L.A.; Berger, C.; Gooley, T.A.; Cherian, S.; Hudecek, M.; Sommermeyer, D.; Melville, K.; Pender, B.; Budiarto, T.M.; et al. Cd19 car-t cells of defined cd4+:Cd8+ composition in adult b cell all patients. *J. Clin. Investig.* **2016**, *126*, 2123–2138. [CrossRef]
12. Eshhar, Z.; Waks, T.; Gross, G.; Schindler, D.G. Specific activation and targeting of cytotoxic lymphocytes through chimeric single chains consisting of antibody-binding domains and the gamma or zeta subunits of the immunoglobulin and t-cell receptors. *Proc. Natl. Acad. Sci. USA* **1993**, *90*, 720–724. [CrossRef] [PubMed]
13. Jensen, M.C.; Popplewell, L.; Cooper, L.J.; DiGiusto, D.; Kalos, M.; Ostberg, J.R.; Forman, S.J. Antitransgene rejection responses contribute to attenuated persistence of adoptively transferred cd20/cd19-specific chimeric antigen receptor redirected t cells in humans. *Biol. Blood Marrow Trans.* **2010**, *16*, 1245–1256. [CrossRef] [PubMed]
14. Stancovski, I.; Schindler, D.G.; Waks, T.; Yarden, Y.; Sela, M.; Eshhar, Z. Targeting of t lymphocytes to neu/her2-expressing cells using chimeric single chain fv receptors. *J. Immunol.* **1993**, *151*, 6577–6582. [PubMed]
15. Till, B.G.; Jensen, M.C.; Wang, J.; Qian, X.; Gopal, A.K.; Maloney, D.G.; Lindgren, C.G.; Lin, Y.; Pagel, J.M.; Budde, L.E.; et al. Cd20-specific adoptive immunotherapy for lymphoma using a chimeric antigen receptor with both cd28 and 4-1bb domains: Pilot clinical trial results. *Blood* **2012**, *119*, 3940–3950. [CrossRef] [PubMed]
16. Finney, H.M.; Lawson, A.D.G.; Bebbington, C.R.; Weir, A.N.C. Chimeric receptors providing both primary and costimulatory signaling in t cells from a single gene product. *J. Immunol.* **1998**, *161*, 2791. [PubMed]
17. Wang, E.; Wang, L.C.; Tsai, C.Y.; Bhoj, V.; Gershenson, Z.; Moon, E.; Newick, K.; Sun, J.; Lo, A.; Baradet, T.; et al. Generation of potent t-cell immunotherapy for cancer using dap12-based, multichain, chimeric immunoreceptors. *Cancer Immunol. Res.* **2015**, *3*, 815–826. [CrossRef] [PubMed]
18. Hombach, A.A.; Chmielewski, M.; Rappl, G.; Abken, H. Adoptive immunotherapy with redirected t cells produces ccr7- cells that are trapped in the periphery and benefit from combined cd28-ox40 costimulation. *Hum. Gene Ther.* **2013**, *24*, 259–269. [CrossRef]
19. Guedan, S.; Chen, X.; Madar, A.; Carpenito, C.; McGettigan, S.E.; Frigault, M.J.; Lee, J.; Posey, A.D., Jr.; Scholler, J.; Scholler, N.; et al. Icos-based chimeric antigen receptors program bipolar th17/th1 cells. *Blood* **2014**, *124*, 1070–1080. [CrossRef]
20. Zhao, Y.; Wang, Q.J.; Yang, S.; Kochenderfer, J.N.; Zheng, Z.; Zhong, X.; Sadelain, M.; Eshhar, Z.; Rosenberg, S.A.; Morgan, R.A. A herceptin-based chimeric antigen receptor with modified signaling domains leads to enhanced survival of transduced t lymphocytes and antitumor activity. *J. Immunol.* **2009**, *183*, 5563–5574. [CrossRef]
21. Savoldo, B.; Ramos, C.A.; Liu, E.; Mims, M.P.; Keating, M.J.; Carrum, G.; Kamble, R.T.; Bollard, C.M.; Gee, A.P.; Mei, Z.; et al. Cd28 costimulation improves expansion and persistence of chimeric antigen receptor-modified t cells in lymphoma patients. *J. Clin. Investig.* **2011**, *121*, 1822–1826. [CrossRef]
22. Han, E.Q.; Li, X.L.; Wang, C.R.; Li, T.F.; Han, S.Y. Chimeric antigen receptor-engineered t cells for cancer immunotherapy: Progress and challenges. *J. Hematol. Oncol.* **2013**, *6*, 47. [CrossRef] [PubMed]

23. Long, A.H.; Haso, W.M.; Shern, J.F.; Wanhainen, K.M.; Murgai, M.; Ingaramo, M.; Smith, J.P.; Walker, A.J.; Kohler, M.E.; Venkateshwara, V.R.; et al. 4-1bb costimulation ameliorates t cell exhaustion induced by tonic signaling of chimeric antigen receptors. *Nat. Med.* **2015**, *21*, 581–590. [CrossRef] [PubMed]
24. Ruella, M.; Barrett, D.M.; Kenderian, S.S.; Shestova, O.; Hofmann, T.J.; Perazzelli, J.; Klichinsky, M.; Aikawa, V.; Nazimuddin, F.; Kozlowski, M.; et al. Dual cd19 and cd123 targeting prevents antigen-loss relapses after cd19-directed immunotherapies. *J. Clin. Investig.* **2016**, *126*, 3814–3826. [CrossRef] [PubMed]
25. Wilkie, S.; van Schalkwyk, M.C.; Hobbs, S.; Davies, D.M.; van der Stegen, S.J.; Pereira, A.C.; Burbridge, S.E.; Box, C.; Eccles, S.A.; Maher, J. Dual targeting of erbb2 and muc1 in breast cancer using chimeric antigen receptors engineered to provide complementary signaling. *J. Clin. Immunol.* **2012**, *32*, 1059–1070. [CrossRef] [PubMed]
26. Zah, E.; Lin, M.Y.; Silva-Benedict, A.; Jensen, M.C.; Chen, Y.Y. T cells expressing cd19/cd20 bispecific chimeric antigen receptors prevent antigen escape by malignant b cells. *Cancer Immunol. Res.* **2016**, *4*, 498–508. [CrossRef] [PubMed]
27. Perna, F.; Berman, S.H.; Soni, R.K.; Mansilla-Soto, J.; Eyquem, J.; Hamieh, M.; Hendrickson, R.C.; Brennan, C.W.; Sadelain, M. Integrating proteomics and transcriptomics for systematic combinatorial chimeric antigen receptor therapy of aml. *Cancer Cell* **2017**, *32*, 506–519. [CrossRef] [PubMed]
28. Dotti, G.; Gottschalk, S.; Savoldo, B.; Brenner, M.K. Design and development of therapies using chimeric antigen receptor-expressing t cells. *Immunol. Rev.* **2014**, *257*, 107–126. [CrossRef]
29. Available online: https://clinicaltrials.gov/ct2/results?cond=aml&term=car&cntry=&state=&city=&dist= (accessed on 12 December 2018).
30. Griffin, J.D.; Linch, D.; Sabbath, K.; Larcom, P.; Schlossman, S.F. A monoclonal antibody reactive with normal and leukemic human myeloid progenitor cells. *Leuk. Res.* **1984**, *8*, 521–534. [CrossRef]
31. Nguyen, D.H.; Ball, E.D.; Varki, A. Myeloid precursors and acute myeloid leukemia cells express multiple cd33-related siglecs. *Exp. Hematol.* **2006**, *34*, 728–735. [CrossRef]
32. Hauswirth, A.W.; Florian, S.; Printz, D.; Sotlar, K.; Krauth, M.T.; Fritsch, G.; Schernthaner, G.H.; Wacheck, V.; Selzer, E.; Sperr, W.R.; et al. Expression of the target receptor cd33 in cd34+/cd38-/cd123+ aml stem cells. *Eur. J. Clin. Investig.* **2007**, *37*, 73–82. [CrossRef]
33. Thol, F.; Schlenk, R.F. Gemtuzumab ozogamicin in acute myeloid leukemia revisited. *Expert Opin. Biol. Ther.* **2014**, *14*, 1185–1195. [CrossRef] [PubMed]
34. Giles, F.J.; Kantarjian, H.M.; Kornblau, S.M.; Thomas, D.A.; Garcia-Manero, G.; Waddelow, T.A.; David, C.L.; Phan, A.T.; Colburn, D.E.; Rashid, A.; et al. Mylotarg (gemtuzumab ozogamicin) therapy is associated with hepatic venoocclusive disease in patients who have not received stem cell transplantation. *Cancer* **2001**, *92*, 406–413. [CrossRef]
35. Walter, R.B.; Appelbaum, F.R.; Estey, E.H.; Bernstein, I.D. Acute myeloid leukemia stem cells and cd33-targeted immunotherapy. *Blood* **2012**, *119*, 6198. [CrossRef] [PubMed]
36. Hills, R.K.; Castaigne, S.; Appelbaum, F.R.; Delaunay, J.; Petersdorf, S.; Othus, M.; Estey, E.H.; Dombret, H.; Chevret, S.; Ifrah, N.; et al. Addition of gemtuzumab ozogamicin to induction chemotherapy in adult patients with acute myeloid leukaemia: A meta-analysis of individual patient data from randomised controlled trials. *Lancet Oncol.* **2014**, *15*, 986–996. [CrossRef]
37. Wang, Q.-S.; Wang, Y.; Lv, H.-Y.; Han, Q.-W.; Fan, H.; Guo, B.; Wang, L.-L.; Han, W.-D. Treatment of cd33-directed chimeric antigen receptor-modified t cells in one patient with relapsed and refractory acute myeloid leukemia. *Mol. Ther.* **2015**, *23*, 184–191. [CrossRef]
38. Kenderian, S.S.; Ruella, M.; Shestova, O.; Klichinsky, M.; Aikawa, V.; Morrissette, J.J.; Scholler, J.; Song, D.; Porter, D.L.; Carroll, M.; et al. Cd33-specific chimeric antigen receptor t cells exhibit potent preclinical activity against human acute myeloid leukemia. *Leukemia* **2015**, *29*, 1637–1647. [CrossRef]
39. Kim, M.Y.; Yu, K.-R.; Kenderian, S.S.; Ruella, M.; Chen, S.; Shin, T.-H.; Aljanahi, A.A.; Schreeder, D.; Klichinsky, M.; Shestova, O.; et al. Genetic inactivation of cd33 in hematopoietic stem cells to enable car t cell immunotherapy for acute myeloid leukemia. *Cell* **2018**, *173*, 1439–1453. [CrossRef]
40. Westwood, J.A.; Murray, W.K.; Trivett, M.; Haynes, N.M.; Solomon, B.; Mileshkin, L.; Ball, D.; Michael, M.; Burman, A.; Mayura-Guru, P.; et al. The lewis-y carbohydrate antigen is expressed by many human tumors and can serve as a target for genetically redirected t cells despite the presence of soluble antigen in serum. *J. Immunother.* **2009**, *32*, 292–301. [CrossRef]

41. Sakamoto, J.; Furukawa, K.; Cordon-Cardo, C.; Yin, B.W.T.; Rettig, W.J.; Oettgen, H.F.; Old, L.J.; Lloyd, K.O. Expression of Lewisa, X, and Y blood group antigens in human colonic tumors and normal tissue and in human tumor-derived cell lines. *Cancer Res.* **1986**, *46*, 1553.
42. Peinert, S.; Prince, H.M.; Guru, P.M.; Kershaw, M.H.; Smyth, M.J.; Trapani, J.A.; Gambell, P.; Harrison, S.; Scott, A.M.; Smyth, F.E.; et al. Gene-modified t cells as immunotherapy for multiple myeloma and acute myeloid leukemia expressing the lewis y antigen. *Gene Ther.* **2010**, *17*, 678. [CrossRef]
43. Kobayashi, K.; Sakamoto, J.; Kito, T.; Yamamura, Y.; Koshikawa, T.; Fujita, M.; Watanabe, T.; Nakazato, H. Lewis blood group-related antigen expression in normal gastric epithelium, intestinal metaplasia, gastric adenoma, and gastric carcinoma. *Am. J. Gastroenterol.* **1993**, *88*, 919–924. [PubMed]
44. Neeson, P.; Shin, A.; Tainton, K.M.; Guru, P.; Prince, H.M.; Harrison, S.J.; Peinert, S.; Smyth, M.J.; Trapani, J.A.; Kershaw, M.H.; et al. Ex vivo culture of chimeric antigen receptor t cells generates functional cd8+ t cells with effector and central memory-like phenotype. *Gene Ther.* **2010**, *17*, 1105. [CrossRef]
45. Jordan, C.T.; Upchurch, D.; Szilvassy, S.J.; Guzman, M.L.; Howard, D.S.; Pettigrew, A.L.; Meyerrose, T.; Rossi, R.; Grimes, B.; Rizzieri, D.A.; et al. The interleukin-3 receptor alpha chain is a unique marker for human acute myelogenous leukemia stem cells. *Leukemia* **2000**, *14*, 1777–1784. [CrossRef] [PubMed]
46. Jin, L.; Lee, E.M.; Ramshaw, H.S.; Busfield, S.J.; Peoppl, A.G.; Wilkinson, L.; Guthridge, M.A.; Thomas, D.; Barry, E.F.; Boyd, A.; et al. Monoclonal antibody-mediated targeting of cd123, il-3 receptor α chain, eliminates human acute myeloid leukemic stem cells. *Cell Stem Cell* **2009**, *5*, 31–42. [CrossRef]
47. Thokala, R.; Olivares, S.; Mi, T.; Maiti, S.; Deniger, D.; Huls, H.; Torikai, H.; Singh, H.; Champlin, R.E.; Laskowski, T.; et al. Redirecting specificity of t cells using the sleeping beauty system to express chimeric antigen receptors by mix-and-matching of vl and vh domains targeting cd123+ tumors. *PLoS ONE* **2016**, *11*, e0159477. [CrossRef] [PubMed]
48. Levis, M.; Small, D. Flt3: Itdoes matter in leukemia. *Leukemia* **2003**, *17*, 1738–1752. [CrossRef]
49. Chien, C.D.; Sauter, C.T.; Ishii, K.; Nguyen, S.M.; Shen, F.; Tasian, S.K.; Chen, W.; Dimitrov, D.S.; Fry, T.J. Preclinical development of flt3-redirected chimeric antigen receptor t cell immunotherapy for acute myeloid leukemia. *Blood* **2016**, *128*, 1072.
50. Wang, Y.; Xu, Y.; Li, S.; Liu, J.; Xing, Y.; Xing, H.; Tian, Z.; Tang, K.; Rao, Q.; Wang, M.; et al. Targeting flt3 in acute myeloid leukemia using ligand-based chimeric antigen receptor-engineered t cells. *J. Hematol. Oncol.* **2018**, *11*, 60. [CrossRef]
51. Bakker, A.B.H.; van den Oudenrijn, S.; Bakker, A.Q.; Feller, N.; van Meijer, M.; Bia, J.A.; Jongeneelen, M.A.C.; Visser, T.J.; Bijl, N.; Geuijen, C.A.W.; et al. C-type lectin-like molecule-1. *Cancer Res.* **2004**, *64*, 8443. [CrossRef]
52. Laborda, E.; Mazagova, M.; Shao, S.; Wang, X.; Quirino, H.; Woods, A.K.; Hampton, E.N.; Rodgers, D.T.; Kim, C.H.; Schultz, P.G.; et al. Development of a chimeric antigen receptor targeting c-type lectin-like molecule-1 for human acute myeloid leukemia. *Int. J. Mol. Sci.* **2017**, *18*, 2259. [CrossRef]
53. Kenderian, S.S.; Habermann, T.M.; Macon, W.R.; Ristow, K.M.; Ansell, S.M.; Colgan, J.P.; Johnston, P.B.; Inwards, D.J.; Markovic, S.N.; Micallef, I.N.; et al. Large b-cell transformation in nodular lymphocyte-predominant hodgkin lymphoma: 40-year experience from a single institution. *Blood* **2016**, *127*, 1960–1966. [CrossRef] [PubMed]
54. Tashiro, H.; Sauer, T.; Shum, T.; Parikh, K.; Mamonkin, M.; Omer, B.; Rouce, R.H.; Lulla, P.; Rooney, C.M.; Gottschalk, S.; et al. Treatment of acute myeloid leukemia with t cells expressing chimeric antigen receptors directed to c-type lectin-like molecule 1. *Mol. Ther. J. Am. Soc. Gene Ther.* **2017**, *25*, 2202–2213. [CrossRef] [PubMed]
55. Wang, J.; Chen, S.; Xiao, W.; Li, W.; Wang, L.; Yang, S.; Wang, W.; Xu, L.; Liao, S.; Liu, W.; et al. Car-t cells targeting cll-1 as an approach to treat acute myeloid leukemia. *J. Hematol. Oncol.* **2018**, *11*, 7. [CrossRef] [PubMed]
56. Legras, S.; Gunthert, U.; Stauder, R.; Curt, F.; Oliferenko, S.; Kluin-Nelemans, H.C.; Marie, J.P.; Proctor, S.; Jasmin, C.; Smadja-Joffe, F. A strong expression of cd44-6v correlates with shorter survival of patients with acute myeloid leukemia. *Blood* **1998**, *91*, 3401–3413. [PubMed]
57. Günthert, U.; Hofmann, M.; Rudy, W.; Reber, S.; Zöller, M.; Haußmann, I.; Matzku, S.; Wenzel, A.; Ponta, H.; Herrlich, P. A new variant of glycoprotein cd44 confers metastatic potential to rat carcinoma cells. *Cell* **1991**, *65*, 13–24. [CrossRef]

58. Neu, S.; Geiselhart, A.; Sproll, M.; Hahn, D.; Kuçi, S.; Niethammer, D.; Handgretinger, R. Expression of cd44 isoforms by highly enriched cd34-positive cells in cord blood, bone marrow and leukaphereses. *Bone Marrow Trans.* **1997**, *20*, 593. [CrossRef] [PubMed]
59. Casucci, M.; Nicolis di Robilant, B.; Falcone, L.; Camisa, B.; Norelli, M.; Genovese, P.; Gentner, B.; Gullotta, F.; Ponzoni, M.; Bernardi, M.; et al. Cd44v6-targeted t cells mediate potent antitumor effects against acute myeloid leukemia and multiple myeloma. *Blood* **2013**, *122*, 3461–3472. [CrossRef] [PubMed]
60. Ciceri, F.; Bonini, C.; Stanghellini, M.T.; Bondanza, A.; Traversari, C.; Salomoni, M.; Turchetto, L.; Colombi, S.; Bernardi, M.; Peccatori, J.; et al. Infusion of suicide-gene-engineered donor lymphocytes after family haploidentical haemopoietic stem-cell transplantation for leukaemia (the tk007 trial): A non-randomised phase i-ii study. *Lancet Oncol.* **2009**, *10*, 489–500. [CrossRef]
61. Di Stasi, A.; Tey, S.K.; Dotti, G.; Fujita, Y.; Kennedy-Nasser, A.; Martinez, C.; Straathof, K.; Liu, E.; Durett, A.G.; Grilley, B.; et al. Inducible apoptosis as a safety switch for adoptive cell therapy. *N. Engl. J. Med.* **2011**, *365*, 1673–1683. [CrossRef] [PubMed]
62. Shen, D.; Jiang, M.; Hao, W.; Tao, L.; Salazar, M.; Fong, H.K. A human opsin-related gene that encodes a retinaldehyde-binding protein. *Biochemistry* **1994**, *33*, 13117–13125. [CrossRef]
63. Ross, J.F.; Wang, H.; Behm, F.G.; Mathew, P.; Wu, M.; Booth, R.; Ratnam, M. Folate receptor type beta is a neutrophilic lineage marker and is differentially expressed in myeloid leukemia. *Cancer* **1999**, *85*, 348–357. [CrossRef]
64. Wang, H.; Zheng, X.; Behm, F.G.; Ratnam, M. Differentiation-independent retinoid induction of folate receptor type beta, a potential tumor target in myeloid leukemia. *Blood* **2000**, *96*, 3529–3536. [PubMed]
65. Pan, X.Q.; Zheng, X.; Shi, G.; Wang, H.; Ratnam, M.; Lee, R.J. Strategy for the treatment of acute myelogenous leukemia based on folate receptor beta-targeted liposomal doxorubicin combined with receptor induction using all-trans retinoic acid. *Blood* **2002**, *100*, 594–602. [CrossRef] [PubMed]
66. Lynn, R.C.; Poussin, M.; Kalota, A.; Feng, Y.; Low, P.S.; Dimitrov, D.S.; Powell, D.J., Jr. Targeting of folate receptor beta on acute myeloid leukemia blasts with chimeric antigen receptor-expressing t cells. *Blood* **2015**, *125*, 3466–3476. [CrossRef] [PubMed]
67. Lynn, R.C.; Feng, Y.; Schutsky, K.; Poussin, M.; Kalota, A.; Dimitrov, D.S.; Powell, D.J., Jr. High-affinity frbeta-specific car t cells eradicate aml and normal myeloid lineage without hsc toxicity. *Leukemia* **2016**, *30*, 1355–1364. [CrossRef] [PubMed]
68. Terstappen, L.W.; Safford, M.; Unterhalt, M.; Konemann, S.; Zurlutter, K.; Piechotka, K.; Drescher, M.; Aul, C.; Buchner, T.; Hiddemann, W.; et al. Flow cytometric characterization of acute myeloid leukemia: Iv. Comparison to the differentiation pathway of normal hematopoietic progenitor cells. *Leukemia* **1992**, *6*, 993–1000. [PubMed]
69. Konopleva, M.; Rissling, I.; Andreeff, M. Cd38 in hematopoietic malignancies. *Chem. Immunol.* **2000**, *75*, 189–206. [PubMed]
70. Yoshida, T.; Mihara, K.; Takei, Y.; Yanagihara, K.; Kubo, T.; Bhattacharyya, J.; Imai, C.; Mino, T.; Takihara, Y.; Ichinohe, T. All-trans retinoic acid enhances cytotoxic effect of t cells with an anti-cd38 chimeric antigen receptor in acute myeloid leukemia. *Clin. Transl. Immunol.* **2016**, *5*, e116. [CrossRef]
71. Rabinowich, H.; Vitolo, D.; Altarac, S.; Herberman, R.B.; Whiteside, T.L. Role of cytokines in the adoptive immunotherapy of an experimental model of human head and neck cancer by human il-2-activated natural killer cells. *J. Immunol.* **1992**, *149*, 340–349.
72. Campana, D.; van Dongen, J.J.; Mehta, A.; Coustan-Smith, E.; Wolvers-Tettero, I.L.; Ganeshaguru, K.; Janossy, G. Stages of t-cell receptor protein expression in t-cell acute lymphoblastic leukemia. *Blood* **1991**, *77*, 1546–1554.
73. Campana, D.; Behm, F.G. Immunophenotyping of leukemia. *J. Immunol. Methods* **2000**, *243*, 59–75. [CrossRef]
74. Tiftik, N.; Bolaman, Z.; Batun, S.; Ayyildiz, O.; Isikdogan, A.; Kadikoylu, G.; Muftuoglu, E. The importance of cd7 and cd56 antigens in acute leukaemias. *Int. J. Clin. Pract.* **2004**, *58*, 149–152. [CrossRef]
75. Miwa, H.; Nakase, K.; Kita, K. Biological characteristics of cd7(+) acute leukemia. *Leuk Lymphoma* **1996**, *21*, 239–244. [PubMed]
76. Gomes-Silva, D.; Atilla, E.; Atilla, P.A.; Mo, F.; Tashiro, H.; Srinivasan, M.; Lulla, P.; Rouce, R.H.; Cabral, J.M.S.; Ramos, C.A.; et al. Cd7 car t cells for the therapy of acute myeloid leukemia. *Mol. Ther.* **2018**, *27*, 272–280. [CrossRef]

77. Gomes-Silva, D.; Srinivasan, M.; Sharma, S.; Lee, C.M.; Wagner, D.L.; Davis, T.H.; Rouce, R.H.; Bao, G.; Brenner, M.K.; Mamonkin, M. Cd7-edited t cells expressing a cd7-specific car for the therapy of t-cell malignancies. *Blood* **2017**, *130*, 285–296. [CrossRef]
78. Silva, D.; Tashiro, H.; Srinivasan, M.; Brenner, M.K.; Mamonkin, M. Cd7 car for the treatment of acute myeloid and lymphoid leukemia. *Blood* **2016**, *128*, 4555.
79. Molldrem, J.; Dermime, S.; Parker, K.; Jiang, Y.Z.; Mavroudis, D.; Hensel, N.; Fukushima, P.; Barrett, A.J. Targeted t-cell therapy for human leukemia: Cytotoxic t lymphocytes specific for a peptide derived from proteinase 3 preferentially lyse human myeloid leukemia cells. *Blood* **1996**, *88*, 2450–2457.
80. Molldrem, J.J.; Clave, E.; Jiang, Y.Z.; Mavroudis, D.; Raptis, A.; Hensel, N.; Agarwala, V.; Barrett, A.J. Cytotoxic t lymphocytes specific for a nonpolymorphic proteinase 3 peptide preferentially inhibit chronic myeloid leukemia colony-forming units. *Blood* **1997**, *90*, 2529–2534. [PubMed]
81. Ma, Q.; Garber, H.R.; Lu, S.; He, H.; Tallis, E.; Ding, X.; Sergeeva, A.; Wood, M.S.; Dotti, G.; Salvado, B.; et al. A novel tcr-like car with specificity for pr1/hla-a2 effectively targets myeloid leukemia in vitro when expressed in human adult peripheral blood and cord blood t cells. *Cytotherapy* **2016**, *18*, 985–994. [CrossRef] [PubMed]
82. Rafiq, S.; Purdon, T.J.; Daniyan, A.F.; Koneru, M.; Dao, T.; Liu, C.; Scheinberg, D.A.; Brentjens, R.J. Optimized t-cell receptor-mimic chimeric antigen receptor t cells directed toward the intracellular wilms tumor 1 antigen. *Leukemia* **2017**, *31*, 1788–1797. [CrossRef]
83. Rezvani, K.; Grube, M.; Brenchley, J.M.; Sconocchia, G.; Fujiwara, H.; Price, D.A.; Gostick, E.; Yamada, K.; Melenhorst, J.; Childs, R.; et al. Functional leukemia-associated antigen-specific memory cd8+ t cells exist in healthy individuals and in patients with chronic myelogenous leukemia before and after stem cell transplantation. *Blood* **2003**, *102*, 2892–2900. [CrossRef] [PubMed]
84. Krug, L.M.; Dao, T.; Brown, A.B.; Maslak, P.; Travis, W.; Bekele, S.; Korontsvit, T.; Zakhaleva, V.; Wolchok, J.; Yuan, J.; et al. Wt1 peptide vaccinations induce cd4 and cd8 t cell immune responses in patients with mesothelioma and non-small cell lung cancer. *Cancer Immunol. Immunother.* **2010**, *59*, 1467–1479. [CrossRef] [PubMed]
85. Gao, L.; Bellantuono, I.; Elsässer, A.; Marley, S.B.; Gordon, M.Y.; Goldman, J.M.; Stauss, H.J. Selective elimination of leukemic CD34+ progenitor cells by cytotoxic t lymphocytes specific for wt1. *Blood* **2000**, *95*, 2198. [PubMed]
86. Chang, A.Y.; Dao, T.; Gejman, R.S.; Jarvis, C.A.; Scott, A.; Dubrovsky, L.; Mathias, M.D.; Korontsvit, T.; Zakhaleva, V.; Curcio, M.; et al. A therapeutic t cell receptor mimic antibody targets tumor-associated prame peptide/hla-i antigens. *J. Clin. Investig.* **2017**, *127*, 2705–2718. [CrossRef] [PubMed]
87. Press, M.F.; Cordon-Cardo, C.; Slamon, D.J. Expression of the her-2/neu proto-oncogene in normal human adult and fetal tissues. *Oncogene* **1990**, *5*, 953–962. [PubMed]
88. Morgan, R.A.; Yang, J.C.; Kitano, M.; Dudley, M.E.; Laurencot, C.M.; Rosenberg, S.A. Case report of a serious adverse event following the administration of t cells transduced with a chimeric antigen receptor recognizing erbb2. *Mol. Ther.* **2010**, *18*, 843–851. [CrossRef]
89. Bonini, C.; Ferrari, G.; Verzeletti, S.; Servida, P.; Zappone, E.; Ruggieri, L.; Ponzoni, M.; Rossini, S.; Mavilio, F.; Traversari, C.; et al. Hsv-tk gene transfer into donor lymphocytes for control of allogeneic graft-versus-leukemia. *Science* **1997**, *276*, 1719–1724. [CrossRef] [PubMed]
90. Straathof, K.C.; Pulè, M.A.; Yotnda, P.; Dotti, G.; Vanin, E.F.; Brenner, M.K.; Heslop, H.E.; Spencer, D.M.; Rooney, C.M. An inducible caspase 9 safety switch for t-cell therapy. *Blood* **2005**, *105*, 4247. [CrossRef]
91. Liu, X.; Jiang, S.; Fang, C.; Yang, S.; Olalere, D.; Pequignot, E.C.; Cogdill, A.P.; Li, N.; Ramones, M.; Granda, B.; et al. Affinity-tuned erbb2 or egfr chimeric antigen receptor t cells exhibit an increased therapeutic index against tumors in mice. *Cancer Res.* **2015**, *75*, 3596–3607. [CrossRef]

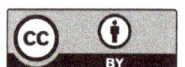

© 2019 by the authors. Licensee MDPI, Basel, Switzerland. This article is an open access article distributed under the terms and conditions of the Creative Commons Attribution (CC BY) license (http://creativecommons.org/licenses/by/4.0/).

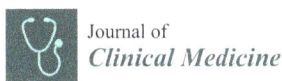

Review

Antigenic Targets for the Immunotherapy of Acute Myeloid Leukaemia

Ghazala Naz Khan [1], Kim Orchard [2] and Barbara-ann Guinn [1,*]

1. Department of Biomedical Sciences, University of Hull, Hull HU7 6RX, UK; G.Khan@hull.ac.uk
2. Department of Haematology, University Hospital Southampton NHS Foundation Trust, Southampton SO16 6YD, UK; kho@soton.ac.uk
* Correspondence: B.Guinn@hull.ac.uk; Tel: +44-1482-466543

Received: 25 December 2018; Accepted: 20 January 2019; Published: 23 January 2019

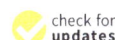

Abstract: One of the most promising approaches to preventing relapse is the stimulation of the body's own immune system to kill residual cancer cells after conventional therapy has destroyed the bulk of the tumour. In acute myeloid leukaemia (AML), the high frequency with which patients achieve first remission, and the diffuse nature of the disease throughout the periphery, makes immunotherapy particularly appealing following induction and consolidation therapy, using chemotherapy, and where possible stem cell transplantation. Immunotherapy could be used to remove residual disease, including leukaemic stem cells from the farthest recesses of the body, reducing, if not eliminating, the prospect of relapse. The identification of novel antigens that exist at disease presentation and can act as targets for immunotherapy have also proved useful in helping us to gain a better understand of the biology that belies AML. It appears that there is an additional function of leukaemia associated antigens as biomarkers of disease state and survival. Here, we discuss these findings.

Keywords: Acute myeloid leukaemia; cancer-testis antigen; human; clinical trial; immunotherapy

---

1. Introduction

Acute Myeloid Leukaemia (AML) is rare in children, but is more commonly observed in adults over the age of 65. For context, in the United Kingdom (UK) there were 3126 new cases of AML in 2015 and 2601 deaths from AML in 2016, in a population of 65 million. AML incidence has increased more than 30% since the 1990s and the mortality rate has increased more than 79% since the early 1970s (https://www.cancerresearchuk.org/health-professional/cancer-statistics/statistics-by-cancer-type/leukaemia-aml/incidence) [1]. This likely reflects the ageing population and prior exposure to treatments for cancer, radiation, benzene, and pre-conditions, such as Down Syndrome (www.nhs.uk/conditions.acute-myeloid-leukaemia) [2]. Typically, at diagnoses, the bone marrow sample comprises of about 1×10^{12} blast cells and prognosis depends on the severity of the illness at the point of diagnosis. Patients with AML usually present with complications of disordered haematopoiesis: bleeding, fatigue, refractory infections, or the clinical consequences of an extremely high white blood cell count: difficulty breathing, confusion, or other symptoms of organ failure [3]. We have been interested in identifying the antigens that are expressed by AML cells for three reasons. They can (i) act as targets for immunotherapy, (ii) provide new information about the biology of the disease, and (iii) act as biomarkers for the best treatment options or survival.

Immunotherapy stimulates the body's own immune system to recognise and kill cancer cells and potentially protect against cancer development in the future. It is known that one of the functions of the immune system is to prevent tumour growth, and this is exemplified by the increased tumour frequencies seen in immunocompromised patients following organ transplantation, those with acquired immune deficiency syndrome (AIDS), and in patients with severe combined immunodeficiency (SCID) syndrome [4]. A range of immunotherapy strategies that engage the innate and more often the adaptive immune system have been developed to treat AML (recently reviewed in [5]).

Survival for patients with AML has the potential to be greatly impacted by immunotherapy. Similar to all leukaemias, AML rapidly spreads throughout the body making localised treatments used for solid tumours, such as radiotherapy, of no real benefit. In addition, almost all AML patients will achieve first remission where minimal residual disease (MRD) can be monitored in anticipation of an all too frequent relapse. Around 70–80% of AML patients that were aged less than 65 achieve remission through chemotherapy treatment [6], but around half relapse in the absence of stem cell transplantation (SCT). During this period the immune system can recover and residual disease in difficult to reach places could be eliminated by immunotherapy. Indeed, we already use immunotherapy to treat AML patients through allo-SCT [7]. To boost this anti-tumour response, patients are given donor leukocyte infusions (DLIs) as follow-up treatments post-transplant to maximise the chances of the transplant being successful. Even with SCT, over one-third of patients will relapse [8], and we know that the mortality rates that are associated with SCT, though decreased with the advent of peripheral blood (PB) based haematopoietic-SCT (HSCT), still remain high. Indeed, patients are often exempted from SCT due to a lack of a suitable donor or because they are too fragile to cope with the rigours of SCT, although reduced intensity regimens have made SCT available to a broader base of older patients [9].

We already know a lot about how the immune system works from transplantation studies for AML patients, especially around the importance of graft-versus-host disease (GvHD) to achieve graft-versus-leukaemia (GvL) through twin studies and T cell depletions [10], the boosting of GvHD through repeated DLI transfusions [11] and the role of reduced intensity conditioning allo-transplants to improve the outcomes for older patients [12]. However many patients, especially those who are ineligible to have a HSCT transplant, will relapse after first remission and require further chemotherapeutic treatments [13]. Ideally, patients could be treated with immunotherapy in first remission, to delay or hopefully prevent relapse.

Currently, the median survival for AML is around one year; however, there has been a steady increase in the overall survival in younger patients [14]. The shift from bone marrow SCTs to PB SCTs has increased donor availability and MRD allows for the prediction of relapse and prophylactic care. However, to date, the largest improvements in survival remain due to improvements in palliative and supportive care [3].

2. Immunotherapy

Although conventional treatments can be successful for patients with leukaemia, with five-year survival rates for those patients treated with conventional chemotherapeutics (e.g., cytarabine and daunorubicin), being at 27.4% (National Cancer Institute, https://seer.cancer.gov/statfacts/html/amyl.html) [15] in comparison to those who were treated with SCTs being at 44.1%, at five-years post-diagnosis [16]. The success of SCTs needs to be considered in a background of 15–25% mortality [17], due to the treatment itself. On the whole aggressive types and stages are still particularly challenging to diagnose and treat. The future of cancer treatment is increasingly focussed on immunotherapy [18] used in combination with conventional treatments, which is seen as the best opportunity for personalised and more effective treatments that could significantly increase survival rates [19], and in the case of liquid tumours, could remove residual disease at diffuse sites in the body.

The ideal immunotherapy targets should play a role in tumour progression [20], so that tumour destruction targets those cells that are responsible for the tumours aggression as well as starting a cascade of activation induced cell death (AICD), immune stimulation in the context of 'danger' and inflammation, and epitope spreading. To ensure monies from National Institute of Health (NIH) grants prioritised immunotherapeutic treatments that focussed on a limited number of antigenic targets, maximising the speed with which treatments reached clinical trials, Cheever and colleagues [21] identified 75 cancer antigens and evaluated them based on nine characteristics that were identified as being essential for effective treatment. p53 [22] was identified as one of the most desirable targets for immunotherapy as targeting p53 can kill both the evolving tumour cell population and any cancer "stem" cell that harbours this as an early stage aberration. By targeting p53, you prevent its support of further tumour growth and genomic instability [23]. However p53, like many other antigens is found to be expressed in solid tumours, but is absent or expressed at low frequencies in haematological malignancies [24]. Indeed, of the antigens considered, those that have been found with any frequency in AML were limited to Wilms' Tumour protein (WT1) (3rd out of 75) and survivin (12th out of 75), reflecting the authors' need to provide a shortlist of antigens relevant to as many solid and haematological malignancies as possible. However, the re-expression of some of the antigens listed has been demonstrated through demethylation agents, such as 5′aza-2′-deoxy-cytidine, in recent studies, including, but not limited to, melanoma antigen (MAGE)-A3 (29th of 75), NY-ESO-1 (34th of 75) [25], and synovial sarcoma X breakpoint 2 (SSX2) (53rd of 75) [26].

3. The Role of Immunotherapy to Prevent or Delay Relapse in AML Patients in Remission

Treatment for leukaemia is often successful and a first remission achieved [27] however, recurrence is seen in about 50% of younger patients and 90% of older patients [28]. MRD monitoring can predict relapse 2–3 months prior to the development of clinical symptoms [29], enabling prophylactic treatment to give patients the best chance of remaining in remission. The death of patients with leukaemia are generally due to disease relapse and patients in first complete remission who are positive for MRD prior to SCT were more likely to die (2.61 times) or relapse (4.9 times) a second time than patients who were MRD negative [30].

Immunotherapy provides an opportunity to remove MRD from cancer patients in first remission, when the burden of disease is low and their immune system is recovering from induction and consolidation therapies. In addition, immunotherapy can be specific to the diseased cells, unlike chemotherapy [31], and destroy leukaemic blast cells in the PB and organs throughout the body. There are a number of different types of antigens [32], including differentiation, mutated, overexpressed, and cancer-testis antigens (CTAs), some of which have been found in AML, including antigens from mutated genes such as Nucleophosmin 1 (NPM1), DNA methyltansferase 3A (DNMT3A), Fms Related Tyrosine Kinase 3 (FLT3), and Ten–Eleven Translocation 2 (TET2) (recently reviewed by [33]). The CTAs category includes some of the oldest and best characterized families, and although MAGE family members were not found to be expressed in presentation AML patient samples with any notable frequency [34], helicase antigen (HAGE) and Per ARNT SIM domain containing 1 (PASD1) antigens have been [34,35]. The differentiation antigens category is another large group of molecules that includes, among many others, the well-known Carcinoembryonic antigen (CEA), glycoprotein 100 (gp100), melan A/melanoma antigen recognized by T cells (MART-1), prostate specific antigen (PSA), and tyrosinase antigens, but relatively few AML antigens have come from this category. The myeloid differentiation antigen CD65 is found at low levels in the least differentiated forms of AML (M0, M1), and usually appears as CD34 disappears during normal myeloid development, reflecting the lack of differentiation in the blast cells in these disease states. The largest group are the overexpressed antigens that include human epidermal growth factor receptor 2 (ErbB-2), human telomerase reverse transcriptase (hTERT), Mucin1 (MUC1), mesothelin, PSA, prostate specific membrane antigen (PSMA), survivin, WT1, p53 and cyclin B1, some of whom are discussed below.

4. CTAs

We are particularly interested in CTAs, whose expression is usually restricted to healthy major histocompatability complex (MHC) class I-deficient germline cells (reviewed by [32]). This feature makes them appealing targets for immunotherapeutic strategies because they provide tumour-specific antigens for MHC class I-restricted CD8+ T cells [36]. Developing immunogenic cancer vaccines that target these antigens has become a priority in how cancer is diagnosed and treated. Boon and colleagues were the first to clone a human tumour antigen, named MAGE-1 [37], through the analyses of responses of cytotoxic T cells to melanoma cells. Subsequently, other CTAs were discovered by the group namely the B melanoma antigen (BAGE) and G antigen (GAGE) gene families. Common characteristics of CTAs include mostly being encoded by multigene families, often mapping to the X chromosome and having their expression level epigenetically regulated with drugs, such as 5-aza-2-deoxycytidine [25,26], and although the functions of many are still unidentified, they have been shown to be involved in tumourigenesis [36]. A large number CTAs have been discovered using serological analysis of recombinant cDNA expression libraries (SEREX) [38] showing much promise as biomarkers for disease and providing targets for immunotherapy. Examples include PASD1 in AML [35], LY6K in lung and oesophageal carcinomas [39], sperm protein 17 (Sp17) in head and neck squamous cell carcinoma [40] and transmembrane protein 31 (TMEM31) in metastatic melanoma [41]. The problem is that CTAs are often expressed in less patients (23% for HAGE [34] and 33% for PASD1 [35]) at AML presentation as compared with leukaemia associated antigens (LAAs), such as Survivin [42] and WT1 [43], which are found in most patients and can act as MRD markers in their own right. However CTAs are restricted in their expression to cancer/leukaemia cells and they offer an opportunity to circumvent the initiation of auto-immune responses that could destroy healthy tissues in vulnerable patients.

It has been increasingly apparent that immunotherapy works best when patients have a healthy immune system and low tumour burden. This is exemplified by the increased cancer incidence observed in patients who have been immune suppressed by Human Immunodeficiency virus (HIV) [44], organ transplantation [45], or cancer treatments, such as radiotherapy and/or chemotherapy [46]. It appears likely that immunotherapy will require use in combination with other treatments, such as hypomethylating agents i.e., SGI-110, a derivative of decitabine [47], which has been shown to lead to the re-expression of MAGE-A and NY-ESO-1 in AML blasts, or more recently treatment in a Phase II clinical trial of AML patients with azacitidine and vorinostat, which led to an increased expression of MAGE, renal cell carcinoma antigen (RAGE), LAGE, SSX2, and taxol resistance associated gene-3 (TRAG3) in blasts, which can be recognised when presented to circulating T cells [48]. In addition, anti-CTLA4 or anti-PD-L1 have been shown to enable the memory of the immune system to recognise tumour antigens (reviewed in [49]).

There has been some suggestion of using CTAs vaccines in a preventative manner at the earliest stages before the cancer advances [50], but predicting which patients are at risk of cancer is often limited to inherited cancers, which account for approximately 5% of all of those affected by cancer and predisposing factors such as exposure to carcinogens that may or may not lead to cancer development.

5. CTAs and AML

HAGE is part of the DEAD-box RNA helicases that implies that its function may include RNA metabolism in malignant cells [51]. It has been shown to be expressed in a number of tumour types but not healthy tissues [52]. In 2002, Adams et al. [34] investigated the expression of 10 CTAs in presentation samples from 26 AML and 42 CML. They found little or no expression of MAGE-A1, -A3, -A6, -A12, BAGE, GAGE, LAGE-1, NY-ESO-1 or RAGE. In contrast to previous studies of CTAs in AML, Adams et al. found that HAGE was expressed in 23% of AML patient samples by RT-PCR while it was detected in 14.8% (11/74) AML patients by qPCR analysis by Chen et al. [53]. HAGE has been found to be induced in a dose dependent manner by 5-aza-2'-deoxycytidine [54], a treatment now being used in Phase II clinical trials to overcome T cell exhaustion that is caused by AML blast arginase II activity [48].

The PASD1 gene was identified through the immunoscreening of testes cDNA libraries [35,55] using the SEREX technique [56]. A number of investigations have demonstrated PASD1 expression in haematological malignancies, including 4/12 (33%) AML samples [35]. In a cohort of haematological malignancy derived cell lines, the sub-cellular localisation of PASD1, as determined by immunostaining with monoclonal antibodies, was variable [57]. The detection of nuclear staining was not unexpected and it likely reflected the presence of a nuclear localisation signal in the common region of the PASD1-1 and PASD1-2 proteins and the role of PASD1 as a transcription factor [58].

Immunogenic T-cell epitopes within PASD1a and PASD1b have proved to be more difficult to identify [59,60]. In AML, Hardwick et al. [60] modified HLA-A*02:01 binding PASD1-specific peptides to generate effective T cell responses. One epitope, Pa14, caused limited expansion in CD8+ T cell numbers from two of three HLA-A*02:01 positive, PASD1-positive AML patient samples. This corresponds with the findings of Rezvani et al. [61], who also found AML T cells have limited capacity to respond to stimulation ex vivo. A 2–3 week limited expansion is the maximum that has been achieved prior to AML T cell death. Reasons for the limited responses may be due to the presence of myeloid suppressor cells in mixed lymphocyte assays [62], interleukin-6 (IL-6) secretion by myeloid leukaemia cells [63], and/or defects in T cell populations in myeloid leukaemia patients [61,64]. However, the stimulation of T cells from a colon cancer patient, by Hardwick et al, led to a substantial increase in the number of Pa14-specific T cells to 13.6% of the CD8+ cell population after four rounds of stimulation, with Pa14-specific IFNγ responses being evidenced [60].

PASD1 expression has not been described in solid tumours although the issues around publishing negative results [65] means that there is little record of which solid tumour have been investigated for PASD1 expression. However the absence of PASD1 expression in solid tumours, including basal cell cancer [66] and ovarian cancer [67], has been published suggesting low expression where it has been described.

6. The Role of Tumour Antigens as Biomarkers for Survival

Although tumour antigens were identified for their potential to act as targets for immunotherapy, using the patient immune response for their identification, a number of subsequent studies showed that some, but not all of these antigens could also act as biomarkers [68]. Indeed, despite their known role in cancer initiation and progression, some antigens with elevated expression correlated with improved survival.

Greiner and Guinn theorised that when leukaemia cells with elevated levels of LAAs are destroyed by chemotherapy the clean-up of the dead/dying cancer cells by the immune system leads to the presentation of antigens in an immunogenic and inflammatory context, leading to improved post-treatment immune responses. In acute promyelocytic leukaemia (APL) patients who harbour the t(15;17) translocation, had a decreased expression of Preferentially Expressed Antigen In Melanoma (PRAME) that correlated with a shorter overall survival [69], whereas the typically favourable t(8;21) translocation was associated with a higher level of PRAME in AML M2 patients [70]. Greiner et al. [71] had shown a significant correlation between high G250 mRNA expression levels and a longer overall survival ($p = 0.022$) based on DNA microarray data from 116 AML patients. In addition, the SSX2 interacting protein (SSX2IP) has been found to be a marker of improved survival in AML patients who had no cytogenetic aberrations [72], while also being elevated in patients with t(15;17), associated with poor prognosis until the advent of (treatment) and decreased in patients harbouring the more favourable t(8;21) [73]. Guinn et al. found a positive correlation between the expression of SSX2IP and the poor prognostic indicator FLT-3-ITD ($p = 0.008$, t test), but not between SSX2IP and other poor prognostic markers, such as cytogenetic abnormalities associated with poor survival, white cell count, age, sex, or survival [73].

However this has not been the case with all antigens. Liberante et al. [74] suggested a 'Goldilocks' effect of the relative levels of PRAME expression in terms of its role as a biomarker for survival. It was found that 'very high' and 'very low' levels of PRAME expression correlated with poor survival. Low levels of PRAME expression may reflect a situation where leukaemia cells are able to escape immune surveillance, while higher levels of PRAME could reflect a higher tumour load and/or the presence of more aberrant leukaemia cells [74]. In addition, elevated survivin expression has been shown to correlate with chemoresistance [42] and poor outcomes [75,76] in AML. This is more commonly the case in solid tumours, where the elevated expression of antigens tends to be associated with a worse clinical outcome, if there is an association. Examples include **survivin** in different solid tumours, including renal cell carcinoma [76] and HAGE in breast cancer [77]. In addition, differences between survival and antigen expression can vary with AML subtype, patient age, and cytogenetics perhaps reflecting the heterogeneity of AML. For example, RAGE-1 and MGEA6 were both found to have elevated expression in the less lineage restricted forms of AML [78], while microarray analysis showed elevated SSX2IP in patients with the t(15;17) and significantly decreased levels of SSX2IP in patients harbouring the t(8;21) [73].

Bergmann et al. showed that high levels of WT1 mRNA in AML were associated with poor long-term outcome [79], while others found no correlation [71,80,81]. However Bergmann's findings reflected the situation in non-small cell lung cancer, where low WT1 mRNA expression has been associated with poor survival and lymph node metastases [82]. This may demonstrate the need to further sub-group patients based on age or other demographics. Indeed, the expression of BCL-2 and WT1 has been associated with a reduced rate of achieving complete remission and overall survival in patients that were younger than 60 years, and no effect on survival rates in patients older than 60 years [83].

7. Antigens that Have Been Shown to Play a Role in the Biological Basis of AML

A number of proteins were identified by virtue of an antibody response against them and were then shown to have an important role in the biological basis of AML. Greiner discussed the role of a number of LAAs in cell cycle proliferation (BAGE, BCL-2, OFA-iLRP, FLT3-ITD, G250, hTERT, PRAME, Hyaluronan-mediated motility receptor (HMMR, also known as RHAMM), proteinase 3, survivin, and WT1), meaning that immunotherapy strategies targeting them would also destroy leukaemic cells that are proliferating abnormally under the control of overexpressed or mutated antigens.

In AML patients with the t(15;17) translocation, SSX2IP levels were associated with gene expression of proteins involved in regulating cyclin dependent kinases (CDK) activity (p57Kip2, cdk7, cyclins D2, D3, E2, and B2), DNA replication (CDC6) and mitosis (survivin and CENPJ) [73]. We also found a very significant correlation between AML patients harbouring a t(8;21) and low cdc20 expression [73]. Boyapati et al. [84] had described a mouse model of AML M2 whose cells had a C-terminal truncated AML-ETO product and developed aneuploidy through the attenuation of the spindle checkpoint. Using microarray datasets for associations between SSX2IP and the genes involved in spindle checkpoints described by Boyapati et al., Guinn et al. [73] found a strong correlation between low-CDC20 expression, one of the substrate-targeting subunits of the anaphase-promoting complex and low-SSX2IP expression in patients harbouring a t(8;21) translocation when compared with AML patients without a t(8;21) translocation and normal donors.

In 2007, Denniss observed the variable expression of PASD1 in synchronised K562 cells over time [85], but could not demonstrate an association with the phases of the cell cycle. Others also noted that only a subset of K562 cells expressed PASD1 (around 17% of the cell population) [60,86] and they could be reproducibly killed by PASD1-specific T cells [60]. PASD1, a homologue to the mouse CLOCK gene, has now been shown to suppress circadian rhythms. The circadian clock regulates and responds to the physiological and environmental changes by regulating transcription in a roughly 24 h cycle. PASD1 through its interaction with CLOCK:BMAL1 reduces transcription regulation, leading to the transformation of cells. PASD1 C-terminal CC1 domain bears homology to the essential regulatory region encoded by CLOCK exon 19. Using molecular mimicry, PASD1 can restrict the activation of CLOCK exon 19 to disrupt the CLOCK:BMAL1 function, therefore supressing transcription [87].

Survivin, coded by the baculoviral IAP repeat-containing 5 (BIRC5) gene, has been shown to be involved in several central pathways that control cell proliferation and viability (reviewed recently by Garg et al. [88]). Of particular note, survivin is a key player of the survivin-Borealin-INCENP core complex that regulates important proteins that are involved in cell division, like aurora B kinase or polo-like kinase 1 [89,90]. Several pathways, such as mTOR- and ran-GTP, are regulated by survivin [91,92], and survivin is involved in spindle formation and anti-apoptosis [91]. While in normal differentiated adult tissues little or no expression of survivin is found, high expression has been described in a number of different solid tumors and hematological malignancies [91]. Attempts to antagonize survivin using antisense molecules are ongoing, including immuno-targeting by vaccination and tyrosine kinase inhibition [93–95]. Notably, a repressor of survivin recently produced encouraging results in heavily pretreated cancer patients [96].

WT1 has emerged as one of the most promising targets for AML immunotherapy, because of its oncogenic role in leukaemogenesis, its high expression in the majority of AML cells, and its ability to function as a tumour rejection antigen [97]. Concomitantly, many other haematological [98–100] and solid [99–101] tumours could benefit from WT1-directed therapy. Despite its ubiquitous expression during embryogenesis, WT1 expression in normal individuals is limited to renal podocytes, gonadal cells, and CD34$^+$ bone marrow cells [102,103], where expression is significantly lower than in leukaemia cells (10–100 fold) [103], making it an excellent target for immunotherapy.

8. Clinical Trials–State-of-The-Art

As T cells are able to recognise and kill cancer cells [104], it was thought that T cell therapies would be the most effective form of immunotherapy. T cells are believed to have an exquisite specificity for epitopes within tumour antigens and they are able to effectively kill cancer cells in a controlled manner. Cytotoxic T-lymphocytes (CTLs) can be stimulated through the use of dendritic cells (DCs) [105], peptide vaccines [106], DNA vaccines [107], and natural killer (NK) cells [108].

DCs are antigen presenting cells that are able to cross present by ingesting and processing extracellular antigens and presenting them on Major Histocompatability Complex (MHC) class I molecules [109]. DC therapy involves extracting the patient's own monocytes, maturing and activating them to DCs using antigens. The DCs are then injected back into the body to stimulate the immune system to eliminate the antigen expressing cancer cells [110].

AML cell lines were used to show that PRAME is involved in retinoic acid-regulated (RAR) cell proliferation and differentiation by inhibiting RAR signalling [111] and introducing all-trans-retinoic acid (ATRA) may be able to reverse this, especially in patients without the t(15;17) mutation. Combination treatment of targeting PRAME along with ATRA would potentially benefit patients expressing elevated levels of PRAME [111]. The presence of PRAME could be an indicator for relapse, as it was found to be increased, after decreasing during remission, even with multiple relapses [112]. PRAME has been shown to induce specific T-cell responses in both solid tumours and leukaemia [113]. However, in some patients expressing PRAME, the cytotoxic response is too weak but after treatment with a Histone deacetylase (HDAC) inhibitor chidamide enhanced PRAME levels are observed, with further improvement when chidamide is combined with the DNA demethylating agent decitabine resulting in immune cells recognizing the PRAME100–108 or PRAME300–309 peptide presented by HLA-A*02:01 [114].

Monoclonal antibodies are used to treat a number of cancers, including low-grade or follicular non-Hodgkin's lymphoma (NHL) and chronic lymphocytic leukaemia (CLL), through treatment with rituximab, which is a CD20 specific antibody. Rituximab targets CD20 that is present on the surface of the B cells, including the malignant NHL and CLL cells [115].

The best strategy for the effective treatment of cancer may include a combination of conventional and immunotherapy techniques [116], or even a combination of immunotherapy techniques, as demonstrated in increasing numbers of mouse models [117] and clinical trials [118–120]. Subsequently, adoptive T cell therapy has been shown to be very promising with the number of cells being returned to patients [121] and their status–activated but not matured [122], being the main considerations. Chimeric antigen receptors-T cells (CAR-T) are where a patients T cells are genetically engineered to express the CAR receptor on their surface against a specific antigen. Upon expansion, they are injected back into the body to recognise and kill the antigen expressing cancer cells. In a recent novel study, a T-cell receptor-mimic (TCRm) CAR, known as WT1-28z, responded to a peptide portion of the intracellular antigen WT1, as it is presented on the surface of the tumour cell in the context of HLA-A*02:01. T cells genetically modified to recognise WT1-28z specifically targeted and lysed HLA-A*02:01+ WT1+ tumours and improved the survival of mice engrafted with HLA-A*02:01+, WT1+ leukaemia cells [123].

There are a number of excellent reviews in this area of research that aim to identify and discuss effective immunotherapy strategies for the future (Table 1). These include cellular immunotherapy [124], whole cell vaccines [125], multidrug resistance [126], DCs [127], oncolytic viruses [128], and nanotechnology [129]. Targeted therapeutic strategies along with ever improving designs in clinical trials pave the way for further success [130].

Table 1. Some examples of current clinical trials involving antigenic targets in acute myeloid leukaemia (AML).

Target Antigen(s)	Designated Name	Type of Immunotherapy	Phase	Findings	Refs
CD33 and CLL1	CD123b-CD33b cCAR	CAR-T/cellular immunotherapy	I	1 patient–44 year old female. Liu stated that the CD33 cCAR T cell therapy could be used as a conduit to transplant, in addition to conventional chemotherapy or alone.	[131]
MUC1-C plus decitabine	GO-203-2C	Peptide inhibition of MUC1/targeted therapy	I/Ib	Combination cohort, response was achieved in 57% compared to GO-203-2C alone who had resistant disease. Showed treatment is safe.	[132]
Proteinase 3	PR1	Peptide vaccine	I/II	PR1 vaccine induces specific immunity that correlates with clinical response, including molecular remission	[133]
Bcl-2	Venetoclax	Small molecule inhibitor	II	Measurable reduction in bone marrow blast counts was observed in 53% of patients	[134]
WT1	galinpepimut-S	Peptide vaccine	II	Median disease-free survival from CR1 was 16.9 months, whereas the overall survival from diagnosis is estimated to be ≥67.6 months	[135]
hTERT	AST-VAC1	hTERT expressing autologous DCs	II	58% developed T-cell responses, 58% patients in CR were free of relapse after 52 months, 57% of patients aged ≥60 also were free of relapse after 54 months	[136]

In addition, combinations of immunotherapy could further enhance survival, reducing residual disease where there are escape variants. Combining the antibodies anti-CTLA-4 and anti-4-1BB revealed CD8$^+$ immune responses against advanced MC38 tumours as well as establishment of memory T cells. Combination treatments reduced autoimmunity in comparison to a single antibody therapy [137] and they often offer an opportunity to eliminate escape variants. Combination therapy could be the answer for drug resistant tumours as the resistance mechanisms of the tumour can be identified and targeted alongside standard treatments. Two cell lines (breast and gastric cancer), resistant to sacituzumab govitecan, became susceptible to therapy through the use of an ATP-binding cassette (ABC) transporter inhibitor that is used in combination with antibody treatment [138]. ABC transporters can cause drug resistance by efflux-removal of the drug from the cell [139]. Promising combination therapies utilising antibodies include Lapatinib with trastuzumab in Her2 positive breast cancer [140], Dabrafenib and Trametinib in relapsed ovarian cancer [141], carboplatin and pemetrexed in advanced non-small cell lung cancer [142], pidilizumab and rituximab in follicular lymphoma [143], albumin-bound paclitaxel and gemcitabine in pancreatic cancer [144], nivolumab and ipilimumab in untreated metastatic melanoma [145], cisplatin and topotecan or cisplatin and gemcitabine in advanced colon cancer [146], and bevacizumab plus oral capecitabine plus irinotecan in metastatic colon cancer [147].

9. Summary

We have described the multiplex of insights that novel antigens have provided into how AML develops and how it might be targeted by immunotherapy approaches during disease remission. We have not however discussed novel treatments that we felt were outside the scope of this review and dealt with in detail elsewhere. Obvious examples include CAR-T cells (recently reviewed in [148]), RNA interference (RNAi) targeting, for example, of Brd4 [149], and antibody therapies, including anti-CD33 (recently reviewed in [150])

Poor T cells responses in AML patients [60,61] make gauging anti-tumour responses using ex vivo T cells from AML patients difficult, and expanding immune and leukaemia cells for therapy before patients relapse have struggled to succeed. However, the success of HSCT and DLIs has shown the capacity of the immune system to overcome leukaemia cells when advantaged to do so.

For the monitoring of MRD and effective T cell responses, it is important that proteins specific to the disease are identified and for immunotherapy that cancer specific antigens are the targets of immune responses, including those enacted by B-cell responses (by definition) and their immune counterparts (CD4+ and CD8+ T-cells among others).

The issues remain when to give vaccines against leukaemia to best impact the disease and the effect of treatment on the immune system cannot be underestimated, especially in myeloid leukaemia. Clinical trials, for what is a relatively rare cancer, as compared to many solid tumours, include a limited number of immunotherapy treatments and perhaps a new list of prioritised tumour antigens for haematological malignancies/leukaemia/myeloid leukaemia are required.

Whatever the way forward for AML treatment, it will undoubtedly require the combination of SCT wherever possible, induction and consolidation therapies to achieve MRD, immune recovery, and a lot of trial and error for this heterogenous population.

Funding: This research received no external funding and the Article Processing Charges were paid for by the University of Hull.

Conflicts of Interest: The authors declare no conflict of interest. The funders had no role in the design of the study; in the collection, analyses, or interpretation of data; in the writing of the manuscript, or in the decision to publish the results.

Abbreviations

AML: acute myeloid leukaemia; ATRA: all-trans-retinoic acid; BAGE: B melanoma antigen; CAR-T: Chimeric antigen receptors-T cells; CLL: chronic lymphocytic leukaemia; CTA: cancer-testis antigen; DC: dendritic cells; DLI: donor leukocyte infusion; GAGE: G antigen; GvHD: Graft-versus-Host disease; HAGE: helicase antigen;

HSCT: haematopoietic stem cell transplant; hTERT: human telomerase reverse transcriptase; LAA: leukaemia associated antigen; MAGE: Melanoma antigen; MHC: major histocompatability complex; MRD: minimal residual disease; MUC1: Mucin1; NHL: Non-hodgkin's lymphoma; PASD1: Per ARNT SIM domain containing 1; PB: peripheral blood; PRAME: Preferentially Expressed Antigen In Melanoma; PSA: prostate specific antigen; RAGE: Renal cell carcinoma antigen; RAR: retinoic acid-regulated SEREX: serological analysis of recombinant cDNA expression; SSX2IP: synovial sarcoma X breakpoint 2 interacting protein; WT1: Wilms' Tumour protein.

References

1. Cancer Research UK: Acute Myeloid Leukaemia (AML) Incidence Statistics. Available online: https://www.cancerresearchuk.org/health-professional/cancer-statistics/statistics-by-cancer-type/leukaemia-aml/incidence (accessed on 21 January 2019).
2. NHS Overview: Acute Myeloid Leukaemia. Available online: www.nhs.uk/conditions.acute-myeloid-leukaemia (accessed on 21 January 2019).
3. Showel, M.M.; Levis, M. Advances in treating acute myeloid leukemia. *F1000Prime Rep.* **2014**, *6*, 96. [CrossRef] [PubMed]
4. Penn, I. Tumors of the immunocompromised patient. *Annu. Rev. Med.* **1988**, *39*, 63–73. [CrossRef] [PubMed]
5. Geiger, T.L.; Rubnitz, J.E. New approaches for the immunotherapy of acute myeloid leukemia. *Discov. Med.* **2015**, *19*, 275–284. [PubMed]
6. Döhner, H.; Estey, E.H.; Amadori, S.; Appelbaum, F.R.; Büchner, T.; Burnett, A.K.; Dombret, H.; Fenaux, P.; Grimwade, D.; Larson, R.A.; et al. Diagnosis and management of acute myeloid leukemia in adults: Recommendations from an international expert panel, on behalf of the European LeukemiaNet. *Blood* **2010**, *115*, 453–474. [CrossRef] [PubMed]
7. Appelbaum, F.R. Haematopoietic cell transplantation as immunotherapy. *Nature* **2001**, *411*, 385–389. [CrossRef] [PubMed]
8. Cornelissen, J.J.; van Putten, W.L.; Verdonck, L.F.; Theobald, M.; Jacky, E.; Daenen, S.M.; van Marwijk Kooy, M.; Wijermans, P.; Schouten, H.; Huijgens, P.C.; et al. Results of a HOVON/SAKK donor versus no-donor analysis of myeloablative HLA-identical sibling stem cell transplantation in first remission acute myeloid leukemia in young and middle-aged adults: Benefits for whom? *Blood* **2007**, *109*, 3658–3666. [CrossRef] [PubMed]
9. McClune, B.L.; Weisdorf, D.J.; Pedersen, T.L.; Tunes da Silva, G.; Tallman, M.S.; Sierra, J.; Dipersio, J.; Keating, A.; Gale, R.P.; George, B.; et al. Effect of age on outcome of reduced-intensity hematopoietic cell transplantation for older patients with acute myeloid leukemia in first complete remission or with myelodysplastic syndrome. *J. Clin. Oncol.* **2010**, *28*, 1878–1887. [CrossRef] [PubMed]
10. Marmont, A.M.; Horowitz, M.M.; Gale, R.P.; Sobocinski, K.; Ash, R.C.; van Bekkum, D.W.; Champlin, R.E.; Dicke, K.A.; Goldman, J.M.; Good, R.A.; et al. T-cell depletion of HLA-identical transplants in leukemia. *Blood* **1991**, *78*, 2120–2130. [PubMed]
11. Collins, R.H., Jr.; Shpilberg, O.; Drobyski, W.R.; Porter, D.L.; Giralt, S.; Champlin, R.; Goodman, S.A.; Wolff, S.N.; Hu, W.; Verfaillie, C.; et al. Donor leukocyte infusions in 140 patients with relapsed malignancy after allogeneic bone marrow transplantation. *J. Clin. Oncol.* **1997**, *15*, 433–444. [CrossRef] [PubMed]
12. Estey, E.; de Lima, M.; Tibes, R.; Pierce, S.; Kantarjian, H.; Champlin, R.; Giralt, S. Prospective feasibility analysis of reduced-intensity conditioning (RIC) regimens for hematopoietic stem cell transplantation (HSCT) in elderly patients with acute myeloid leukemia (AML) and high-risk myelodysplastic syndrome (MDS). *Blood* **2007**, *109*, 1395–1400. [CrossRef] [PubMed]
13. Dores, G.M.; Devesa, S.S.; Curtis, R.E.; Linet, M.S.; Morton, L.M. Acute leukemia incidence and patient survival among children and adults in the United States, 2001–2007. *Blood* **2012**, *119*, 34–43. [CrossRef] [PubMed]
14. Maynadié, M.; De Angelis, R.; Marcos-Gragera, R.; Visser, O.; Allemani, C.; Tereanu, C.; Capocaccia, R.; Giacomin, A.; Lutz, J.M.; Martos, C.; et al. Survival of European patients diagnosed with myeloid malignancies: A HAEMACARE study. *Haematologica* **2013**, *98*, 230–238. [CrossRef] [PubMed]
15. National Cancer Institute Cancer Stat Facts: Leukaemia–Acute Myeloid Leukaemia (AML). Available online: https://seer.cancer.gov/statfacts/html/amyl.html (accessed on 21 January 2019).
16. Master, S.; Mansour, R.; Devarakonda, S.S.; Shi, Z.; Mills, G.; Shi, R. Predictors of Survival in Acute Myeloid Leukemia by Treatment Modality. *Anticancer Res.* **2016**, *36*, 1719–1727.

17. Estey, E.; Döhner, H. Acute myeloid leukaemia. *Lancet* **2006**, *368*, 1894–1907. [CrossRef]
18. Ryan, J.F.; Hovde, R.; Glanville, J.; Lyu, S.C.; Ji, X.; Gupta, S.; Tibshirani, R.J.; Jay, D.C.; Boyd, S.D.; Chinthrajah, R.S.; et al. Successful immunotherapy induces previously unidentified allergen-specific CD4+ T-cell subsets. *Proc. Natl. Acad. Sci. USA* **2016**, *113*, E1286–E1295. [CrossRef] [PubMed]
19. Schadendorf, D.; Hodi, F.S.; Robert, C.; Weber, J.S.; Margolin, K.; Hamid, O.; Patt, D.; Chen, T.T.; Berman, D.M.; Wolchok, J.D. Pooled Analysis of Long-Term Survival Data from Phase II and Phase III Trials of Ipilimumab in Unresectable or Metastatic Melanoma. *J. Clin. Oncol.* **2015**, *33*, 1889–1894. [CrossRef] [PubMed]
20. Zhang, J.Y.; Looi, K.S.; Tan, E.M. Identification of tumor-associated antigens as diagnostic and predictive biomarkers in cancer. *Methods Mol. Biol.* **2009**, *520*, 1–10. [CrossRef]
21. Cheever, M.A.; Allison, J.P.; Ferris, A.S.; Finn, O.J.; Hastings, B.M.; Hecht, T.T.; Mellman, I.; Prindiville, S.A.; Viner, J.L.; Weiner, L.M.; et al. The prioritization of cancer antigens: A national cancer institute pilot project for the acceleration of translational research. *Clin. Cancer Res.* **2009**, *15*, 5323–5337. [CrossRef]
22. Soussi, T. p53 Antibodies in the sera of patients with various types of cancer: A review. *Cancer Res.* **2000**, *60*, 1777–1788.
23. Bykov, V.J.N.; Eriksson, S.E.; Bianchi, J.; Wiman, K.G. Targeting mutant p53 for efficient cancer therapy. *Nat. Rev. Cancer* **2018**, *18*, 89–102. [CrossRef]
24. Padua, R.A.; Guinn, B.A.; Al-Sabah, A.I.; Smith, M.; Taylor, C.; Pettersson, T.; Ridge, S.; Carter, G.; White, D.; Oscier, D.; et al. RAS, FMS and p53 mutations and poor clinical outcome in myelodysplasias: A 10-year follow-up. *Leukemia* **1998**, *12*, 887–892. [CrossRef] [PubMed]
25. Almstedt, M.; Blagitko-Dorfs, N.; Duque-Afonso, J.; Karbach, J.; Pfeifer, D.; Jager, E.; Lubbert, M. The DNA demethylating agent 5-aza-2′-deoxycytidine induces expression of NY-ESO-1 and other cancer/testis antigens in myeloid leukemia cells. *Leuk. Res.* **2010**, *34*, 899–905. [CrossRef] [PubMed]
26. Atanackovic, D.; Luetkens, T.; Kloth, B.; Fuchs, G.; Cao, Y.; Hildebrandt, Y.; Meyer, S.; Bartels, K.; Reinhard, H.; Lajmi, N.; et al. Cancer-testis antigen expression and its epigenetic modulation in acute myeloid leukemia. *Am. J. Hematol.* **2011**, *86*, 918–922. [CrossRef] [PubMed]
27. Burnett, A.K.; Goldstone, A.H.; Stevens, R.M.; Hann, I.M.; Rees, J.K.; Gray, R.G.; Wheatley, K. Randomised comparison of addition of autologous bone-marrow transplantation to intensive chemotherapy for acute myeloid leukaemia in first remission: Results of MRC AML 10 trial. UK Medical Research Council Adult and Children's Leukaemia Working Parties. *Lancet* **1998**, *351*, 700–708. [CrossRef]
28. Schlenk, R.F.; Döhner, H. Genomic applications in the clinic: Use in treatment paradigm of acute myeloid leukemia. *Hematol. Am. Soc. Hematol. Educ. Program.* **2013**, *2013*, 324–330. [CrossRef]
29. San Miguel, J.F.; Martínez, A.; Macedo, A.; Vidriales, M.B.; López-Berges, C.; González, M.; Caballero, D.; García-Marcos, M.A.; Ramos, F.; Fernández-Calvo, J.; et al. Immunophenotyping investigation of minimal residual disease is a useful approach for predicting relapse in acute myeloid leukemia patients. *Blood* **1997**, *90*, 2465–2470. [PubMed]
30. Walter, R.B.; Buckley, S.A.; Pagel, J.M.; Wood, B.L.; Storer, B.E.; Sandmaier, B.M.; Fang, M.; Gyurkocza, B.; Delaney, C.; Radich, J.P.; et al. Significance of minimal residual disease before myeloablative allogeneic hematopoietic cell transplantation for AML in first and second complete remission. *Blood* **2013**, *122*, 1813–1821. [CrossRef]
31. Liu, H.; Kline, J. Novel Immunotherapy to Eliminate Minimal Residual Disease in AML Patients. *J. Hematol. Thromboemb. Dis.* **2013**, *1*. Available online: https://www.omicsonline.org/open-access/novel-immunotherapy-to-eliminate-minimal-residual-disease-in-aml-patients-2329-8790.1000112.php?aid=12874 (accessed on 21 January 2019). [CrossRef]
32. Coulie, P.G.; Van den Eynde, B.J.; van der Bruggen, P.; Boon, T. Tumour antigens recognized by T lymphocytes: At the core of cancer immunotherapy. *Nat. Rev. Cancer* **2014**, *14*, 135–146. [CrossRef]
33. Saultz, J.N.; Garzon, R. Acute Myeloid Leukemia: A Concise Review. *J. Clin. Med.* **2016**, *5*, 33. [CrossRef]
34. Adams, S.P.; Sahota, S.S.; Mijovic, A.; Czepulkowski, B.; Padua, R.A.; Mufti, G.J.; Guinn, B.A. Frequent expression of HAGE in presentation chronic myeloid leukaemias. *Leukemia* **2002**, *16*, 2238–2242. [CrossRef] [PubMed]
35. Guinn, B.A.; Bland, E.A.; Lodi, U.; Liggins, A.P.; Tobal, K.; Petters, S.; Wells, J.W.; Banham, A.H.; Mufti, G.J. Humoral detection of leukaemia-associated antigens in presentation acute myeloid leukaemia. *Biochem. Biophys. Res. Commun.* **2005**, *335*, 1293–1304. [CrossRef]

36. Smith, H.A.; McNeel, D.G. The SSX family of cancer-testis antigens as target proteins for tumor therapy. *Clin. Dev. Immunol.* **2010**, *2010*, 150591. [CrossRef]
37. van der Bruggen, P.; Traversari, C.; Chomez, P.; Lurquin, C.; De Plaen, E.; Van den Eynde, B.; Knuth, A.; Boon, T. A gene encoding an antigen recognized by cytolytic T lymphocytes on a human melanoma. *Science* **1991**, *254*, 1643–1647. [CrossRef]
38. Chen, Y.T.; Scanlan, M.J.; Sahin, U.; Türeci, O.; Gure, A.O.; Tsang, S.; Williamson, B.; Stockert, E.; Pfreundschuh, M.; Old, L.J. A testicular antigen aberrantly expressed in human cancers detected by autologous antibody screening. *Proc. Natl. Acad. Sci. USA* **1997**, *94*, 1914–1918. [CrossRef]
39. Ishikawa, N.; Takano, A.; Yasui, W.; Inai, K.; Nishimura, H.; Ito, H.; Miyagi, Y.; Nakayama, H.; Fujita, M.; Hosokawa, M.; et al. Cancer-testis antigen lymphocyte antigen 6 complex locus K is a serologic biomarker and a therapeutic target for lung and esophageal carcinomas. *Cancer Res.* **2007**, *67*, 11601–11611. [CrossRef]
40. Schutt, C.A.; Mirandola, L.; Figueroa, J.A.; Nguyen, D.D.; Cordero, J.; Bumm, K.; Judson, B.L.; Chiriva-Internati, M. The cancer-testis antigen, sperm protein 17, a new biomarker and immunological target in head and neck squamous cell carcinoma. *Oncotarget* **2017**, *8*, 100280–100287. [CrossRef]
41. Li, J.; Zou, X.; Li, C.; Zhong, J.; Chen, Y.; Zhang, X.; Qi, F.; Li, M.; Cai, Z.; Tang, A. Expression of novel cancer/testis antigen TMEM31 increases during metastatic melanoma progression. *Oncol. Lett.* **2017**, *13*, 2269–2273. [CrossRef] [PubMed]
42. Invernizzi, R.; Travaglino, E.; Lunghi, M.; Klersy, C.; Bernasconi, P.; Cazzola, M.; Ascari, E. Survivin expression in acute leukemias and myelodysplastic syndromes. *Leuk. Lymphoma* **2004**, *45*, 2229–2237. [CrossRef] [PubMed]
43. Cilloni, D.; Renneville, A.; Hermitte, F.; Hills, R.K.; Daly, S.; Jovanovic, J.V.; Gottardi, E.; Fava, M.; Schnittger, S.; Weiss, T.; et al. Real-time quantitative polymerase chain reaction detection of minimal residual disease by standardized WT1 assay to enhance risk stratification in acute myeloid leukemia: A European LeukemiaNet study. *J. Clin. Oncol.* **2009**, *27*, 5195–5201. [CrossRef]
44. Silverberg, M.J.; Chao, C.; Leyden, W.A.; Xu, L.; Horberg, M.A.; Klein, D.; Towner, W.J.; Dubrow, R.; Quesenberry, C.P., Jr.; Neugebauer, R.S.; et al. HIV infection, immunodeficiency, viral replication, and the risk of cancer. *Cancer Epidemiol. Prev. Biomark.* **2011**, *20*, 2551–2559. [CrossRef]
45. Engels, E.A.; Pfeiffer, R.M.; Fraumeni, J.F., Jr.; Kasiske, B.L.; Israni, A.K.; Snyder, J.J.; Wolfe, R.A.; Goodrich, N.P.; Bayakly, A.R.; Clarke, C.A.; et al. Spectrum of cancer risk among US solid organ transplant recipients. *JAMA* **2011**, *306*, 1891–1901. [CrossRef] [PubMed]
46. Travis, L.B.; Gospodarowicz, M.; Curtis, R.E.; Clarke, E.A.; Andersson, M.; Glimelius, B.; Joensuu, T.; Lynch, C.F.; van Leeuwen, F.E.; Holowaty, E.; et al. Lung cancer following chemotherapy and radiotherapy for Hodgkin's disease. *J. Natl. Cancer Inst.* **2002**, *94*, 182–192. [CrossRef] [PubMed]
47. Srivastava, P.; Paluch, B.E.; Matsuzaki, J.; James, S.R.; Collamat-Lai, G.; Karbach, J.; Nemeth, M.J.; Taverna, P.; Karpf, A.R.; Griffiths, E.A. Immunomodulatory action of SGI-110, a hypomethylating agent, in acute myeloid leukemia cells and xenografts. *Leuk. Res.* **2014**, *38*, 1332–1341. [CrossRef]
48. Mussai, F.; Wheat, R.; Sarrou, E.; Booth, S.; Stavrou, V.; Fultang, L.; Perry, T.; Kearns, P.; Cheng, P.; Keehsan, K.; et al. Targeting the arginine metabolic brake enhances immunotherapy for leukaemia. *Int. J. Cancer* **2018**. [CrossRef] [PubMed]
49. Ribas, A. Tumor immunotherapy directed at PD-1. *N. Engl. J. Med.* **2012**, *366*, 2517–2519. [CrossRef] [PubMed]
50. Finn, O.J. The dawn of vaccines for cancer prevention. *Nat. Rev. Immunol.* **2018**, *18*, 183–194. [CrossRef]
51. Riley, C.L.; Mathieu, M.G.; Clark, R.E.; McArdle, S.E.; Rees, R.C. Tumour antigen-targeted immunotherapy for chronic myeloid leukaemia: Is it still viable? *Cancer Immunol. Immunother.* **2009**, *58*, 1489–1499. [CrossRef]
52. Mathieu, M.G.; Linley, A.J.; Reeder, S.P.; Badoual, C.; Tartour, E.; Rees, R.C.; McArdle, S.E. HAGE, a cancer/testis antigen expressed at the protein level in a variety of cancers. *Cancer Immun.* **2010**, *10*, 2.
53. Chen, Q.; Lin, J.; Qian, J.; Yao, D.M.; Qian, W.; Li, Y.; Chai, H.Y.; Yang, J.; Wang, C.Z.; Zhang, M.; et al. Gene expression of helicase antigen in patients with acute and chronic myeloid leukemia. *Zhongguo Shi Yan Xue Ye Xue Za Zhi* **2011**, *19*, 1171–1175.
54. Stankovic, T.; McLarnon, A.; Agathanggelou, A.; Goodyear, O.; Craddock, C.; Moss, P. Epigenetic Manipulation of Cancer Testis Antigen (CTA) Expression: A Strategy for Manipulating the Graft-Versus Leukaemia Response in Patients Allografted for Haematological Malignancies. *Blood* **2008**, *112*, 600.

55. Liggins, A.P.; Guinn, B.A.; Hatton, C.S.; Pulford, K.; Banham, A.H. Serologic detection of diffuse large B-cell lymphoma-associated antigens. *Int. J. Cancer* **2004**, *110*, 563–569. [CrossRef]
56. Sahin, U.; Tureci, O.; Schmitt, H.; Cochlovius, B.; Johannes, T.; Schmits, R.; Stenner, F.; Luo, G.; Schobert, I.; Pfreundschuh, M. Human neoplasms elicit multiple specific immune responses in the autologous host. *Proc. Natl. Acad. Sci. USA* **1995**, *92*, 11810–11813. [CrossRef]
57. Cooper, C.D.; Liggins, A.P.; Ait-Tahar, K.; Roncador, G.; Banham, A.H.; Pulford, K. PASD1, a DLBCL-associated cancer testis antigen and candidate for lymphoma immunotherapy. *Leukemia* **2006**, *20*, 2172–2174. [CrossRef] [PubMed]
58. Xu, Z.S.; Zhang, H.X.; Zhang, Y.L.; Liu, T.T.; Ran, Y.; Chen, L.T.; Wang, Y.Y.; Shu, H.B. PASD1 promotes STAT3 activity and tumor growth by inhibiting TC45-mediated dephosphorylation of STAT3 in the nucleus. *J. Mol. Cell Biol.* **2016**, *8*, 221–231. [CrossRef] [PubMed]
59. Ait-Tahar, K.; Liggins, A.P.; Collins, G.P.; Campbell, A.; Barnardo, M.; Lawrie, C.; Moir, D.; Hatton, C.; Banham, A.H.; Pulford, K. Cytolytic T-cell response to the PASD1 cancer testis antigen in patients with diffuse large B-cell lymphoma. *Br. J. Haematol.* **2009**, *146*, 396–407. [CrossRef] [PubMed]
60. Hardwick, N.; Buchan, S.; Ingram, W.; Khan, G.; Vittes, G.; Rice, J.; Pulford, K.; Mufti, G.; Stevenson, F.; Guinn, B.A. An analogue peptide from the Cancer/Testis antigen PASD1 induces CD8+ T cell responses against naturally processed peptide. *Cancer Immun.* **2013**, *13*, 16.
61. Rezvani, K.; Yong, A.S.; Tawab, A.; Jafarpour, B.; Eniafe, R.; Mielke, S.; Savani, B.N.; Keyvanfar, K.; Li, Y.; Kurlander, R.; et al. Ex vivo characterization of polyclonal memory CD8+ T-cell responses to PRAME-specific peptides in patients with acute lymphoblastic leukemia and acute and chronic myeloid leukemia. *Blood* **2009**, *113*, 2245–2255. [CrossRef]
62. Mougiakakos, D.; Jitschin, R.; von Bahr, L.; Poschke, I.; Gary, R.; Sundberg, B.; Gerbitz, A.; Ljungman, P.; Le Blanc, K. Immunosuppressive CD14+HLA-DRlow/neg IDO+ myeloid cells in patients following allogeneic hematopoietic stem cell transplantation. *Leukemia* **2013**, *27*, 377–388. [CrossRef]
63. Buggins, A.G.; Patten, P.E.; Richards, J.; Thomas, N.S.; Mufti, G.J.; Devereux, S. Tumor-derived IL-6 may contribute to the immunological defect in CLL. *Leukemia* **2008**, *22*, 1084–1087. [CrossRef]
64. Wendelbo, Ø.; Nesthus, I.; Sjo, M.; Paulsen, K.; Ernst, P.; Bruserud, Ø. Functional characterization of T lymphocytes derived from patients with acute myelogenous leukemia and chemotherapy-induced leukopenia. *Cancer Immunol. Immunother.* **2004**, *53*, 740–747. [CrossRef] [PubMed]
65. Guinn, B. The future of publishing scientific data: Is it time to accept the wider publication of null data? *EC Cancer* **2014**, *1*, 1–2.
66. Ghafouri-Fard, S.; Abbasi, A.; Moslehi, H.; Faramarzi, N.; Taba Taba Vakili, S.; Mobasheri, M.B.; Modarressi, M.H. Elevated expression levels of testis-specific genes TEX101 and SPATA19 in basal cell carcinoma and their correlation with clinical and pathological features. *Br. J. Dermatol.* **2010**, *162*, 772–779. [CrossRef]
67. Khan, G.; Brooks, S.E.; Mills, K.I.; Guinn, B.A. Infrequent Expression of the Cancer-Testis Antigen, PASD1, in Ovarian Cancer. *Biomark. Cancer* **2015**, *7*, 31–38. [CrossRef]
68. Schumacher, T.N.; Schreiber, R.D. Neoantigens in cancer immunotherapy. *Science* **2015**, *348*, 69–74. [CrossRef]
69. Santamaría, C.; Chillón, M.C.; García-Sanz, R.; Balanzategui, A.; Sarasquete, M.E.; Alcoceba, M.; Ramos, F.; Bernal, T.; Queizán, J.A.; Peñarrubia, M.J.; et al. The relevance of preferentially expressed antigen of melanoma (PRAME) as a marker of disease activity and prognosis in acute promyelocytic leukemia. *Haematologica* **2008**, *93*, 1797–1805. [CrossRef]
70. van Baren, N.; Chambost, H.; Ferrant, A.; Michaux, L.; Ikeda, H.; Millard, I.; Olive, D.; Boon, T.; Coulie, P.G. PRAME, a gene encoding an antigen recognized on a human melanoma by cytolytic T cells, is expressed in acute leukaemia cells. *Br. J. Haematol.* **1998**, *102*, 1376–1379. [CrossRef] [PubMed]
71. Greiner, J.; Schmitt, M.; Li, L.; Giannopoulos, K.; Bosch, K.; Schmitt, A.; Dohner, K.; Schlenk, R.F.; Pollack, J.R.; Dohner, H.; et al. Expression of tumor-associated antigens in acute myeloid leukemia: Implications for specific immunotherapeutic approaches. *Blood* **2006**, *108*, 4109–4117. [CrossRef]
72. Guinn, B.; Greiner, J.; Schmitt, M.; Mills, K.I. Elevated expression of the leukemia-associated antigen SSX2IP predicts survival in acute myeloid leukemia patients who lack detectable cytogenetic rearrangements. *Blood* **2009**, *113*, 1203–1204. [CrossRef] [PubMed]

73. Guinn, B.A.; Bullinger, L.; Thomas, N.S.; Mills, K.I.; Greiner, J. SSX2IP expression in acute myeloid leukaemia: An association with mitotic spindle failure in t(8;21), and cell cycle in t(15;17) patients. *Br. J. Haematol.* **2008**, *140*, 250–251. [CrossRef] [PubMed]
74. Liberante, F.G.; Pellagatti, A.; Boncheva, V.; Bowen, D.T.; Mills, K.I.; Boultwood, J.; Guinn, B.A. High and low, but not intermediate, PRAME expression levels are poor prognostic markers in myelodysplastic syndrome at disease presentation. *Br. J. Haematol.* **2013**, *162*, 282–285. [CrossRef] [PubMed]
75. Carter, B.Z.; Qiu, Y.; Huang, X.; Diao, L.; Zhang, N.; Coombes, K.R.; Mak, D.H.; Konopleva, M.; Cortes, J.; Kantarjian, H.M.; et al. Survivin is highly expressed in CD34(+)38(-) leukemic stem/progenitor cells and predicts poor clinical outcomes in AML. *Blood* **2012**, *120*, 173–180. [CrossRef]
76. Tamm, I.; Richter, S.; Oltersdorf, D.; Creutzig, U.; Harbott, J.; Scholz, F.; Karawajew, L.; Ludwig, W.D.; Wuchter, C. High expression levels of x-linked inhibitor of apoptosis protein and survivin correlate with poor overall survival in childhood de novo acute myeloid leukemia. *Clin. Cancer Res.* **2004**, *10*, 3737–3744. [CrossRef]
77. Abdel-Fatah, T.M.; McArdle, S.E.; Johnson, C.; Moseley, P.M.; Ball, G.R.; Pockley, A.G.; Ellis, I.O.; Rees, R.C.; Chan, S.Y. HAGE (DDX43) is a biomarker for poor prognosis and a predictor of chemotherapy response in breast cancer. *Br. J. Cancer* **2014**, *110*, 2450–2461. [CrossRef]
78. Guinn, B.A.; Gilkes, A.F.; Mufti, G.J.; Burnett, A.K.; Mills, K.I. The tumour antigens RAGE-1 and MGEA6 are expressed more frequently in the less lineage restricted subgroups of presentation acute myeloid leukaemia. *Br. J. Haematol.* **2006**, *134*, 238–239. [CrossRef] [PubMed]
79. Bergmann, L.; Miething, C.; Maurer, U.; Brieger, J.; Karakas, T.; Weidmann, E.; Hoelzer, D. High levels of Wilms' tumor gene (wt1) mRNA in acute myeloid leukemias are associated with a worse long-term outcome. *Blood* **1997**, *90*, 1217–1225. [PubMed]
80. Yanada, M.; Terakura, S.; Yokozawa, T.; Yamamoto, K.; Kiyoi, H.; Emi, N.; Kitamura, K.; Kohno, A.; Tanaka, M.; Tobita, T.; et al. Multiplex real-time RT-PCR for prospective evaluation of WT1 and fusion gene transcripts in newly diagnosed de novo acute myeloid leukemia. *Leuk. Lymphoma* **2004**, *45*, 1803–1808. [CrossRef]
81. Gaiger, A.; Schmid, D.; Heinze, G.; Linnerth, B.; Greinix, H.; Kalhs, P.; Tisljar, K.; Priglinger, S.; Laczika, K.; Mitterbauer, M.; et al. Detection of the WT1 transcript by RT-PCR in complete remission has no prognostic relevance in de novo acute myeloid leukemia. *Leukemia* **1998**, *12*, 1886–1894. [CrossRef] [PubMed]
82. Hayashi, S.; Oji, Y.; Kanai, Y.; Teramoto, T.; Kitaichi, M.; Kawaguchi, T.; Okada, M.; Sugiyama, H.; Matsumura, A. Low Wilms' tumor gene expression in tumor tissues predicts poor prognosis in patients with non-small-cell lung cancer. *Cancer Investig.* **2012**, *30*, 165–171. [CrossRef]
83. Karakas, T.; Miething, C.C.; Maurer, U.; Weidmann, E.; Ackermann, H.; Hoelzer, D.; Bergmann, L. The coexpression of the apoptosis-related genes bcl-2 and wt1 in predicting survival in adult acute myeloid leukemia. *Leukemia* **2002**, *16*, 846–854. [CrossRef]
84. Boyapati, A.; Yan, M.; Peterson, L.F.; Biggs, J.R.; Le Beau, M.M.; Zhang, D.E. A leukemia fusion protein attenuates the spindle checkpoint and promotes aneuploidy. *Blood* **2007**, *109*, 3963–3971. [CrossRef] [PubMed]
85. Denniss, F. The Protein Expression of Two Leukaemia Associated Antigens in AML: PASD1 and SSX2IP and Their Potential as Targets for Immunotherapy. MSc Thesis, King's College London, London, UK, 2006.
86. Denniss, F.A.; Breslin, A.; Ingram, W.; Hardwick, N.R.; Mufti, G.J.; Guinn, B.A. The leukaemia-associated antigen, SSX2IP, is expressed during mitosis on the surface of myeloid leukaemia cells. *Br. J. Haematol.* **2007**, *138*, 668–669. [CrossRef] [PubMed]
87. Michael, A.K.; Harvey, S.L.; Sammons, P.J.; Anderson, A.P.; Kopalle, H.M.; Banham, A.H.; Partch, C.L. Cancer/Testis Antigen PASD1 Silences the Circadian Clock. *Mol. Cell* **2015**, *58*, 743–754. [CrossRef]
88. Garg, H.; Suri, P.; Gupta, J.C.; Talwar, G.P.; Dubey, S. Survivin: A unique target for tumor therapy. *Cancer Cell Int.* **2016**, *16*, 49. [CrossRef] [PubMed]
89. Jeyaprakash, A.A.; Klein, U.R.; Lindner, D.; Ebert, J.; Nigg, E.A.; Conti, E. Structure of a Survivin-Borealin-INCENP core complex reveals how chromosomal passengers travel together. *Cell* **2007**, *131*, 271–285. [CrossRef] [PubMed]
90. Ruchaud, S.; Carmena, M.; Earnshaw, W.C. The chromosomal passenger complex: One for all and all for one. *Cell* **2007**, *131*, 230–231. [CrossRef]
91. Altieri, D.C. Survivin, cancer networks and pathway-directed drug discovery. *Nat. Rev. Cancer* **2008**, *8*, 61–70. [CrossRef] [PubMed]

92. Xia, F.; Canovas, P.M.; Guadagno, T.M.; Altieri, D.C. A survivin-ran complex regulates spindle formation in tumor cells. *Mol. Cell. Biol.* **2008**, *28*, 5299–5311. [CrossRef] [PubMed]
93. Chang, M.L.; Chen, J.C.; Alonso, C.R.; Kornblihtt, A.R.; Bissell, D.M. Regulation of fibronectin splicing in sinusoidal endothelial cells from normal or injured liver. *Proc. Natl. Acad. Sci. USA* **2004**, *101*, 18093–18098. [CrossRef] [PubMed]
94. Pennati, M.; Folini, M.; Zaffaroni, N. Targeting survivin in cancer therapy. *Expert Opin. Ther. Targets* **2008**, *12*, 463–476. [CrossRef] [PubMed]
95. Sung, B.; Pandey, M.K.; Ahn, K.S.; Yi, T.; Chaturvedi, M.M.; Liu, M.; Aggarwal, B.B. Anacardic acid (6-nonadecyl salicylic acid), an inhibitor of histone acetyltransferase, suppresses expression of nuclear factor-kappaB-regulated gene products involved in cell survival, proliferation, invasion, and inflammation through inhibition of the inhibitory subunit of nuclear factor-kappaBalpha kinase, leading to potentiation of apoptosis. *Blood* **2008**, *111*, 4880–4891. [PubMed]
96. Nakahara, T.; Takeuchi, M.; Kinoyama, I.; Minematsu, T.; Shirasuna, K.; Matsuhisa, A.; Kita, A.; Tominaga, F.; Yamanaka, K.; Kudoh, M.; et al. YM155, a novel small-molecule survivin suppressant, induces regression of established human hormone-refractory prostate tumor xenografts. *Cancer Res.* **2007**, *67*, 8014–8021. [CrossRef] [PubMed]
97. Sugiyama, H. WT1 (Wilms' tumor gene 1): Biology and cancer immunotherapy. *Jpn. J. Clin. Oncol.* **2010**, *40*, 377–387. [CrossRef] [PubMed]
98. Oka, Y.; Tsuboi, A.; Murakami, M.; Hirai, M.; Tominaga, N.; Nakajima, H.; Elisseeva, O.A.; Masuda, T.; Nakano, A.; Kawakami, M.; et al. Wilms tumor gene peptide-based immunotherapy for patients with overt leukemia from myelodysplastic syndrome (MDS) or MDS with myelofibrosis. *Int. J. Hematol.* **2003**, *78*, 56–61. [CrossRef] [PubMed]
99. Tsuboi, A.; Oka, Y.; Udaka, K.; Murakami, M.; Masuda, T.; Nakano, A.; Nakajima, H.; Yasukawa, M.; Hiraki, A.; Oji, Y.; et al. Enhanced induction of human WT1-specific cytotoxic T lymphocytes with a 9-mer WT1 peptide modified at HLA-A*2402-binding residues. *Cancer Immunol. Immunother.* **2002**, *51*, 614–620. [CrossRef] [PubMed]
100. Oka, Y.; Tsuboi, A.; Oji, Y.; Kawase, I.; Sugiyama, H. WT1 peptide vaccine for the treatment of cancer. *Curr. Opin. Immunol.* **2008**, *20*, 211–220. [CrossRef]
101. Oka, Y.; Tsuboi, A.; Taguchi, T.; Osaki, T.; Kyo, T.; Nakajima, H.; Elisseeva, O.A.; Oji, Y.; Kawakami, M.; Ikegame, K.; et al. Induction of WT1 (Wilms' tumor gene)-specific cytotoxic T lymphocytes by WT1 peptide vaccine and the resultant cancer regression. *Proc. Natl. Acad. Sci. USA* **2004**, *101*, 13885–13890. [CrossRef] [PubMed]
102. Inoue, K.; Ogawa, H.; Sonoda, Y.; Kimura, T.; Sakabe, H.; Oka, Y.; Miyake, S.; Tamaki, H.; Oji, Y.; Yamagami, T.; et al. Aberrant overexpression of the Wilms tumor gene (WT1) in human leukemia. *Blood* **1997**, *89*, 1405–1412. [PubMed]
103. Hosen, N.; Sonoda, Y.; Oji, Y.; Kimura, T.; Minamiguchi, H.; Tamaki, H.; Kawakami, M.; Asada, M.; Kanato, K.; Motomura, M.; et al. Very low frequencies of human normal CD34+ haematopoietic progenitor cells express the Wilms' tumour gene WT1 at levels similar to those in leukaemia cells. *Br. J. Haematol.* **2002**, *116*, 409–420. [CrossRef]
104. Wolfel, T.; Klehmann, E.; Muller, C.; Schutt, K.H.; Meyer zum Buschenfelde, K.H.; Knuth, A. Lysis of human melanoma cells by autologous cytolytic T cell clones. Identification of human histocompatibility leukocyte antigen A2 as a restriction element for three different antigens. *J. Exp. Med.* **1989**, *170*, 797–810. [CrossRef]
105. Zizzari, I.G.; Veglia, F.; Taurino, F.; Rahimi, H.; Quaglino, E.; Belleudi, F.; Riccardo, F.; Antonilli, M.; Napoletano, C.; Bellati, F.; et al. HER2-based recombinant immunogen to target DCs through FcγRs for cancer immunotherapy. *J. Mol. Med.* **2011**, *89*, 1231–1240. [CrossRef] [PubMed]
106. Bae, J.; Smith, R.; Daley, J.; Mimura, N.; Tai, Y.T.; Anderson, K.C.; Munshi, N.C. Myeloma-specific multiple peptides able to generate cytotoxic T lymphocytes: A potential therapeutic application in multiple myeloma and other plasma cell disorders. *Clin. Cancer Res.* **2012**, *18*, 4850–4860. [CrossRef] [PubMed]
107. Nguyen-Hoai, T.; Baldenhofer, G.; Ahmed, M.S.; Pham-Duc, M.; Gries, M.; Lipp, M.; Dörken, B.; Pezzutto, A.; Westermann, J. CCL19 (ELC) improves TH1-polarized immune responses and protective immunity in a murine Her2/neu DNA vaccination model. *J. Gene Med.* **2012**, *14*, 128–137. [CrossRef] [PubMed]

108. Anderson, M.W.; Zhao, S.; Freud, A.G.; Czerwinski, D.K.; Kohrt, H.; Alizadeh, A.A.; Houot, R.; Azambuja, D.; Biasoli, I.; Morais, J.C.; et al. CD137 is expressed in follicular dendritic cell tumors and in classical Hodgkin and T-cell lymphomas: Diagnostic and therapeutic implications. *Am. J. Pathol.* **2012**, *181*, 795–803. [CrossRef] [PubMed]
109. Nierkens, S.; Tel, J.; Janssen, E.; Adema, G.J. Antigen cross-presentation by dendritic cell subsets: One general or all sergeants? *Trends Immunol.* **2013**, *34*, 361–370. [CrossRef] [PubMed]
110. Sabado, R.L.; Bhardwaj, N. Dendritic cell immunotherapy. *Ann. N. Y. Acad. Sci.* **2013**, *1284*, 31–45. [CrossRef] [PubMed]
111. Bullinger, L.; Schlenk, R.F.; Götz, M.; Botzenhardt, U.; Hofmann, S.; Russ, A.C.; Babiak, A.; Zhang, L.; Schneider, V.; Döhner, K.; et al. PRAME-induced inhibition of retinoic acid receptor signaling-mediated differentiation—A possible target for ATRA response in AML without t(15;17). *Clin. Cancer Res.* **2013**, *19*, 2562–2571. [CrossRef]
112. Paydas, S.; Tanriverdi, K.; Yavuz, S.; Disel, U.; Baslamisli, F.; Burgut, R. PRAME mRNA levels in cases with acute leukemia: Clinical importance and future prospects. *Am. J. Hematol.* **2005**, *79*, 257–261. [CrossRef]
113. Greiner, J.; Bullinger, L.; Guinn, B.A.; Dohner, H.; Schmitt, M. Leukemia-associated antigens are critical for the proliferation of acute myeloid leukemia cells. *Clin. Cancer Res.* **2008**, *14*, 7161–7166. [CrossRef]
114. Yao, Y.; Zhou, J.; Wang, L.; Gao, X.; Ning, Q.; Jiang, M.; Wang, J.; Yu, L. Increased PRAME-specific CTL killing of acute myeloid leukemia cells by either a novel histone deacetylase inhibitor chidamide alone or combined treatment with decitabine. *PLoS ONE* **2013**, *8*, e70522. [CrossRef]
115. Yang, H.; Rosove, M.H.; Figlin, R.A. Tumor lysis syndrome occurring after the administration of rituximab in lymphoproliferative disorders: High-grade non-Hodgkin's lymphoma and chronic lymphocytic leukemia. *Am. J. Hematol.* **1999**, *62*, 247–250. [CrossRef]
116. Peng, Z. Current status of gendicine in China: Recombinant human Ad-p53 agent for treatment of cancers. *Hum. Gene Ther.* **2005**, *16*, 1016–1027. [CrossRef] [PubMed]
117. Bose, A.; Lowe, D.B.; Rao, A.; Storkus, W.J. Combined vaccine+axitinib therapy yields superior antitumor efficacy in a murine melanoma model. *Melanoma Res.* **2012**, *22*, 236–243. [CrossRef] [PubMed]
118. Karan, D.; Van Veldhuizen, P. Combination immunotherapy with prostate GVAX and ipilimumab: Safety and toxicity. *Immunotherapy* **2012**, *4*, 577–580. [CrossRef] [PubMed]
119. Ciccarese, C.; Nobili, E.; Grilli, D.; Casolari, L.; Rihawi, K.; Gelsomino, F.; Tortora, G.; Massari, F. The safety and efficacy of enzalutamide in the treatment of advanced prostate cancer. *Expert Rev. Anticancer Ther.* **2016**, *16*, 681–696. [CrossRef] [PubMed]
120. Daniels, G.A.; McKinney, M.; Ongkeko, W.; Wang-Rodriguez, J.; Sakamoto, K.; Elliott, R.L.; Head, J.F. A phase 1 clinical trial of a PSA/IL-2/GM-CSF containing prostate cancer vaccine in PSA defined biochemical recurrent prostate cancer patients. *J. Clin. Oncol.* **2016**, *34*, e14584. [CrossRef]
121. Gattinoni, L.; Finkelstein, S.E.; Klebanoff, C.A.; Antony, P.A.; Palmer, D.C.; Spiess, P.J.; Hwang, L.N.; Yu, Z.; Wrzesinski, C.; Heimann, D.M.; et al. Removal of homeostatic cytokine sinks by lymphodepletion enhances the efficacy of adoptively transferred tumor-specific CD8+ T cells. *J. Exp. Med.* **2005**, *202*, 907–912. [CrossRef] [PubMed]
122. Klebanoff, C.A.; Gattinoni, L.; Palmer, D.C.; Muranski, P.; Ji, Y.; Hinrichs, C.S.; Borman, Z.A.; Kerkar, S.P.; Scott, C.D.; Finkelstein, S.E.; et al. Determinants of successful CD8+-cell adoptive immunotherapy for large established tumors in mice. *Clin. Cancer Res.* **2011**, *17*, 5343–5352. [CrossRef]
123. Rafiq, S.; Purdon, T.J.; Daniyan, A.F.; Koneru, M.; Dao, T.; Liu, C.; Scheinberg, D.A.; Brentjens, R.J. Optimized T-cell receptor-mimic chimeric antigen receptor T cells directed toward the intracellular Wilms Tumor 1 antigen. *Leukemia* **2017**, *31*, 1788–1797. [CrossRef]
124. Smits, E.L.; Lee, C.; Hardwick, N.; Brooks, S.; Van Tendeloo, V.F.; Orchard, K.; Guinn, B.A. Clinical evaluation of cellular immunotherapy in acute myeloid leukaemia. *Cancer Immunol. Immunother.* **2011**, *60*, 757–769. [CrossRef]
125. Keenan, B.P.; Jaffee, E.M. Whole cell vaccines–past progress and future strategies. *Semin. Oncol.* **2012**, *39*, 276–286. [CrossRef]
126. Curiel, T.J. Immunotherapy: A useful strategy to help combat multidrug resistance. *Drug Resist. Updat.* **2012**, *15*, 106–113. [CrossRef] [PubMed]
127. Palucka, K.; Banchereau, J. Cancer immunotherapy via dendritic cells. *Nat. Rev. Cancer* **2012**, *12*, 265–277. [CrossRef] [PubMed]

128. Guo, Z.S.; Liu, Z.; Bartlett, D.L. Oncolytic Immunotherapy: Dying the Right Way is a Key to Eliciting Potent Antitumor Immunity. *Front. Oncol.* **2014**, *4*, 74. [CrossRef] [PubMed]
129. Goldberg, M.S. Immunoengineering: How nanotechnology can enhance cancer immunotherapy. *Cell* **2015**, *161*, 201–204. [CrossRef]
130. Mellman, I.; Coukos, G.; Dranoff, G. Cancer immunotherapy comes of age. *Nature* **2011**, *480*, 480–489. [CrossRef]
131. Liu, F.; Pinz, K.; Ma, Y.; Wada, M.; Chen, K.; Ma, G.; Su, Y.; Zhang, S.; He, G.; Ma, Y. First-in-human CLL1-CD33 compound CAR Tcells as a two-pronged approach for the treatment of refactory acute myeloid leukemia. In Proceedings of the 23rd Congress of the European Hematology Association, Stockholm, Sweden, 14–17 June 2018.
132. Liegel, J.; Rosenblatt, J.; Stone, R.M.; McMasters, M.; Levine, J.D.; Nahas, M.; Joyce, R.M.; Jain, S.; DeAngelo, D.J.; Garcia, J.S.; et al. Phase I/Ib Trial of the MUC1 Inhibitor GO-203-2C Alone and in Combination with Decitabine for Acute Myeloid Leukemia. *Blood* **2017**, *130*, 2659.
133. Qazilbash, M.H.; Wieder, E.; Thall, P.F.; Wang, X.; Rios, R.; Lu, S.; Kanodia, S.; Ruisaard, K.E.; Giralt, S.A.; Estey, E.H.; et al. PR1 peptide vaccine induces specific immunity with clinical responses in myeloid malignancies. *Leukemia* **2017**, *31*, 697–704. [CrossRef]
134. Chyla, B.; Daver, N.; Doyle, K.; McKeegan, E.; Huang, X.; Ruvolo, V.; Wang, Z.; Chen, K.; Souers, A.; Leverson, J.; et al. Genetic Biomarkers of Sensitivity and Resistance to Venetoclax Monotherapy in Patients With Relapsed Acute Myeloid Leukemia. *Am. J. Hematol.* **2018**. [CrossRef]
135. Maslak, P.G.; Dao, T.; Bernal, Y.; Chanel, S.M.; Zhang, R.; Frattini, M.; Rosenblat, T.; Jurcic, J.G.; Brentjens, R.J.; Arcila, M.E.; et al. Phase 2 trial of a multivalent WT1 peptide vaccine (galinpepimut-S) in acute myeloid leukemia. *Blood Adv.* **2018**, *2*, 224–234. [CrossRef]
136. Khoury, H.J.; Collins, R.H., Jr.; Blum, W.; Stiff, P.S.; Elias, L.; Lebkowski, J.S.; Reddy, A.; Nishimoto, K.P.; Sen, D.; Wirth, E.D., 3rd; et al. Immune responses and long-term disease recurrence status after telomerase-based dendritic cell immunotherapy in patients with acute myeloid leukemia. *Cancer* **2017**, *123*, 3061–3072. [CrossRef]
137. Kocak, E.; Lute, K.; Chang, X.; May, K.F.; Exten, K.R.; Zhang, H.; Abdessalam, S.F.; Lehman, A.M.; Jarjoura, D.; Zheng, P.; et al. Combination therapy with anti-CTL antigen-4 and anti-4-1BB antibodies enhances cancer immunity and reduces autoimmunity. *Cancer Res.* **2006**, *66*, 7276–7284. [CrossRef]
138. Chang, C.H.; Wang, Y.; Zalath, M.; Liu, D.; Cardillo, T.M.; Goldenberg, D.M. Combining ABCG2 Inhibitors with IMMU-132, an Anti-Trop-2 Antibody Conjugate of SN-38, Overcomes Resistance to SN-38 in Breast and Gastric Cancers. *Mol. Cancer Ther.* **2016**, *15*, 1910–1919. [CrossRef]
139. Borges-Walmsley, M.I.; McKeegan, K.S.; Walmsley, A.R. Structure and function of efflux pumps that confer resistance to drugs. *Biochem. J.* **2003**, *376*, 313–338. [CrossRef]
140. Baselga, J.; Bradbury, I.; Eidtmann, H.; Di Cosimo, S.; de Azambuja, E.; Aura, C.; Gómez, H.; Dinh, P.; Fauria, K.; Van Dooren, V.; et al. Lapatinib with trastuzumab for HER2-positive early breast cancer (NeoALTTO): A randomised, open-label, multicentre, phase 3 trial. *Lancet* **2012**, *379*, 633–640. [CrossRef]
141. Robert, C.; Karaszewska, B.; Schachter, J.; Rutkowski, P.; Mackiewicz, A.; Stroiakovski, D.; Lichinitser, M.; Dummer, R.; Grange, F.; Mortier, L.; et al. Improved overall survival in melanoma with combined dabrafenib and trametinib. *N. Engl. J. Med.* **2015**, *372*, 30–39. [CrossRef]
142. Zukin, M.; Barrios, C.H.; Pereira, J.R.; Ribeiro, R.e.A.; Beato, C.A.; do Nascimento, Y.N.; Murad, A.; Franke, F.A.; Precivale, M.; Araujo, L.H.; et al. Randomized phase III trial of single-agent pemetrexed versus carboplatin and pemetrexed in patients with advanced non-small-cell lung cancer and Eastern Cooperative Oncology Group performance status of 2. *J. Clin. Oncol.* **2013**, *31*, 2849–2853. [CrossRef]
143. Westin, J.R.; Chu, F.; Zhang, M.; Fayad, L.E.; Kwak, L.W.; Fowler, N.; Romaguera, J.; Hagemeister, F.; Fanale, M.; Samaniego, F.; et al. Safety and activity of PD1 blockade by pidilizumab in combination with rituximab in patients with relapsed follicular lymphoma: A single group, open-label, phase 2 trial. *Lancet Oncol.* **2014**, *15*, 69–77. [CrossRef]
144. Von Hoff, D.D.; Ervin, T.; Arena, F.P.; Chiorean, E.G.; Infante, J.; Moore, M.; Seay, T.; Tjulandin, S.A.; Ma, W.W.; Saleh, M.N.; et al. Increased survival in pancreatic cancer with nab-paclitaxel plus gemcitabine. *N. Engl. J. Med.* **2013**, *369*, 1691–1703. [CrossRef]
145. Larkin, J.; Hodi, F.S.; Wolchok, J.D. Combined Nivolumab and Ipilimumab or Monotherapy in Untreated Melanoma. *N. Engl. J. Med.* **2015**, *373*, 1270–1271. [CrossRef]

146. Leath, C.A.; Straughn, J.M. Chemotherapy for advanced and recurrent cervical carcinoma: Results from cooperative group trials. *Gynecol. Oncol.* **2013**, *129*, 251–257. [CrossRef]
147. Ducreux, M.; Adenis, A.; Pignon, J.P.; François, E.; Chauffert, B.; Ichanté, J.L.; Boucher, E.; Ychou, M.; Pierga, J.Y.; Montoto-Grillot, C.; et al. Efficacy and safety of bevacizumab-based combination regimens in patients with previously untreated metastatic colorectal cancer: Final results from a randomised phase II study of bevacizumab plus 5-fluorouracil, leucovorin plus irinotecan versus bevacizumab plus capecitabine plus irinotecan (FNCLCC ACCORD 13/0503 study). *Eur. J. Cancer* **2013**, *49*, 1236–1245. [CrossRef]
148. Jurcic, J.G. Novel Immunotherapy Approaches in AML: Focus on Monoclonal Antibodies. *Clin. Lymphoma Myeloma Leuk.* **2017**, *17*, S115–S119. [CrossRef]
149. Zuber, J.; Shi, J.; Wang, E.; Rappaport, A.R.; Herrmann, H.; Sison, E.A.; Magoon, D.; Qi, J.; Blatt, K.; Wunderlich, M.; et al. RNAi screen identifies Brd4 as a therapeutic target in acute myeloid leukaemia. *Nature* **2011**, *478*, 524–528. [CrossRef]
150. Laing, A.A.; Harrison, C.J.; Gibson, B.E.S.; Keeshan, K. Unlocking the potential of anti-CD33 therapy in adult and childhood acute myeloid leukemia. *Exp. Hematol.* **2017**, *54*, 40–50. [CrossRef]

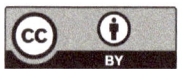

© 2019 by the authors. Licensee MDPI, Basel, Switzerland. This article is an open access article distributed under the terms and conditions of the Creative Commons Attribution (CC BY) license (http://creativecommons.org/licenses/by/4.0/).

MDPI
St. Alban-Anlage 66
4052 Basel
Switzerland
Tel. +41 61 683 77 34
Fax +41 61 302 89 18
www.mdpi.com

Journal of Clinical Medicine Editorial Office
E-mail: jcm@mdpi.com
www.mdpi.com/journal/jcm